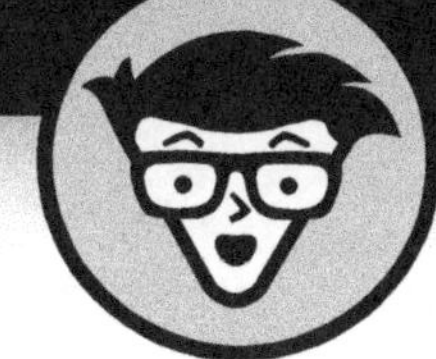

Breathing Exercises

by Shamash Alidina

FOREWORD BY Patrick McKeown

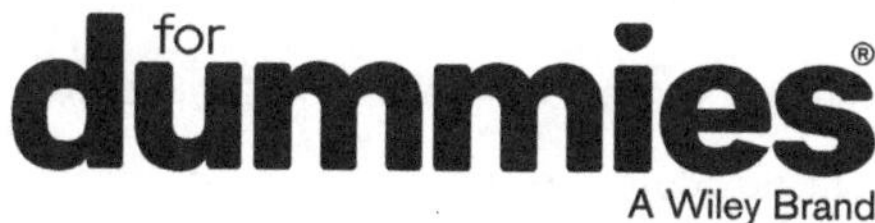

Breathing Exercises For Dummies®

Published by: **John Wiley & Sons, Inc.,** 111 River Street, Hoboken, NJ 07030-5774, www.wiley.com

For general information on our other products and services, please contact our Customer Care Department within the U.S. at 877-762-2974, outside the U.S. at 317-572-3993, or fax 317-572-4002. For technical support, please visit https://hub.wiley.com/community/support/dummies.

Wiley publishes in a variety of print and electronic formats and by print-on-demand. Some material included with standard print versions of this book may not be included in e-books or in print-on-demand. If this book refers to media that is not included in the version you purchased, you may download this material at http://booksupport.wiley.com. For more information about Wiley products, visit www.wiley.com.

Library of Congress Control Number: 2025946117

ISBN 978-1-394-33103-1 (pbk); ISBN 978-1-394-33105-5 (ebk); ISBN 978-1-394-33104-8 (ebk)

Printed and bound by CPI Group (UK) Ltd, Croydon, CR0 4YY

C9781394331031_301025

The manufacturer's authorized representative according to the EU General Product Safety Regulation is Wiley-VCH GmbH, Boschstr. 12, 69469 Weinheim, Germany, e-mail: Product_Safety@wiley.com.

Contents at a Glance

Table of Contents

Foreword

Breathing. Everyone does it. Everyone talks about it. But what does it really mean to you?

Some think breathing practice is all about taking deep, full breaths to calm the nerves when the world gets a little too loud. Others imagine it's about fast, forceful breathing to chase a euphoric high. Then there's the classic: "Breathe in through your nose, out through your mouth." It's a bit of a Wild West out there. Everyone has an opinion, but few have taken the time to truly understand the landscape.

I've been exploring this terrain for more than two decades, and I can tell you this: Breathing goes far deeper than most people imagine. It's not just about more air, bigger breaths, or louder exhales. In fact, the most powerful shift I ever made, one that changed the entire direction of my life, was this: I learned to breathe less. Not more. Not deeper. Just less.

Don't just take my word for it when I say to breathe less. This book looks at what the breath can do for you. Experiment with it. Read the science, which Shamash Alidina presents in a way you can actually understand. Try the exercises. See what resonates with you. Breathing has so many applications, but each of us gets something from the practice that is deeply personal. This doesn't mean you need to try every single exercise. But it does mean you should stay curious about your own breath and not just follow the crowd. Because when it comes to breathing, the crowd isn't often right.

When I first got into breathing, I wasn't following some trend. I wasn't doing it for Instagram or to feel zen. I did it because it worked. I had a permanently blocked nose. I held my breath while gently nodding my head for 20 seconds at a time, and to my surprise, my nose cleared. I began breathing slightly less air than usual, just enough to feel a light hunger for air. And something shifted. My hands warmed up. A calm settled through my body. That was all the proof I needed.

I didn't understand all the science at the time, but what I felt was enough to keep going. Since then, I've come to learn what most people are never taught: that carbon dioxide is not just a waste gas, that oxygen delivery is not just about how much air you suck in, and that how you breathe changes how you sleep, how you move, how you think, and even how safe your brain feels in any given moment.

And that sensation of breathlessness when you exercise? It's not fixed by fitness alone. Most physical training doesn't place enough load on your breathing to fundamentally change it. If you want to improve how you breathe under pressure, you have to go after the very thing that causes breathlessness in the first place.

Let's get practical: If you wake up with a dry mouth, there's a good chance your nose isn't doing its job at night. If you snore, if your sleep feels unrefreshing, if your mind is foggy during the day, breathing is often at the root of it. If you've been told to breathe deeply but you feel more anxious or dizzy, the answer may be to do the opposite: Breathe gently, quietly, and just a little less.

This is not magic. It's science. And once you understand the why, you can practice with purpose and feel real results.

The tools you'll discover in this book aren't just useful. They're life-changing. I say that with full sincerity. These tools will help you sleep better, feel calmer, move with greater efficiency, focus your mind, and build real resilience. They touch everything: respiratory health, mental health, dental health, sleep, movement, yoga, sport, and more. Breathing is simple. Breathing is complex. But done well, it is the closest thing we have to a master key for health and performance.

Here's the truth: You cannot reach your full potential if your breathing is off. But here's the good news: When your breathing improves, everything else can follow.

Breathing Exercises For Dummies is written for you. Whether you're just starting out or you're already deep into your wellness journey, it opens up a world that is both accessible and profound. But don't just let it sit on the shelf. Read it. Try it. Feel it. Let the exercises become your steady companion, your go-to when the pressure is on, when the mind races, when sleep eludes you, or when life simply demands your best self.

Because honestly, what other function can improve so many areas of your life for so little effort?

Now that is a life skill.

Patrick McKeown

Author of *The Oxygen Advantage* and *The Breathing Cure*

Founder of OxygenAdvantage.com and ButeykoClinic.com

Introduction

f you're breathing right now (which I certainly hope you are), congratulations! You're already doing something essential for survival. But here's the twist: Just because you're breathing doesn't mean you're doing it optimally. And that's where this book comes in.

For something so fundamental, breathing is surprisingly misunderstood. It's something we do about 20,000 times a day without much thought. Yet the way we breathe has profound effects on our health, energy, focus, sleep, and even emotions. The good news? With a little awareness and a few simple techniques, you can transform your breathing into a powerful tool for improving your life.

Maybe you've stumbled across breathwork or breathing exercises through yoga or meditation. Perhaps you've heard about elite athletes using breathing techniques to enhance endurance. Maybe you experience chronic stress, and you've noticed that paying attention to your breathing actually makes you feel more anxious rather than calm — which is more common than people think. Or perhaps, like many people, you've found yourself out of breath climbing the stairs and thought, "I should probably do something about this." Whatever your reason for picking up this book, you're about to learn that breathing is far more than just an automatic process — it's a skill you can refine and optimize to work for you.

Learning about breath has certainly changed my life. Even after years of teaching mindfulness, I was surprised to realize how my own breathing habits were quietly draining my energy and impacting my well-being. Taking a deeper dive into understanding breath — and practicing the exercises I share in this book — changed that. I hope it brings the same positive shift for you.

About This Book

This book is designed as a practical, easy-to-follow guide to breathing exercises, whether you're a complete beginner or someone looking to deepen your breathwork practice. You don't need to read it cover to cover — just jump to the sections that interest you. Each chapter stands alone, so whether you're looking for ways to calm down before bed, improve focus during the day, or boost physical performance, you'll find something useful.

You'll discover breathing techniques rooted in science, ancient wisdom, and modern research. This book covers everything from foundational breathing habits to advanced breathwork practices used by athletes, mindfulness experts, and health professionals. Along the way, you'll find simple exercises, fascinating facts, and practical insights to help you get the most out of your breath.

Some sections include extra details for those who like to dig deeper into the science, but if that's not your thing, feel free to skip ahead. This book is about making breathing work for you, not overwhelming you with complex theories.

Within this book, you may note that some web addresses break across two lines of text. If you're reading this book in print and want to visit one of these web pages, simply key in the web address exactly as it's noted in the text, pretending as though the line break doesn't exist. If you're reading this as an e-book, you've got it easy — just click the web address to be taken directly to the web page.

Note: This book is intended as a general guide to breathing exercises and is not a substitute for professional medical advice, diagnosis, or treatment. Breathing exercises can offer many benefits, but it may not be suitable for everyone — particularly if you have an underlying medical condition or respiratory issues or if you're pregnant. If you have any concerns or health conditions, consult a qualified healthcare professional before attempting any of the exercises in this book.

Always listen to your body. If you experience any discomfort or adverse effects, stop immediately and seek medical advice. Not only will this ensure your safety, but it will also allow your healthcare provider to monitor how breathwork impacts your overall well-being. Keeping your healthcare provider in the loop is always a good idea.

Foolish Assumptions

In writing this book, I made a few assumptions about you, dear reader. For instance, I assume you:

>> Are open to trying out different breathing exercises

>> Want to improve your well-being, whether that's by reducing stress, sleeping better, improving focus, or increasing energy levels

>> Are curious about how breathwork can enhance your daily life but don't necessarily have prior experience

>> Prefer practical techniques over heavy scientific jargon (although I love science, I keep things straightforward and practical)

If any of these assumptions apply to you, you're in the right place. And if none of these assumptions fit, you're still welcome to stick around — after all, who *couldn't* benefit from better breathing?

Icons Used in This Book

To help you navigate this book, I've sprinkled in a few handy icons along the way:

Paragraphs marked by the Tip icon offer practical advice to make your breathing practice easier and more effective.

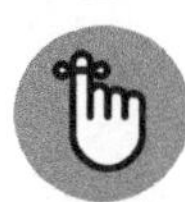

The Remember icon highlights key takeaways to keep in mind as you learn.

The Warning icon flags things to watch out for, such as when certain techniques may not be suitable for everyone.

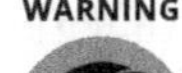

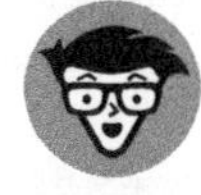

Sometimes I get into the weeds on a subject and offer more information than you absolutely need to know. When I do, I flag those paragraphs with the Technical Stuff icon.

I use the Play This icon to highlight breathing exercises with a recorded audio that you can listen to online at www.dummies.com/go/breathingexercisesfd.

I use the Try This icon for shorter breathing exercises that don't have an audio component.

Beyond the Book

In addition to everything you'll find in these pages, this book also comes with some great companion resources to help you put your breathing practice into action.

First, you have access to an exclusive Cheat Sheet, which provides quick-reference tips on key breathing exercises, common mistakes to avoid, and simple ways to integrate breathwork into your daily routine. To access the Cheat Sheet, simply go to `www.dummies.com` and type **Breathing Exercises For Dummies Cheat Sheet** in the Search box.

Next, you find two bonus chapters: Ten Common Myths about Breathing and Ten Ways Breathing Exercises Improve Your Well-Being.

But that's not all! You'll also find online audio tracks featuring guided breathing exercises from the book. These recordings will help you follow along with techniques for relaxation, focus, energy, and sleep — without having to constantly check the book. To access the audio tracks, visit `www.dummies.com/go/breathingexercisesfd`.

Where to Go from Here

Unlike a novel, this book isn't meant to be read from beginning to end. You can start wherever makes the most sense for you. If you're new to breathwork, Part 1 is a great place to begin — it covers the fundamentals of breathing, how it affects your body and mind, and how to assess your own breathing habits.

If stress relief is your priority and you know the basics of breathing, skip ahead to the chapters that call to you in Part 2. If you're an athlete or looking for a performance edge, Chapters 15 and 16 on advanced breathwork and endurance training will be right up your alley. And if you're just here for some quick and easy breathing exercises, check out Chapter 19 for ten powerful techniques you can start using today.

Wherever you begin, remember that better breathing starts with awareness. So, take a slow, deep breath in through your nose, let it out slowly, and get ready to explore the incredible power of your breath.

1

Getting Started with Breathing Exercises

This part introduces you to the fascinating world of breathing, highlighting why breathing well is one of the simplest yet most powerful ways to enhance your health, happiness, and focus. You begin by appreciating how your breath directly affects your body and mind, understanding the basics of breathing exercises, and uncovering how breathwork has been practiced over the centuries.

Next, you dive into the science of breathing, exploring the essential anatomy of your respiratory system and seeing how breathing nourishes your body with oxygen while managing carbon dioxide levels. You also discover the crucial role of your autonomic nervous system and how targeted breathing exercises can either energize your day or promote relaxation and calm.

You unravel the powerful mind-body connection that breathing fosters. You explore how breath impacts your emotions, reduces stress, and helps you achieve greater mindfulness and mental clarity. Practical exercises in mindful breathing equip you with the tools to gently shift emotional states and sharpen your focus whenever you need.

Finally, you assess your own breathing habits to discover if you're breathing optimally or if you have room for improvement. Through simple self-assessment techniques and practical exercises, you become aware of common breathing mistakes and how to correct them. You also explore how modern technology — such as apps and wearable devices — can provide immediate feedback and support as you continue your breathing journey.

Chapter **1**

Breathing: The Key to Health, Happiness, and Focus

f you're like most people, you've probably never thought much about how you breathe. You just do it — on autopilot.

But what if I told you that this unconscious act, done more than 20,000 times a day, could be the missing key to your energy, focus, sleep, and even emotional well-being? What if your breathing is actually *holding you back?*

In this chapter, I show you how the simple act of breathing — when done consciously and skillfully — can unlock a cascade of physical, mental, and emotional benefits. You take a deep breath with me and explore why your breath is not just a background process, but the foundation of a healthier, calmer, and more vibrant life.

Appreciating How Breathing Impacts Your Body and Mind

Let's start with a quick experiment right away. Take a nice deep breath in, and really slowly let it out. Did you notice anything? Perhaps your shoulders relaxed a bit. Maybe your mind cleared momentarily. That's just a tiny glimpse of what proper breathing can do for you.

Your breath is the remote control for your nervous system. No joke! When you breathe rapidly, you're essentially pressing the "stress button" on your body, triggering your sympathetic nervous system (the one responsible for the fight-or-flight response). When you breathe slowly and deeply, you're hitting the "calm button," activating your parasympathetic nervous system (the one responsible for the rest-and-digest mode). Pretty neat, right?

Years ago, during my training to become a science teacher, I found myself in front of 35 lively teenagers — and an inspector sitting at the back of the classroom with a clipboard. No pressure, right? My heart started pounding, my palms turned clammy, and I could feel that familiar rush of nerves creeping in. I had just a couple of minutes before the lesson began, and I knew I had to get centered or risk spiraling. I noticed my breath was fast and shallow — the classic stress response.

So, I turned to a technique I'd recently learned: 4:6 breathing. I inhaled slowly to a count of 4 and then exhaled even more slowly to a count of 6. With each out breath, I silently said the word *calm.* Within a minute, I felt more grounded. The nerves didn't disappear entirely, but they softened. I stepped into the classroom with a steady presence, taught the lesson, and passed the inspection. I went on to teach for ten years before shifting into mindfulness and breathwork full time — but I'll never forget how that one simple breathing technique helped me keep my cool when it mattered most.

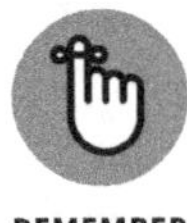

REMEMBER

Your breathing affects virtually every system in your body. Here's a short list of what happens when you breathe properly:

>> Your blood pressure normalizes.

>> Your heart rate steadies.

>> Your immune system gets a boost.

>> Your digestion improves.

>> Your stress hormones decrease.

>> Your brain receives optimal oxygen.

On the flip side, poor breathing habits can contribute to anxiety, fatigue, poor concentration, and sleep problems. They can even worsen conditions like asthma and high blood pressure.

One member of my community got in touch with me complaining of feeling anxious and struggling with insomnia. She was a manager who prided herself on "pushing through" challenges. When we had a video coaching call, it was clear to me that she was taking shallow, rapid breaths exclusively in her upper chest. After just two weeks of practicing proper deep breathing (called *diaphragmatic breathing*) for five minutes daily, she reported sleeping better than she had in years and feeling "strangely calm" during meetings. "I just breathe differently now," she told me, "and everything else follows."

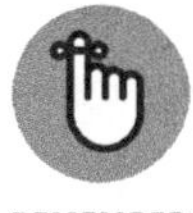

REMEMBER

Your breath is your secret superpower. You can't will your heart to slow down or ask your immune system to fight harder. But your breath? It listens. In seconds, you begin to regulate your nervous system, lower your blood pressure, and calm a racing mind. It's one of the only parts of your body's automatic system you can consciously steer — anytime, anywhere.

This isn't just relaxation. It's rewiring. When you understand how to breathe *on purpose,* you unlock a built-in tool for focus, resilience, energy, and peace. And the best part? You've had it with you all along.

Introducing Breathing Exercises

This book is about breath in general and breathing exercises in particular. So, what do I mean by breathing exercises?

Defining breathing exercises

Simply put, *breathing exercises* are specific techniques that help you control how you breathe to positively impact your physical, mental, and emotional state.

Think of breathing exercises as workouts for your respiratory system. Just as you may do bicep curls to strengthen your arms or stretches to improve flexibility, breathing exercises train your breathing muscles and adjust your patterns to work more efficiently.

But breathing exercises go beyond physical training. They're also a form of mental and emotional training that helps you become more aware of and regulate your physiological and psychological states. They're like having a built-in stress management system that you can activate anytime, anywhere.

One afternoon during a particularly chaotic workshop I was leading for a corporate client in London, the fire alarm went off. As 30 stressed executives and I evacuated to the street, I noticed everyone checking their phones and looking anxious. The manager asked if we could do a quick exercise outside. I agreed. "While we wait," I announced with perhaps too much enthusiasm, "let's practice box breathing!" There were some eye rolls, but after a minute of guided practice, the mood noticeably shifted. By the time we returned inside (it was a false alarm), one participant joked, "Can we pull the alarm again when I have my performance review next week?!"

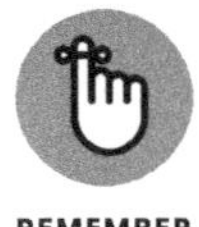

Conscious breathing is a small thing that can make a big difference in your life.

Identifying the three essential ingredients of all breathing exercises

Most breathing exercises — whether they're ancient pranayama yoga techniques, modern heart rate variability (HRV) biofeedback methods, or anything in between — are constructed from three core components. Think of these as the essential ingredients in a recipe: Adjust one element, and you completely transform the experience and outcome.

Heart rate variability is a measure of your overall well-being.

As shown in Figure 1-1, three components work together to create the complete breathing exercise experience:

>> **Breath Pattern (How You Breathe):** This is the mechanical foundation — what you actually do with your inhale, exhale, and any pauses in between. The breath pattern encompasses several key variables:

- **Pace:** Breathing rapidly can energize you, whereas breathing slowly can help you calm down.

- **Depth:** Shallow breathing affects different parts of your nervous system than deep, diaphragmatic breathing.

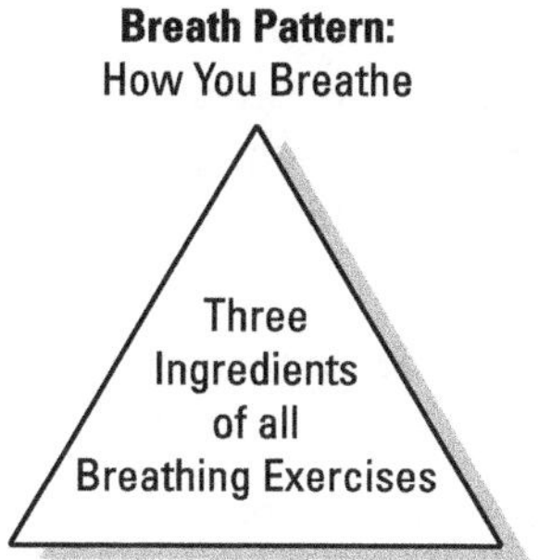

FIGURE 1-1: The three components of the breathing experience.

- **Ratio:** The mathematical relationship between different phases of breath. For example, a 4-6-2 pattern means inhaling for four counts, exhaling for six counts, and holding for two counts.

- **Breath route:** Whether you breathe through your nose, mouth, or alternate between them significantly impacts the physiological effects.

A classic example of a breathing pattern is box breathing, which follows a precise 4-4-4-4 pattern: Inhale for four counts, hold for four, exhale for four, hold for four. This creates a "box" of equal timing that promotes balance and focus.

>> **Intention (Why You're Doing It):** Your intention acts as the compass that guides the entire exercise. It determines not just what technique you choose, but how you approach it. Different intentions require different breathing strategies:

- Calming the nervous system may call for extended exhale breathing, where your out breath is longer than your in breath, activating your parasympathetic nervous system.

- Boosting alertness and energy could involve techniques like *kapalabhati* (skull-shining breath), with its rapid, forceful exhales (see Chapter 12).

- Releasing stress and tension may be best served by cyclic sighing or resonant breathing at your body's optimal frequency (see Chapters 3 and 8).

The intention shapes everything from the pace and depth of your breathing to how long you practice and what you focus on during the exercise.

>> **Attention (Where Your Mind Is):** This is what transforms mechanical breathing into mindful breathing — the difference between simply moving air in and out of your lungs and creating a meditative experience. Your attention can focus on various aspects:

- **Physical sensations:** The feeling of cool air entering your nostrils, the expansion of your rib cage, or the gentle rise and fall of your belly

- **Counting or rhythm:** Using numbers to maintain your chosen pattern while keeping your mind anchored

- **Visualization:** Imagining light flowing in with each inhale, or stress leaving with each exhale

- **Present-moment awareness:** Simply observing the breath without trying to change or control it

You can think of these three components like going to a live pop concert. The pattern is the beat — it keeps everything moving in time, just like the steady rhythm of the music. The intention is the vibe — are you here for fun, to feel something deep, to let go? That sets the emotional tone, like the mood of the performance. And attention? That's you in the crowd — not just passively watching, but fully immersed, singing along, lights flashing, heart syncing with the music. You're both audience and participant, shaping the experience with your presence.

When all three elements work in harmony, even the simplest breathing exercise becomes a powerful tool for transformation. Change any one element, and you create an entirely different experience — just as changing the beat, the reason for being there, or your listening focus transforms how you experience the music.

This framework will help you understand and modify any breathing exercise you encounter throughout this book, giving you the tools to customize practices for your specific needs and goals.

Exploring various breathing exercises

The world of breathing exercises is wonderfully diverse. Here's a quick tour of some popular techniques I explore more deeply later in this book:

>> **Diaphragmatic breathing (see Chapter 7):** Also known as belly breathing, abdominal breathing, or simply deep breathing, this fundamental technique focuses on using your *diaphragm* (the dome-shaped muscle below your lungs) rather than your chest muscles when breathing. It's the foundation of most other breathing practices.

- **>> Box breathing (see Chapter 8):** A simple but powerful technique where you inhale, hold your breath, exhale, and hold again, each for the same count. Navy SEALs famously use this technique to stay calm under pressure. If it works for them during combat, it can probably help you handle your in-laws during the holidays!

- **>> 4-7-8 breathing (see Chapter 8):** Made popular by Dr. Andrew Weil, this technique involves inhaling for four seconds, holding for seven seconds, and exhaling for eight seconds in a specific way. It's particularly helpful for falling asleep and managing anxiety.

- **>> Alternate-nostril breathing (see Chapter 15):** A yogic practice where you inhale and exhale through one nostril at a time. It's like having your own internal balancing system — perfect for when you feel scattered or overwhelmed.

- **>> Coherent or resonant breathing (see Chapter 8):** This technique involves breathing at a specific rate (typically, five to six breaths per minute) to maximize HRV and promote focus and calm. Think of it as finding your breathing "sweet spot" where everything in your body hums along harmoniously.

- **>> Cyclic sighing (see Chapter 3):** This technique involves a long, slow inhale followed by a second short top-up breath, and then an extended, relaxed sigh out through the mouth. It's like giving your nervous system a gentle nudge to settle down. Research shows that just a few minutes of this kind of sighing can significantly reduce anxiety and shift you into a more relaxed, parasympathetic state.

I cover many more techniques in this book! Each of them has specific benefits and optimal situations for use. The beauty is that you can choose different breathing exercises for different needs — like having a toolbox where each tool serves a specific purpose.

Discovering the connection between breathing exercises and breathwork

You may hear the terms *breathing exercises* and *breathwork* used interchangeably, but there's a subtle difference that's useful to understand.

Breathing exercises, sometimes also called *conscious breathing*, are specific techniques that help you guide your breath for a desired effect — calming your nerves, energizing your body, improving sleep, and more. These are typically short, practical tools you can use anytime, anywhere. They're like the building blocks of breathwork: quick, focused, and often aimed at managing stress or boosting your physical and mental well-being.

Breathwork is the act of doing breathing exercises — for example, "I did some breathwork this morning — box breathing, to be precise." Breathwork can also refer to a broader practice that includes one or more breathing exercises, often combined in a deliberate sequence. A breathwork session may be a five-minute self-guided routine or a longer experience led by a teacher. Some sessions dive deep — bringing up strong emotions, promoting healing, or creating altered states of consciousness. Others are gentle, quiet, and grounding.

Think of it this way: Breathing exercises are like daily movement (stretching, walking, a quick yoga flow), while breathwork sessions can be anything from a regular workout to a full-body retreat. They're both part of the same world.

From ancient yogic *pranayama* to modern therapeutic techniques, cultures throughout history have used conscious breathing to shift health, mood, and even awareness.

As one participant in my community shared after a guided session: "I came for stress relief but found parts of myself I didn't know were lost."

That's the power of breath. Start simple, and it may just take you somewhere profound.

Taking the First Step: Being Aware of Your Breath

Before diving into specific techniques, the most important first step is simply becoming aware of your current breathing patterns. This awareness itself can be transformative.

TRY THIS

Right now, without changing anything, notice:

>> Are you breathing through your nose or mouth?

>> Is your breath shallow or deep?

>> Which parts of your body move when you breathe? Your chest? Your belly?

>> What's the rhythm of your breath? Fast or slow? Even or uneven?

>> How does your breathing change as you pay attention to it?

This simple act of observation is powerful. *Remember:* Awareness precedes change. You can't improve what you don't notice.

One simple exercise to build this awareness is what I call the "Hand on Heart, Hand on Belly" technique:

1. **Place one hand on your chest and the other hand on your abdomen, just below your rib cage.**

2. **Close your eyes and breathe normally for a minute.**

3. **Notice which hand moves more.**

Most people discover they're shallow, chest breathers rather than deep, diaphragmatic breathers — a pattern associated with stress and anxiety. I show you how to fix this in Chapter 7 on diaphragmatic breathing.

I remember teaching this exercise during a workshop where a skeptical staff member grudgingly participated. After just one minute, he admitted, "I've been holding my breath unconsciously, without noticing. No wonder I get headaches by lunchtime every day." Small awareness, big revelation.

When you're under stress, your breathing naturally becomes more shallow and rapid — part of your body's fight-or-flight response. This pattern was useful when our ancestors needed quick bursts of energy to escape predators, but it's less helpful when you're stuck in traffic or facing a tight deadline. Being aware of this pattern gives you the opportunity to interrupt it.

Simply becoming aware of your breath doesn't mean you need to control it immediately. Begin by observing with curiosity rather than harsh self-judgement. Your breath has been with you since your first moment in this world, and it will be with you until your last.

Befriending your breath is the start of a beautiful relationship. That's what this book is all about.

THE RICH HISTORY OF BREATHWORK ACROSS AGES AND CULTURES

Breathing exercises aren't a modern wellness trend — they're one of humanity's oldest healing practices. Virtually every major spiritual and healing tradition throughout history has incorporated some form of conscious breathing.

In India, *pranayama* (breath control) has been a core component of yoga for thousands of years. The very word *pranayama* reveals how central breath was to ancient

(continued)

(continued)

understanding: *Prana* means life force, and *ayama* means to extend or draw out. Through controlled breathing, practitioners believed they could extend their life force and vitality.

In ancient China, Taoist practitioners developed breathing techniques as part of their pursuit of longevity and spiritual development. These practices were integrated into movement-based exercises called *qigong* and *tai chi,* which continue to be practiced worldwide today.

Indigenous cultures across continents have used rhythmic breathing in ceremonial and healing contexts. From Native American purification ceremonies to Australian Aboriginal didgeridoo playing (which requires circular breathing), the breath has been recognized as a gateway to healing and altered consciousness.

Interest in breathwork surged in the modern age. Practices like the Buteyko Breathing Method, Oxygen Advantage, Sudarshan Kriya Yoga, the Wim Hof Method, and Holotropic Breathwork emerged, bringing attention to the therapeutic, health, and performance enhancement potential of conscious breathing.

Today, scientific research is catching up with ancient wisdom. Studies are confirming what practitioners have known for centuries: that specific slow breathing patterns can influence HRV, brain activity, immune function, and emotional regulation

Envisioning Your Breathing Journey

Picture this: You're standing at the edge of a swimming pool for the first time. The water looks inviting, but also a little intimidating. You've heard swimming is great exercise, wonderful for your health, and incredibly relaxing. But right now? You're not entirely convinced you need to get wet.

This may be how you feel about breathing exercises and breathwork. You may have picked up this book because someone told you breathing exercises could change your life, or perhaps you've read about the benefits online. Maybe you're dealing with stress, anxiety, or just feeling like you need something more in your toolkit for handling life's ups and downs. But like standing at that pool's edge, you may be wondering: "Is this really for me?"

The journey from skepticism to mastery of breath follows a similar path to learning how to swim. And just like swimming, when you learn the basics, you'll have a skill that will serve you for life.

Overcoming your initial fears or skepticism

Remember being a child and perhaps feeling nervous about jumping into water? That hesitation is perfectly natural — it's your brain's way of keeping you safe around something new and potentially overwhelming. The same thing happens with breathing exercises.

You may be thinking, "I already know how to breathe — I do it automatically without thinking!" And you're absolutely right. But here's the thing: There's a world of difference between the *automatic* breathing that keeps you alive and the *conscious* breathing that can transform how you feel, think, and live.

Concerns I hear include the following:

>> "Is this all a bunch of mumbo jumbo?"

>> "What if it feels weird or uncomfortable?"

>> "What if I do it wrong?"

>> "What if feeling my breathing makes me more anxious?"

These worries are like being concerned about getting water up your nose when learning to swim — valid concerns that dissolve when you know what you're doing. The beauty of breathing exercises is that, unlike swimming, you can't actually drown! Your body has incredible built-in safety mechanisms that will keep you breathing normally if you ever feel uncomfortable.

I still remember my first experience with conscious breathing. I was in my twenties, feeling overwhelmed with my studies, and somehow I ended up in a local meditation class. When the teacher started talking about breathing meditation, I thought, "This is ridiculous — I could be at home watching TV." But then something unexpected happened. As I followed the guidance and focused on my breath, I experienced a surprising shift. For the first time, I realized I wasn't just my racing thoughts or anxious mind. It was as if I'd been staring at the choppy surface of a lake and suddenly caught a glimpse of the stillness underneath. It shocked me — in the best possible way.

Keep well away from water when doing breathing exercises.

WARNING

Try this simple exercise right now:

1. **Place one hand on your chest.**

2. **Don't change anything — just notice how you're breathing naturally.**

TRY THIS

   If your breathing happens to change, that's fine, too.

3. **Count three natural breaths in and out.**

   Be conscious of your experience, as best you can.

4. **Say to yourself: "I've just done a breathing exercise!"**

That's an example of conscious breathing. You've already started. Everything that follows simply builds from here.

Deciding to begin your journey

There's usually a moment when someone decides to learn to swim. Maybe they're tired of sitting on the sidelines at pool parties, or they want to feel confident around water, or they've fallen in accidentally and realized this is a skill they actually need. With breathing, there's often a similar catalyst moment.

For you, perhaps it's stress. Modern life has a way of leaving us feeling like we're constantly struggling to keep our heads above water. Or maybe you come to breathwork after experiencing anxiety, where it feels like your breath has suddenly become your enemy rather than your friend. Some people discover it after a health scare, or when they realize they want to feel more connected to their body and mind.

The decision to begin your breathing journey is really a decision to befriend your breath. Right now, you may barely notice it most of the time — it's like that reliable friend who's always there but you take for granted. Learning breathing exercises is like deciding to really get to know this friend, to discover what they're capable of, and to develop a much deeper relationship.

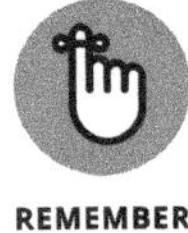

You're never alone. Imagine having a friend always by your side, ready to help you feel better in seconds. That's the friend your breath can be. This book aims to help you build that meaningful connection.

I'll never forget the day I truly committed to making breathwork a regular practice. I was dealing with a particularly stressful period — deadlines mounting, relationship challenges, the usual life stuff that can feel overwhelming. I'd been dabbling with breathing exercises for a while, but not really taking them seriously.

Then one evening, I was lying awake at 2 a.m., mind racing, feeling like my breath was shallow and unsatisfying. That's when I had my "pool edge" moment. I thought, "I've read about this stuff. Why am I not using it for myself?" I started doing coherent breathing and, within minutes, fell asleep peacefully. The next morning, I decided that breathing exercises weren't just going to be something I tried now and then — they were going to be something I lived and shared with everyone who was interested in learning more.

Discovering and practicing the basics

When you first learn to swim, you don't start by attempting the butterfly stroke or diving from the high board. You begin in the shallow end, learning to float, getting comfortable with putting your face in the water, and mastering basic movements. Breathing exercises work the same way.

The fundamentals of breathwork are deceptively simple, just like the basics of swimming. You learn to float before you learn strokes, and in breathing, you learn awareness before you learn techniques. These basics become the foundation for everything else you'll do, no matter how advanced you become.

Think of the following fundamentals as your "water safety" skills — the essential knowledge that keeps you feeling secure and confident.

Breath awareness

Just like learning to float, breath awareness is about noticing what's already happening. You're not forcing anything. You're simply becoming conscious of the natural rhythm that's been there all along.

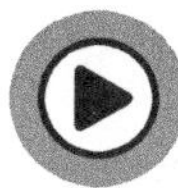

This is your first "lesson in the shallow end" (listen to Track 2):

1. **Sit comfortably or lie down somewhere you won't be disturbed.**

2. **Close your eyes or soften your gaze downward.**

3. **No need to change your breathing — just notice it.**

4. **Become aware of where you feel the breath most clearly.**

   Is it in your nose? Your chest? Your belly?

5. **Notice the natural pause between inhale and exhale.**

6. **Count five breaths, starting over if you lose count.**

7. **Take a moment to notice how you feel.**

This exercise is like learning to float — you're discovering that you can be supported by something that's already there. You don't need to create anything new. You just need to pay attention.

Gentle control

This is like learning your first swimming stroke — you're beginning to guide your breath intentionally, but gently. No forcing, no strain, just conscious direction.

Try your first "swimming stroke," called slow-motion breathing (listen to Track 3):

1. **Start with the breath awareness from the previous section.**

2. **On your next inhale, use your nose and slow it down just slightly — like swimming in slow motion.**

3. **Pause briefly at the top of the inhale.**

4. **Exhale slowly and smoothly using your nose.**

    Aim to make your breathing as quiet as you comfortably can.

5. **Pause briefly at the bottom of the exhale as much as feels natural.**

6. **Repeat for five to ten breaths.**

7. **Return to natural breathing and notice any changes.**

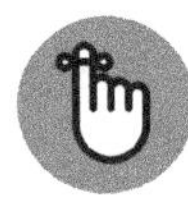

This should feel easy and comfortable. If you feel strain, you're trying too hard – like someone thrashing in the water instead of gliding smoothly.

Rhythm and pacing

In swimming, you learn to coordinate your movements. In breathing, you learn to create sustainable, comfortable rhythms that you can maintain without effort.

Discover your natural rhythm:

1. **Sit or lie down somewhere comfortable and quiet.**

2. **Begin by simply watching your breath for a few moments.**

3. **When you're ready, start to count the length of your natural inhale.**

    How many seconds does it take, without effort?

4. **Now count the length of your natural exhale.**

    Is it the same? Longer? Shorter? Just notice.

5. **Try this for a few more breaths.**

    Let your breath stay as quiet as possible — as if you're breathing through silk.

6. **After a few minutes, see if you can gently settle into a rhythm that feels natural.**

    Perhaps breathe in for four and out for five or six. No need to be precise — this is about feeling your natural flow.

7. **Let the rhythm carry you for five to ten more breaths.**

8. **Return to natural breathing and notice how you feel.**

Finding exercises that work best for you

After you've learned basic swimming strokes, you may discover that you love the freestyle but find the backstroke challenging, or that you're naturally gifted at breaststroke but struggle with butterfly. Everyone has their preferences and natural tendencies. The same is true with breathing exercises.

Some people (like me!) fall in love with coherent breathing — that steady, rhythmic practice that creates heart coherence (see Chapter 8). It's like a comfortable, sustainable freestyle stroke that you can do for long periods. Others prefer the energizing effects of breath-holding techniques (see Chapter 9), which are more like powerful sprints that leave you feeling invigorated. Still others find their home in gentle, flowing practices that feel more like a peaceful backstroke through calm waters (see Chapter 8).

The key is experimentation without judgment. Just as a swimming instructor may have you try different strokes to see what feels natural, you'll want to explore various breathing techniques to discover your favorites.

In my workshops, I love watching people discover their "breathing personality." I remember a busy executive who was convinced she needed energizing breathing techniques to help with her demanding schedule. But when we tried 4-6 breathing, something in her whole system just relaxed. "This feels like coming home," she said. Meanwhile, her colleague found the same exercise too slow and loved the more dynamic box breathing practices. Neither was right nor wrong — they just had different constitutions and needs.

LETTING GO OF PERFECT BREATHING

If you've ever felt more anxious after reading about breathing techniques, worrying you're "doing it wrong" or not breathing "perfectly," you're not alone. Many people experience this at first. Ironically, the more you try to control the breath perfectly, the more tension you may create. So let's clear the air: You don't need to be a breathing expert to benefit from conscious breathing.

Think of the different breathing exercises in this book like seeds. You try planting them and see what grows. Some may flourish quickly; others may take time or not take at all.

(continued)

(continued)

Some flowers you'll enjoy more than others. Your life is like your garden, and you get to choose which seeds to sow. Over time, with a bit of patience and care, you'll grow a mix of plants and flowers that feels right for you. And remember, you're free to find your own seeds, too, or even create a new mix that's uniquely yours. Your garden won't look like anyone else's and that's exactly how it should be. Feel free to gently play, experiment, and adapt to find out what sort of breathing exercises work best for you.

Going deeper if you want

When you're comfortable swimming in the shallow end and you've mastered the basic strokes, you may find yourself curious about deeper waters. In swimming, this may mean longer distances, different diving techniques, or perhaps training for more challenging goals. In breathwork, "going deeper" can mean several different things.

Some people are drawn to longer practice sessions — instead of 10 minutes of breathing exercises, they may enjoy 30 minutes or even hour-long sessions. It's like deciding to swim laps for fitness rather than just splashing around for fun. Others are interested in more advanced techniques that work with breath retention, or practices that combine breathing with movement or visualization.

Here are some options for advanced exploration:

>> **Extended practice sessions:** Just as marathon swimmers build up their endurance gradually, you can slowly extend your breathing sessions. Start by adding just five minutes to your regular practice and see how it feels.

>> **Breath retention practices:** These are the "deep end" practices — working with holding your breath for periods, which can be incredibly powerful for building mental resilience and accessing deeper states of consciousness.

>> **Combining breath with movement:** This may involve walking meditation with conscious breathing, or yoga practices that coordinate breath and movement.

>> **Breathwork in daily life:** The ultimate goal is to take your breathing skills out of the "practice pool" and into the "open water" of daily life — using conscious breathing during stressful meetings, while stuck in traffic, or when you need to center yourself quickly.

Just as you wouldn't attempt to swim across a lake before you're ready, don't rush into advanced breathing practices. Your breath is powerful, and respect for that power keeps the practice safe and beneficial. If you're interested in more intensive breathwork, consider working with a qualified instructor, just as you might hire a swimming coach for advanced techniques.

In the zone: Finding flow

There's a moment every experienced swimmer knows, when technique melts away and you're simply moving through water like you were born to it. Your stroke becomes effortless, your breathing perfectly synchronized, your mind clear and present. You're not *doing* swimming anymore. Swimming is simply happening *through* you. This is what athletes call *being in the zone* or what psychologists term *flow state*.

The exact same thing happens with breathing practices. After weeks or months of learning techniques, paying attention to counts and rhythms, and consciously directing your breath, something magical shifts. Suddenly, you're not *doing* a breathing exercise — the breath is simply flowing perfectly on its own, and you're along for the ride.

In this state, the breathing breathes you. Your body knows exactly what it needs, your mind settles into profound stillness, and there's a sense of connection to something larger than yourself. Time seems to disappear. The boundary between you and your breath dissolves. It's incredibly peaceful and, paradoxically, incredibly energizing at the same time.

Here's what flow state feels like in breathing practice:

>> Effortless rhythm that seems to sustain itself

>> A deep sense of presence and connection

>> Time distortion (5 minutes feels like 30, or 30 feels like 5)

>> Profound stillness in both mind and body

>> Feeling as if your body is naturally being "breathed" rather than your having to do the "breathing"

I remember the first time this happened to me. I was about six months into regular daily practice, sitting in my garden one morning. I started with my usual coherent breathing routine, expecting to do my normal 20 minutes. But something was different that day. About five minutes in, my breathing seemed to take on a life of its own. The rhythm became so natural and perfect that I stopped counting, stopped trying, stopped doing anything at all.

When I finally opened my eyes, almost 40 minutes had passed, but it felt like just a few minutes. I wasn't tired or stiff. Instead, I felt like I'd been recharged at the deepest level. The effects lasted the entire day — I moved through challenges with deep calm, my thinking was clearer, and I felt more connected to the people around me. It was like I'd discovered a completely new way of being in the world.

Over time, I learned a quiet truth: Flow can't be forced. It comes and goes like a breeze — never on demand, but often when least expected. Think of it as a gift that the breath occasionally brings, not a goal to chase. When you cling too tightly to those peak moments, they slip through your fingers, leaving behind frustration instead of freedom. But when you breathe without grasping, joy has a way of sneaking in through the side door.

The following flow-state practice isn't really a technique — it's more of an invitation to not-technique:

1. **Begin with any breathing practice in this chapter.**

2. **After a few minutes, gradually release any effort or control.**

3. **Let your breath find its own perfect rhythm.**

   If your mind tries to "help," gently return to simply receiving whatever the breath wants to do.

4. **Trust completely in your body's wisdom and stay as long as feels natural.**

5. **When you're ready to finish, take a moment to appreciate what just happened.**

Appreciating the ripple effect: Beyond the pool

Here's where the swimming metaphor becomes even more beautiful. When you truly learn to swim, the confidence and skills don't stay in the pool. You feel differently around all bodies of water. You're more confident on boats, more relaxed at the beach, and more willing to explore new aquatic adventures. The skills ripple out into a general sense of capability and confidence.

The same thing happens with breathing practices, but the ripple effect is even more profound because your breath is with you every moment of every day. When you develop a deep, friendly relationship with your breathing, it changes how you handle stress, how you fall asleep, how you wake up, how you approach difficult conversations, and how you experience your own body and emotions.

Students often tell me things like: "I never realized I was holding my breath during difficult phone calls, but now I notice and consciously breathe instead" or "When my child was having a meltdown, instead of getting triggered, I took three conscious breaths and was able to stay calm and helpful" or "I use my breathing to transition between work mode and home mode — it's like having a reset button."

Continuing your journey

As you embark on this breathing journey, remember that, like learning to swim, it's not about perfection — it's about developing a skill that serves you for life. Some days, your "swimming" will feel effortless and beautiful. Other days, you may feel like you're just keeping your head above water. Both are perfectly normal and part of the process.

The wonderful thing about breathing exercises is that, unlike swimming, you don't need a pool, special equipment, or perfect weather conditions. Your breath is always with you, ready to be your friend, your teacher, your refuge, and your pathway to greater well-being.

Start in the shallow end, be patient with yourself, practice regularly but gently, and trust that your body already knows how to do this. Before you know it, you'll be swimming in the vast, beautiful ocean of your own breath — confident, capable, and deeply at peace.

The water's perfect. Come on in!

Chapter **2**

The Science of Breathing

Breathing is so natural, it's easy to forget how incredible it is. You're somehow getting the oxygen that's floating around in the air into your blood and then into each of the tiny cells in your body. That's pretty amazing! And not only that, but somehow your lungs are also removing the unwanted gases from your body and expelling them out into the air.

You have your nose, lungs, and diaphragm to thank for this magic. In this chapter, I explain how they work and what their functions are. When you understand the science of breathing, the breathing exercises in this book will make a lot more sense.

Breathing Anatomy 101

Your breathing is primarily controlled by three key structures: the nose, the lungs, and the diaphragm. Each of these plays a unique and crucial role in the oxygenation of your body and the removal of carbon dioxide.

By understanding how these parts work together, you can breathe your way to better health, performance, and calm.

The nose: Nature's air filter and flow regulator

Your nose is more than just an airway — it's a highly sophisticated organ with more than 30 functions that support your health and breathing efficiency.

But how does the nose do all this? Well, when air is drawn into the nose, it enters the nasal cavity, a labyrinth of passageways. These passages are lined with tiny hairlike structures called *cilia* and a protective mucous membrane. These tiny hairs work together to filter, humidify, and warm the air before it reaches your lungs, ensuring it's just the right temperature and moisture level.

At the top of this cavity are the *olfactory nerves* — your direct link to a part of the brain that governs memory and emotion. These nerves are responsible for your sense of smell, but they also play a role in mood, taste, and even danger detection (like smelling smoke). As shown in Figure 2-1, the nasal cavity is far more complex than it may appear from the outside, and its structure is key to understanding why nasal breathing is so beneficial.

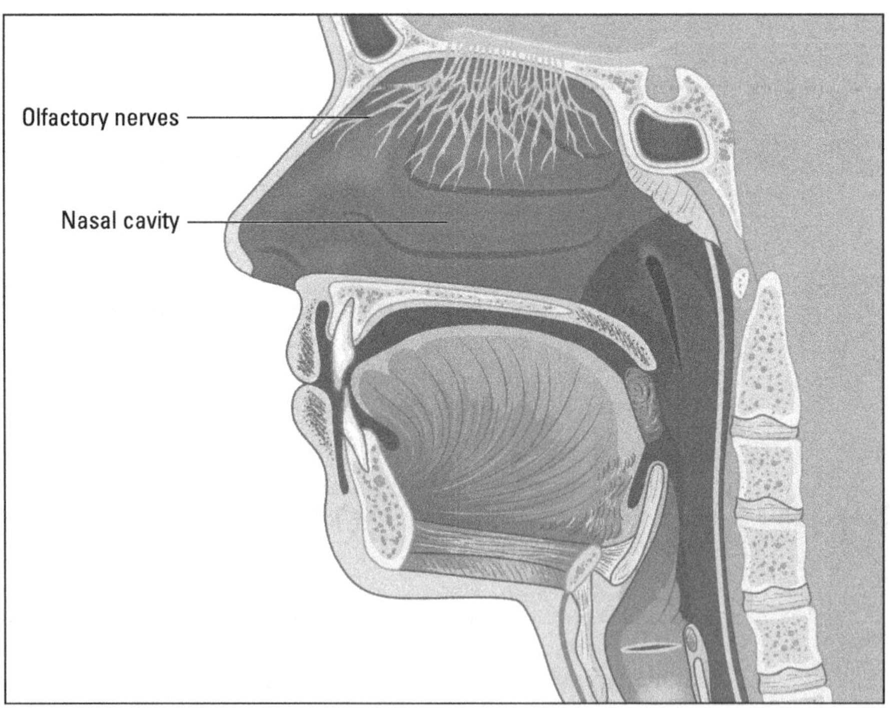

FIGURE 2-1: The structure of the nose.

Breathing through the nose offers many benefits, including the following:

>> **Filtration and protection:** Nasal hairs and mucous membranes trap dust, *allergens* (substances that trigger an allergic reaction), and *pathogens* (disease-causing agents, such as viruses or bacteria), reducing infections and allergies.

>> **Humidification and warming:** The nose adds moisture and warms the air before it reaches the lungs, preventing irritation.

>> **Nitric oxide production:** Nasal breathing generates nitric oxide, which improves circulation, reduces inflammation, fights bacteria and viruses, and enhances oxygen uptake.

>> **Better breathing rhythm:** Breathing through the nose slows and deepens breathing, improving the balance of oxygen and carbon dioxide (see "Balancing Oxygen and Carbon Dioxide," later in this chapter).

>> **Enhanced sleep:** Nasal breathing can reduce snoring, *sleep apnea* (a sleep disorder in which you repeatedly stop and start breathing while sleeping), and mouth dryness, promoting deeper rest.

>> **Stronger diaphragmatic breathing:** Nasal breathing engages the diaphragm, increasing lung capacity and reducing stress.

>> **Immune system support:** The nasal passages contain immune cells that neutralize harmful microbes.

One of the key lessons of this book is to learn to use your nose to breathe more often, both during the day, when doing low to moderate exercise, and at night while you sleep. You can find the benefits of nasal breathing and methods to keep your nose unblocked in Chapter 6.

THE EXPLORER WHO UNLOCKED THE SECRET OF NASAL BREATHING

In the 1800s, George Catlin, an American artist and explorer, spent years living among more than 50 Native American tribes. He observed their way of life and noted their strength, health, and vitality, despite the absence of modern medicine.

As Catlin observed the Indians' way of life, one unusual habit stood out: They all breathed through their noses — day and night. It wasn't just a coincidence. Parents would gently press their babies' lips shut as they slept, ensuring that they learned to breathe through their noses from infancy. The tribes believed that "the mouth is for

(continued)

(continued)

eating and the nose is for breathing" — a simple yet powerful philosophy that kept them strong and disease-free.

Catlin was so amazed by what he saw that he wrote a book about it in 1869, titled *Shut Your Mouth and Save Your Life,* in which he warned that mouth breathing was ruining people's health in Western society, leading to weaker immune systems, poor facial development, and chronic illness.

At the time, most people ignored Catlin's advice. But today, modern science confirms what these tribes instinctively knew: Nasal breathing is the key to better health, deeper sleep, and stronger lungs.

So, next time you catch yourself breathing through your mouth, remember George Catlin's discovery, and shut your mouth to save your life!

The lungs: The oxygen exchange center

Your lungs work 24/7 to keep you alive — bringing in fresh oxygen and getting rid of carbon dioxide. But they're more than just big air bags in your chest. The lungs have a smart design that makes breathing smooth, efficient, and automatic.

Think of the lungs like an upside-down tree — with a strong trunk (windpipe), big branches (bronchi), and thousands of tiny twigs (bronchioles) that end in tiny air sacs (alveoli). Here's how all these pieces work (see Figure 2-2):

>> **Trachea (windpipe):** The trachea is the main tube that carries air from your nose and mouth into your lungs. It has tiny hairlike cilia that trap dust and germs so they don't get into your lungs.

>> **Bronchi:** The trachea splits into two big tubes, called *bronchi* — one for each lung.

>> **Bronchioles:** Each bronchus branches into smaller and smaller tubes, called *bronchioles* (which are like tiny tree branches). You have about 30,000 bronchioles in each lung, spreading air everywhere.

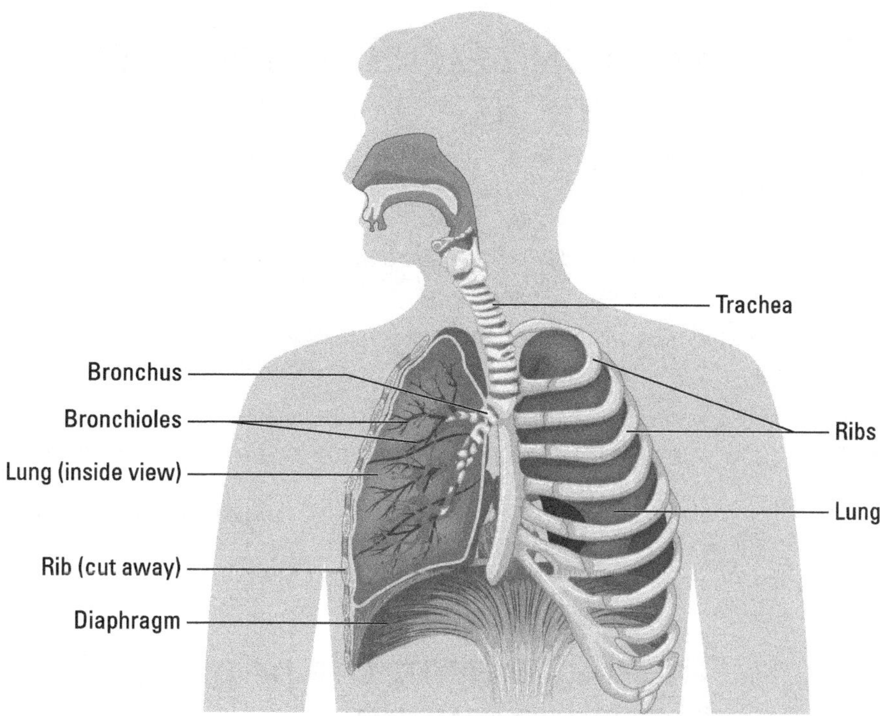

FIGURE 2-2:
The structure of
the lungs.

© *John Wiley & Sons, Inc.*

>> **Alveoli:** At the very end of the bronchioles are about 600 million tiny air sacs called *alveoli.* This is where oxygen gets into your blood and carbon dioxide is removed. The alveoli are covered in tiny blood vessels that take oxygen into your body and send carbon dioxide out.

>> **Diaphragm:** The diaphragm is a big, dome-shaped muscle sitting under your lungs. When you breathe in, the diaphragm moves down, making room for your lungs to fill with air. When you breathe out, the diaphragm moves up, pushing air out of your lungs. (See the next section for more on the diaphragm.)

Despite being vital for survival, most people don't use their lungs efficiently, often engaging in shallow, upper-chest breathing that limits oxygen absorption and contributes to fatigue, stress, and poor overall health. Understanding how your lungs work and how to optimize their function can lead to better energy levels, improved endurance, and greater resistance to illness. (Check out the nearby sidebar for more on why lung efficiency matters.)

Your lungs hold up to 6 liters of air, but most people use only a small fraction of their lung capacity. Shallow, rapid breathing limits oxygen intake and carbon dioxide regulation, leading to:

- **Fatigue and brain fog:** Less oxygen reaches the brain and muscles, reducing mental clarity and energy.

- **Increased stress and anxiety:** Shallow breathing triggers the body's stress response, keeping you in a state of tension.

- **Poor posture and musculoskeletal tension:** Chest breathing overworks the neck and shoulder muscles, contributing to tension headaches and poor posture.

By maximizing lung efficiency, you can dramatically improve your energy, mental focus, endurance, and overall health.

The diaphragm: The primary breathing muscle

The diaphragm (refer to Figure 2-2) is the most important muscle in breathing, yet most people don't use it efficiently. Located just below your lungs, it's a large, dome-shaped muscle that separates your chest cavity from your abdomen. Every breath you take is powered by the diaphragm, which controls the volume of air entering and exiting your lungs.

Many people rely too much on their chest and neck muscles for breathing, leading to shallow, inefficient respiration. Training your diaphragm to work properly can transform your breathing, increase oxygen efficiency, lower stress, and improve endurance.

How the diaphragm works

The diaphragm functions like a bellows, controlling airflow into and out of your lungs. Here's how it works:

1. **When you inhale, the diaphragm contracts and moves downward, creating more space in your chest cavity.**

   A vacuum is created inside your lungs, causing air to rush in. Ideally, this movement should expand your belly instead of lifting your chest.

2. **When you exhale, the diaphragm relaxes and moves back up, reducing space in the chest cavity.**

Air is pushed out of the lungs, expelling carbon dioxide and making room for fresh oxygen in the next breath.

This automatic movement happens thousands of times a day, but many people unknowingly develop dysfunctional breathing patterns that limit the diaphragm's efficiency.

The problem with shallow chest breathing

Many people unconsciously breathe using their chest and shoulders rather than their diaphragm. This overuses the neck and chest muscles, leading to:

>> **Reduced oxygen intake:** Shallow breathing limits lung expansion, decreasing oxygen absorption.

>> **Increased stress and anxiety:** Chest breathing activates the sympathetic nervous system, keeping the body in fight-or-flight mode.

>> **Poor posture and neck tension:** Overuse of the neck, shoulders, and upper chest muscles leads to stiffness and headaches.

>> **Lower endurance and fatigue:** Inefficient breathing makes physical activity feel harder, reducing stamina.

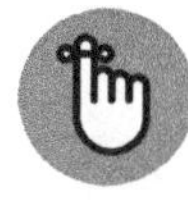

By retraining your diaphragm, you can breathe deeper, absorb more oxygen, and feel calmer and more energized.

REMEMBER

The benefits of diaphragmatic breathing

Training your diaphragm to work efficiently has profound health benefits, including:

TIP

>> **Increased oxygen efficiency:** More air reaches the lower lobes of the lungs, where oxygen exchange is greatest.

>> **Lower heart rate and blood pressure:** Deep, slow breathing signals relaxation to the nervous system.

>> **Reduced anxiety and stress:** Diaphragmatic breathing activates the parasympathetic nervous system (rest and digest mode).

>> **Improved posture and core stability:** Diaphragmatic breathing strengthens the deep core muscles, supporting better spinal alignment.

>> **Enhanced athletic performance:** Diaphragmatic breathing increases endurance by making breathing more efficient and saving energy.

>> **Better sleep:** Diaphragmatic breathing promotes relaxation, reducing snoring and sleep disturbances.

You can find out more about diaphragmatic breathing and how to do it in Chapter 7.

Understanding How Breathing Nourishes the Body

Breathing is more than just taking in air — it's a complex, life-sustaining process that fuels every cell in your body. Every inhale delivers oxygen to your bloodstream, while every exhale removes carbon dioxide, preventing the buildup of harmful waste. This balance is essential for maintaining energy, brain function, and overall health.

Yet many people take shallow, inefficient breaths, limiting oxygen absorption and disrupting the body's delicate oxygen–carbon dioxide exchange. Understanding how breathing nourishes your body can help you optimize your breathing for better health, energy, and mental clarity.

Getting oxygen to your blood

Oxygen is the fuel of life — every cell in your body depends on it to function. However, simply breathing in oxygen isn't enough; it must be efficiently absorbed into the bloodstream and delivered where it's needed.

Here's how oxygen makes its way into your body:

1. **You _inhale_ (breathe in) through the nose or mouth.**

   Air travels down your _trachea_ (windpipe) and into your lungs. Inside your lungs are millions of tiny air sacs called _alveoli,_ which are like microscopic balloons. Wrapped around each one are _capillaries,_ tiny blood vessels that allow oxygen to pass through. This is where the real exchange begins.

2. **Oxygen enters the cells and moves through the blood.**

   In the alveoli, oxygen passes into the capillaries and binds to red blood cells, which act like oxygen taxis. These cells travel through your arteries, delivering oxygen to the organs and muscles that need it most — especially your brain, heart, and muscles, which are always hungry for more.

Inside your cells, oxygen helps create energy, which powers everything your body does: walking, thinking, digesting food, and even healing. But if your breathing is inefficient (say, too fast or shallow), less oxygen reaches your cells. That can leave you feeling tired, foggy, or low on energy.

3. **You *exhale* (breathe out).**

As your cells use oxygen to create energy, they produce a waste gas: carbon dioxide. This gas travels back through your bloodstream to your lungs. Then, as you breathe out, your diaphragm pushes upward, helping you clear out the carbon dioxide through your lungs and out of your mouth or nose — like taking out what you don't need.

Removing excess carbon dioxide from your blood

Carbon dioxide is just as essential as oxygen — in the right amounts. Many people assume that carbon dioxide is just a waste gas, but it actually plays a crucial role in oxygen delivery and *pH* (a measure of acidity and alkalinity) balance in the body.

Here's how breathing regulates carbon dioxide:

1. **The body produces carbon dioxide.**

Every time your cells make energy (which they're doing all the time), they produce carbon dioxide as a by-product. This gas dissolves into your blood and hitches a ride back to your lungs, ready to be released.

2. **Your body uses some of that carbon dioxide to help get oxygen into your cells.**

This is where it gets clever: Carbon dioxide helps control how easily oxygen is released from a substance in your red blood cells called *hemoglobin*. This smart system is known as the *Bohr effect*.

When your carbon dioxide levels are just right, hemoglobin knows when to let go of oxygen, allowing it to enter your cells where it's needed. But if you *over-breathe* (taking in too much air or breathing too fast), you blow off too much carbon dioxide. That makes your red blood cells cling too tightly to oxygen — and ironically, your cells get less of what they need.

This can leave you feeling dizzy, anxious, short of breath, or just off — even though you're breathing more.

3. **You exhale, and excess carbon dioxide is removed from the body.**

Exhaling is how your body gets rid of any extra carbon dioxide it doesn't need. But how you exhale matters. Slow, nasal breathing helps keep your carbon dioxide at just the right level. It prevents over-breathing, supports calmness, and ensures that oxygen gets where it needs to go — efficiently and smoothly.

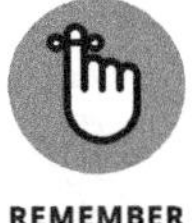

By breathing efficiently, you fuel your body, sharpen your mind, and enhance your overall well-being — one breath at a time.

Your Nervous System and Your Breath

Breathing is one of the few bodily functions that is both automatic and under conscious control. Although your body breathes on its own, you can also intentionally change your breath to influence your nervous system, stress levels, and energy.

Your breath and nervous system are deeply connected — by altering your breathing, you can shift from stressed to calm or from distracted to focused, depending on what you need.

Understanding your autonomic nervous system

Your nervous system is like your body's control center, regulating everything from digestion to heart rate to emotional responses. A key part of this system is the autonomic nervous system, which is divided into two branches:

>> **Sympathetic nervous system (fight-or-flight):** The sympathetic nervous system activates when you're stressed, anxious, or whenever you need energy, such as when exercising or giving a speech. It increases your heart rate, blood pressure, and breathing rate, preparing the body for action. But it can lead to chronic stress if it's overactivated over the long term.

>> **Parasympathetic nervous system (rest-and-digest):** The parasympathetic nervous system activates when you're calm, relaxed, and at ease. It slows down the heart rate and breathing, promoting relaxation and healing. It also helps with digestion, recovery, and deep sleep.

Your breathing directly influences which system is dominant — fast, shallow breathing triggers the sympathetic nervous system, while slow, deep breathing activates the parasympathetic nervous system.

Seeing how breathing exercises can calm and relax

Breathing is one of the most powerful tools we have for reducing stress, calming anxiety, and promoting relaxation as and when you need it. When you're feeling overwhelmed, your sympathetic nervous system (responsible for fight-or-flight responses) is in overdrive. This leads to rapid breathing, increased heart rate, and heightened tension in the body.

By simply slowing down your breath, you can activate the parasympathetic nervous system — also known as the rest-and-digest system. This shift promotes relaxation, lowers blood pressure, reduces stress hormones, and helps restore balance to the body and mind.

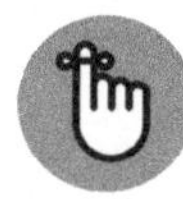

When you breathe slowly and deeply, particularly through the nose, you signal to your body that it's safe to relax.

One simple but powerful technique for relaxation and overall well-being is the 4-6 Breathing technique, which promotes a slower, more controlled breathing pattern, with the longer exhale. This technique helps balance oxygen and carbon dioxide levels, encourages diaphragmatic breathing, and activates your rest-and-digest mode (the parasympathetic nervous system).

Follow these steps and listen to Track 4 to try the 4-6 Breathing technique:

1. **Find a comfortable position.**

    Sit or lie down in a relaxed posture. Close your eyes if it helps you focus.

2. **Breathe in gently through your nose for a count of four.**

    Allow your belly to expand as you inhale gently and deeply, counting to four.

3. **Exhale through your nose for a count of six.**

    Slowly release the air, making the exhale longer than the inhale. Try to stay relaxed and avoid forcing the breath. No effort needed at all.

4. **Repeat for several minutes.**

    Continue this rhythm for however long you've got. It could be just a few cycles, or if you have time, or five to ten minutes, focusing on the steady flow of air in and out.

    If it feels natural, pause briefly after exhaling before starting the next inhale.

This technique helps slow down breathing, reduce anxiety, increase focus, and can give peace of mind.

Practicing regularly, especially before bed or during stressful moments, can significantly enhance your sense of calm and well-being. If the 4-6 Breathing technique doesn't feel comfortable, adjust the timings so they work for you. For example, 3-5 or 5-7 may work better in your case. The key is to breathe gently rather than to over-breathe with large in and out breaths.

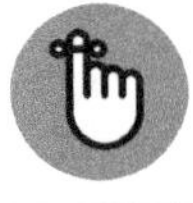

The extended exhale slows the heart rate, helping your body transition into a state of relaxation. It also increases carbon dioxide retention, which can have a calming effect on the nervous system.

Crucially, this slower breathing rhythm stimulates the *vagus nerve* (a major nerve that runs from your brain down through your chest and abdomen, connecting to key organs like the heart, lungs, and digestive system). Activating the vagus nerve helps shift your body into the parasympathetic state —the rest-and-digest mode — which promotes calm, lowers stress hormones, and supports long-term health.

Finding out how breathing exercises energize and focus

Just as slow breathing calms the nervous system, certain breathing techniques can boost energy, sharpen focus, and improve mental clarity. Fast and controlled breathing stimulates the sympathetic nervous system, increasing oxygen intake, circulation, and alertness.

If you're feeling fatigued, sluggish, or mentally foggy, activating your breath can wake up your body and mind naturally — without caffeine.

The best breathing exercises for quick energy and focus either have an equal length of in and out breath or involve breathing in for longer than you breathe out. Energizing breathing exercises can sometimes include breathing much faster than usual, for a short period of time.

The stimulating breath technique, also known as bellows breath (or *Bhastrika Pranayama* in yoga) is a quick and effective method to boost energy and alertness. *Bhastrika* means bellows (as in the device used by a blacksmith to blow air to ignite a fire). This practice, rooted in traditional yoga, invigorates the body and sharpens the mind, making it an excellent tool for combating fatigue and enhancing focus.

Bellows breath is a powerful practice, so it's important to use it with care. Always practice on an empty stomach — ideally, at least two hours after eating. Avoid it during pregnancy. If you ever feel dizzy, pause, slow down, and return to normal breathing. Those with high blood pressure, panic attacks, heart conditions, ulcers, or chronic constipation should consult a healthcare provider or experienced teacher before trying it. Most importantly, go at your own pace. It should feel energizing, not exhausting.

Here's how to do the stimulating breath technique:

1. **Find a comfortable position.**

   Sit upright in a chair with your back straight and shoulders relaxed, or stand with your feet hip-width apart.

2. **Close your mouth, with your lips gently sealed.**

   Focus on breathing through your nose throughout the exercise.

3. **Take a few calm, slow, deep breaths through your nose.**

4. **Begin rapid breathing.**

   Exhale through your nose by contracting your abdominal muscles (as if gently pushing your belly in). Instantly inhale through your nose by relaxing the belly and letting the diaphragm do the work. Each breath is rapid — a bit like a pump. There should be a whooshing sound as you breathe in and out. As a beginner, aim for approximately one breath in and out every two seconds.

5. **Maintain the rhythm.**

   Continue this rapid breathing pattern for 10 breaths during your initial practice sessions. As you become more comfortable, gradually increase to 20 breaths.

6. **Rest and repeat.**

   After completing a round, return to normal breathing. Take a few deep, calming breaths to allow your body to adjust.

   Repeat the rapid breathing exercise for up to three rounds in total, depending on your comfort level.

Over time (weeks or months), you can slowly increase to one breath per second and then two breaths per second. With regular practice, you might work up to 120 breaths in a round, but only if it continues to feel steady and comfortable. The moment it feels forced or dizzying, take a break.

Make sure your spine is relatively straight to allow optimal airflow and prevent strain. If you feel lightheaded or dizzy, stop the exercise and return to regular breathing. Over time, your endurance will improve. After doing this energizing exercise, I recommend you do some 4–6 Breathing, meditation, or another activity to rebalance your nervous system so you're not in an overly stressed state. Finally, practice this technique in the morning or early afternoon to avoid interfering with your sleep patterns.

Balancing Oxygen and Carbon Dioxide

Most people think of oxygen as the hero of breathing and carbon dioxide as just a waste product. But both oxygen and carbon dioxide are essential, and they need to exist in the right balance for your body to function optimally. Your oxygen and carbon dioxide levels need to remain in balance. Your goal is to ensure that both gases are present in just the right amounts.

Discovering why you need some carbon dioxide in your blood

Your body needs the right amount of carbon dioxide in your blood to help it use oxygen properly. When you inhale, oxygen enters your lungs and is carried to your bloodstream by hemoglobin. However, oxygen doesn't readily release itself from hemoglobin. It needs the presence of carbon dioxide to signal when and where it should be delivered. If you breathe too fast, you expel too much carbon dioxide, which makes it harder for oxygen to reach your cells. This means that even if you have plenty of oxygen in your blood, your body struggles to use it efficiently — leading to symptoms like dizziness, brain fog, fatigue, and even anxiety.

Imagine hemoglobin as a delivery truck and oxygen as the cargo. These trucks travel through your bloodstream, carrying oxygen to your body's cells. But they won't unload the cargo unless they get the right signal. That's where carbon dioxide comes in — it's like a GPS signal or unloading instruction. When carbon dioxide levels are balanced, the hemoglobin truck gets the message: "Time to drop off the oxygen here!" But if you don't have enough carbon dioxide (as when you over-breathe), the signal gets too weak. The trucks keep driving around with their cargo still onboard — and your cells miss out on the oxygen they need, even though it's technically there.

This is why breathing too fast doesn't mean more oxygen is reaching your cells. In fact, it can do the opposite.

Understanding how breathing exercises can help you rebalance

If you over-breathe, you lose too much carbon dioxide, throwing off the oxygen–carbon dioxide balance and making your breathing less efficient. Thankfully, you can retrain your body to breathe in a way that preserves just the right amount of carbon dioxide, allowing your oxygen to do its job properly. One way to achieve this goal is to breathe in a quiet and controlled way, using your nose.

Quiet nasal breathing is a simple breathing exercise to help restore the oxygen–carbon dioxide balance. Follow these steps and listen to Track 5 to do it:

1. **Inhale gently and quietly through your nose.**

2. **Exhale softly and quietly through your nose.**

3. **Continue for a minute or so, keeping your breathing light and quiet.**

   Notice your lower abdomen expanding and contracting as you breathe in and out using your diaphragm.

   If you find yourself feeling a bit of *air hunger* (the feeling that you need more air), that's actually a good sign. It means your body is learning to readjust its breathing rate.

   Notice if your hand or feet feel warmer, or if there's more saliva in your mouth. These are signs that your parasympathetic nervous system is engaging — again, good signs you're doing the exercise correctly.

   This simple exercise helps gently increase your carbon dioxide levels, improving how well oxygen reaches your brain and muscles. When it feels comfortable, try practicing for a few minutes at a time, about three times a day. With regular practice, you'll likely notice a positive shift in your energy, focus, and overall well-being.

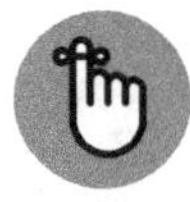

Breathing isn't just about getting more oxygen — it's about using oxygen efficiently, which depends on having the right amount of carbon dioxide in your blood.

Breathe slower, through your nose to maintain a healthy carbon dioxide level. Avoid rapid, shallow breathing, which expels too much carbon dioxide and disrupts oxygen delivery. Use breath-holding techniques to train your body to tolerate carbon dioxide better.

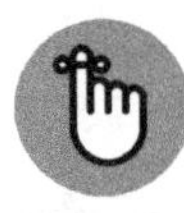

By keeping your oxygen and carbon dioxide levels in balance, you'll breathe more efficiently, feel more energized, and enjoy greater mental clarity — all without needing to take bigger breaths. To help you do this, you'll find simple, science-backed exercises in the following chapters: nasal breathing in Chapter 6, deep breathing in Chapter 7, slow breathing in Chapter 8, and light breathing in Chapter 9. The key takeaway? Breathe through your nose, and aim for a breath that's deep, slow, and light whenever you remember. With regular practice, this gentle shift can boost your energy, sharpen your focus, and bring a sense of calm into your everyday life.

IN THIS CHAPTER

» **Understanding the conversation between the lungs and the brain**

» **Seeing how breathing is linked to your emotions**

» **Finding out how mindful breathing can help manage your energy levels and focus**

Chapter **3**

Breath and the Mind-Body Connection

Breathing isn't just about getting air into your lungs — it's a bridge between mind and body, shaping mood, influencing stress, and supporting well-being. This chapter shows how breath awareness can quickly shift your emotional state, restore clarity, and sharpen focus.

HOW I GOT INTO BREATHING EXERCISES

When I began teaching in my early twenties, stress quickly took over. Large classes and endless workloads left me exhausted. I tried running to cope, but the stress lingered. It wasn't until I noticed how shallow and rushed my breathing had become that things started to shift. My breath reflected my tension — fast and chest-bound — keeping me on edge.

Discovering breathing exercises was a turning point. Unlike physical exercise, breathwork calmed my mind and brought immediate relief. It became a practical tool I could use anytime. With breath awareness, teaching became less about surviving and more about engaging with presence and clarity.

Eavesdropping on the Conversation between Your Lungs and Your Brain

Your lungs and your brain are in constant dialogue, communicating with each other every moment of your life, even though you may not realize it. This ongoing conversation influences your emotional state, stress responses, and overall health. Understanding this relationship can empower you to actively manage your emotional and physical well-being.

Your respiratory system sends vital signals to your brain that affect how you think, feel, and react. Every breath you take acts like a messenger, carrying information from your lungs to your brain via your nervous system.

Your breath communicates directly with your brain through your autonomic nervous system (see Chapter 2), which controls many bodily functions automatically:

>> **Inhalation:** Typically activates your sympathetic nervous system, raising alertness and heart rate slightly, preparing your body for action.

>> **Exhalation:** Usually activates your parasympathetic nervous system, signaling your body to calm down, slowing your heart rate, and helping you feel more relaxed.

To harness the power of your lungs' communication with your brain, try these simple practices:

>> **Observe your breathing.** Check your breathing regularly throughout the day. Notice if it's shallow, rapid, or irregular — this can indicate stress or anxiety.

>> **Use conscious breathing exercises.** Practice slow, controlled breathing to communicate safety to your brain and body, triggering relaxation and focus.

>> **Experiment with rhythmic breathing.** Techniques such as quietly inhaling for five seconds and quietly exhaling for five seconds can powerfully rebalance your nervous system, enhancing your well-being. Learn more about this technique, called coherent breathing, in Chapter 8.

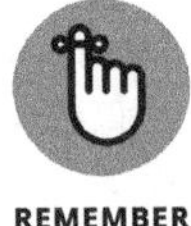

By paying attention to this powerful conversation between your lungs and your brain, you can greatly improve your emotional resilience, cognitive abilities, and overall health. Your lungs aren't just helping you survive — they're guiding you toward thriving.

Your brain and lungs are in constant communication through the autonomic nervous system and the vagus nerve. Stretch receptors in your lungs send signals to the brain stem about how full your lungs are, and the brain responds by adjusting your breathing rate. At the same time, your emotional state — managed by areas like the amygdala and prefrontal cortex — can speed up or slow down your breathing. This two-way feedback loop influences your heart rate, stress response, and emotional regulation. In short, how you breathe can directly affect how you feel — and vice versa.

Discovering the Connection between Breathing and Emotions

Understanding how your emotions and breathing are interconnected can transform your life — from your physical health to your emotional well-being and relationships.

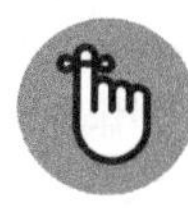

Breathing patterns are not only *indicators* of emotional states — they actively *influence* them. Here's how:

>> **Anxiety and stress:** Rapid, shallow breathing can exacerbate anxiety and stress. It signals to your brain that danger is present, keeping your body in a heightened state of alertness. Conversely, slow, deep breathing communicates safety, reducing anxiety and stress levels.

>> **Calm and relaxation:** Slow, deep breathing activates the parasympathetic nervous system (see Chapter 2), helping you feel calmer. Techniques such as slow diaphragmatic breathing and extended exhalation effectively lower stress and create feelings of relaxation and control.

>> **Mood and emotional balance:** Your breathing patterns directly influence your emotional resilience. Regular breathing exercises can help stabilize your mood and enhance emotional balance.

By learning to notice your breathing rate and depth, you begin to discover how to get better control of your emotions.

Here's a straightforward way to observe how your breath affects your emotions:

1. **Breathe in a rapid and shallow way for a minute or less.**

    Notice how it's making you feel. What emotions does it bring up? Where do you feel the emotion in your body? What thoughts are you having?

2. **Take a break for a minute to write down how the experience was for you.**

3. **Practice slow, quiet, diaphragmatic breathing for a minute.**

    Place your hands gently on the sides of your lower rib cage, just above your
    waist and below your chest. Your thumbs can rest toward your back, with your
    fingers wrapping around the sides toward the front. Breathe slowly in and out
    through your nose. As you inhale, see if you can feel your ribs expanding
    slightly outward into your hands. As you exhale, notice the ribs drawing gently
    back in. If it feels comfortable, try breathing out for slightly longer than you
    breathe in. Stay curious. Observe how your body feels, and notice any
    thoughts or emotions that arise, without needing to change them.

4. **Write about your experience.**

    Jot down your experience. Compare the kinds of thoughts, feelings, and
    sensations you experienced with rapid, shallow breathing, compared to slow,
    deep breathing.

Your breath is like a built-in emotional radar, constantly giving you clues about
how you're feeling. Ever noticed how your breathing changes when you're anxious, relaxed, excited, or angry? By tuning into these subtle shifts, you can become
better at recognizing and understanding your emotional states. Here's what
to look for:

>> **Rapid, shallow breathing:** Usually signals anxiety, stress, or fear, unless
you're doing some intense physical exercise.

>> **Slow, deep breathing:** Often indicates relaxation, calmness, or contentment.

>> **Irregular breathing:** Might suggest feelings of uncertainty, nervousness, or
excitement.

>> **Holding your breath:** Often this happens unconsciously, so it's harder to
spot. Commonly happens when you're tense, scared, or intensely focused.

This is why breathing exercises are powerful tools to manage stress, anxiety, and
emotional upheaval. Deliberate breathing techniques can help reset your nervous
system, shifting your state from stress to calmness.

To practice recognizing emotional states through your breath:

TRY THIS

1. **Set a timer to go off at multiple times in the day, and take a moment to
notice your breathing when the alarm goes off.**

2. **Ask yourself what your breathing pattern is like.**

    Is your breathing fast, slow, shallow, deep, regular, or irregular?

3. **Reflect briefly on your emotions or thoughts at that moment.**

   Can you link the way you're breathing with what you're feeling?

With regular practice, you'll quickly build a reliable way to gauge your emotional state just by checking in with your breathing.

Seeing How the Breath Affects Your Energy Level

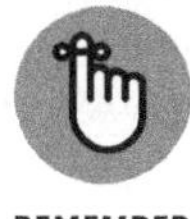

Your heart literally beats faster on your in breath than it does on your out breath. So, if you want to activate more energy, breathe in for longer than you breathe out. If you want to be more calm, breathe out for longer than you breathe in.

In the following sections, I walk you through exercises to calm down and exercises to rev up.

Using breath to calm down

Here are a couple of quick and effective breathing techniques you can use to shift your emotions:

The extended exhale breathing exercise is a simple yet powerful method for calming your mind, reducing stress, and activating the body's natural relaxation response. To do it, follow these steps and listen to Track 6:

1. **Find a comfortable position.**

   Sit or lie down comfortably. Ensure your spine is straight but relaxed. Relax your shoulders, soften your jaw, and gently close your eyes if it feels comfortable.

2. **Slowly inhale through your nose for a comfortable count — typically around three or four seconds.**

   Allow your belly to expand gently instead of breathing into your upper chest.

3. **Gently exhale through your mouth with pursed lips, as if you're gently blowing out a candle or softly sighing; make your exhale longer than your inhale — typically around six to eight seconds.**

   If six to eight seconds feels too long, you can start with shorter times, as long as the exhale is longer than the inhale.

4. Continue breathing this way until you feel calmer and more relaxed.

With each exhale, imagine releasing tension from your body, softening further, and letting go of stress.

You can do this exercise for just three breaths if that's all you have time for, and you may notice the effect. To deepen the effect, practice for five minutes a day, or more.

For a more effective exercise, follow these tips:

>> Breathe gently and softly — don't force the breath.

>> Keep your attention gently focused on the sensation of breathing.

>> If your mind wanders, gently guide your attention back to the breath without judgment.

>> Adjust the length of the exhale as needed — comfortably longer than your inhale is enough.

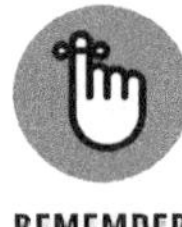

A longer exhale calms your nerves, sending signals to your brain that you're safe, helping to slow down your heart rate, lower blood pressure, and release tension in your body.

Using breath to energize

The calming breathing exercises can have the effect of energizing you, as they recharge your batteries. But what if you want to do an exercise to energize yourself immediately?

The three-part breath (Dirga Pranayama) from yoga is traditionally calming, but you can use it as an energizing breath by gently increasing your breath awareness, fully oxygenating your body, and bringing conscious attention to each inhale and exhale. It's also a great exercise to do at the start of a breathwork session. Follow these steps and listen to Track 7 to practice:

1. Find a comfortable position.

Sit upright with your spine comfortably tall but relaxed. Relax your shoulders, soften your face, and close your eyes gently or leave them open with a soft gaze.

2. Begin by gently exhaling completely through your nose, emptying your lungs to create space.

3. **Gently breathe in through your nose in three stages, without holding your breath:**

- **Lower belly:** Inhale slowly, expanding your belly as it gently moves outward (imagine filling your lower lungs first).

- **Rib cage:** Continue inhaling smoothly, feeling your ribs expanding sideways, front and back.

- **Upper chest:** Draw breath into your upper chest, feeling the upper lungs gently expand, lifting your collarbones slightly.

   The inhale should be smooth and in three parts: belly, ribs, chest.

4. **Exhale slowly through your nose in reverse order.**

   The chest relaxes first, then the ribs soften inward, and finally your belly gently draws back toward your spine, completely emptying the lungs.

5. **Repeat mindfully for three to ten cycles.**

   Keep breathing slowly, smoothly, and deeply, without force. With each cycle, notice your body energizing and becoming more alert and focused.

Full yogic breathing oxygenates your brain and body, naturally boosting energy and alertness, as well as stretching the muscles you use to breathe. The mindful attention required brings increased clarity, reducing feelings of sluggishness and fatigue.

Here are some tips for getting the most out of this exercise:

>> Make sure that each inhale and exhale is comfortable — not overly forced.

>> Focus gently but attentively on the sensation of your breath moving through each stage.

>> Aim for breaths that feel full yet natural, maintaining a steady, energizing rhythm.

Practice this breathing technique whenever you're experiencing a slump to enhance your energy, clarity, and overall vitality.

Breathing for Mental Clarity and Focus

In our fast-paced world, distractions seem endless — notifications pinging, social media scrolling, overflowing inboxes, and even the noisy chatter in our own minds.

Often, the underlying issue isn't the distractions themselves, but rather how the brain reacts to stress, fatigue, or overstimulation. When your brain perceives stress, it shifts into survival mode, limiting your capacity to think clearly and stay attentive. Shallow, rapid breathing — a common response to stress — further compounds the problem, starving your brain of the oxygen it needs for clear thought. And your brain needs lots of oxygen in the right places to be able to focus effectively.

The good news is that by changing your breathing pattern, you can quickly shift your brain back into a calm, clear state, enabling you to reclaim your focus.

Breathing can enhance cognitive performance, helping you make smarter decisions. Rhythmic breathing practices, such as coherent breathing (see Chapter 8), synchronize brain waves, leading to better mental clarity, improved memory, and greater focus. By controlling the rhythm of your breathing, your body helps your brain optimize its function, enhancing your mental efficiency throughout the day.

WHAT ABOUT MINDFULNESS?

Mindfulness is brilliant — I love it, teach it daily, and see its benefits firsthand. It's about noticing the present moment with kindness, curiosity, and openness. But on its own, mindfulness can fall short, especially when you're mentally scattered or anxious. That's when it can feel so hard to focus.

Think of mindfulness as cleaning a window to see clearly. But if your breathing is shallow or erratic, it's like wearing dirty glasses — even a clean window won't help you focus. Poor breathing habits from stress or inattention can make mindfulness harder, as your mind wanders and frustration builds.

That's why combining mindfulness with breathing exercises is so powerful. Breathwork resets your breathing, boosts oxygen to the brain, calms your nervous system, and helps sustain focus and presence.

Better breathing isn't just for the day. Gentle evening breathwork and nasal breathing during sleep improves overnight oxygen flow, helping you wake up clearer and calmer.

So, before you polish the mindful window, check your breath. Together, mindful awareness and healthy breathing elevate clarity, energy, and presence.

Sometimes, when we're overwhelmed, distracted, or struggling to focus, our breathing becomes shallow, rapid, and irregular. This subtle shift can imbalance the oxygen and carbon dioxide levels in the body, making us feel even more foggy or stressed. This is because not enough oxygen can get into your brain cells. One solution to this is quiet, slow, deep breathing or mini breath holds (see Chapter 9). Box breathing is also great for improving focus (see Chapter 8).

Another simple yet powerful breathing technique, known as *cyclic sighing* or *physiological sighing*, can rapidly restore focus and mental clarity.

First studied in neuroscience labs and popularized by Dr. Andrew Huberman, the physiological sigh is a natural reflex that humans (and even animals) use to self-regulate stress. It involves a double inhale followed by a long, controlled exhale, helping to recalibrate oxygen and carbon dioxide levels in the body. You may have noticed yourself unconsciously sighing after an emotional moment or deep concentration — this is your body's way of resetting. Now, you can intentionally use this breath to enhance focus and performance.

Early research from Stanford shows that cyclic sighing may help calm the nervous system, but more studies are needed to know for whom it works best. If you experience panic attacks, avoid this technique for now (see Chapter 10 for safer breath practices). And as always, consult your doctor before trying new breathing exercises.

Follow these steps and listen to Track 8 to practice cyclic sighing:

1. **Take a deep breath in through your nose, and then, just before exhaling, take a second, smaller inhale to fully expand your lungs.**

   The second inhale allows the lungs to fully inflate, preventing the alveoli (see Chapter 2) from collapsing, and improving oxygen absorption.

2. **Exhale fully and slowly through your mouth, as if gently blowing out a candle. Add a sighing sound if you want.**

   The key is the extended exhale, which helps offload excess carbon dioxide, lowering physiological stress, calms the nervous system, and promotes mental clarity.

3. **Repeat one to three times.**

This simple pattern helps reset your nervous system and sharpen your focus within seconds. It works within 30 seconds, making it one of the fastest ways to regain focus in the middle of a task. If you enjoy the practice and find it helpful, practice for five minutes a day.

Here are some tips for maximizing the benefits:

>> **Use it before high-focus activities.** For example, try this breath before writing, public speaking, or making important decisions.

>> **Pair it with intention.** As you exhale, mentally let go of distractions and refocus on your next step.

>> **Practice throughout the day.** If you feel scattered, take a moment to pause and do two to three cycles of the cyclic sighing.

>> **Combine it with movement.** Walking while breathing this way can amplify its effects, keeping both the body and the mind engaged.

Chapter 4

Assessing Your Own Breathing

Before diving into too many fancy breathing techniques, it's important to understand how you breathe right now. Think of this chapter as a friendly checkup for your lungs and breathing habits. You start by figuring out what kind of breather you are. Then you explore some cool tech tools that can help you tune up your breathing. I also give you a few practical exercises to try at home. After reading this chapter, you'll know your breathing style, your breathing pitfalls, and how to start breathing better every day.

Diagnosing What Kind of Breather You Are

Everybody breathes (that part is nonnegotiable), but *how* we breathe can vary a lot from person to person. Some people take slow, deep breaths that use the diaphragm; others take quick, shallow puffs using the chest and shoulders. In this section, you figure out where you stand and what that information means for your health.

Assessing your breathing habits

Is your breathing deep or shallow? Do you breathe through your nose or your mouth? Do you ever unconsciously hold your breath? These habits can tell you a lot about your "breathing personality."

Shallow versus deep breathing

There are two main styles of breathing — shallow and deep — and understanding the difference is key. Most people think of shallow breathing as a small breath and deep breathing as a big breath. But this error causes all sorts of problems.

Think of shallow breathing versus deep breathing as the difference between chest breathing and diaphragmatic breathing:

>> **Chest breathing:** When you inhale, do your shoulders and chest rise, or does your belly expand? If your shoulders are doing the cha-cha with every inhale, you're likely a chest breather. In chest breathing (also known as shallow breathing), you're drawing air mainly into the upper lungs. It's the kind of breath you might take when startled or stressed — quick and high.

>> **Diaphragmatic breathing:** In diaphragmatic breathing (also known as belly breathing, abdominal breathing, or deep breathing), your *diaphragm* (see Chapter 7) moves downward and your abdomen and lower ribs gently expand. This lets you fill the lower parts of your lungs more fully. Diaphragmatic breathing is how babies naturally breathe and how adults tend to breathe when relaxed or sleeping. It's more efficient and calming.

This simple exercise invites you to gently tune in to the movement of your lower ribs as you breathe, helping you activate your diaphragm and move away from shallow chest breathing. This is one of the best tests to find out whether you're breathing diaphragmatically.

1. **Sit up or stand.**

2. **Place your fingers and thumb on your lower two ribs.**

   Point your thumbs behind you and your fingers in front of you. You should be able to feel your lower ribs with your hands.

3. **Breathe in.**

   Did you notice the lower ribs pushing outwards slightly?

4. **Breathe out.**

   Did you notice the lower ribs going back inward slightly?

If you notice your lower ribs going out as you breathe in, and your lower ribs moving in as you breathe out, congrats! You're doing diaphragmatic breathing. If not, that means you need to do some of the exercises in this book to learn to do diaphragmatic breathing.

Diaphragmatic breathing is the healthier default for resting breathing because it pulls air deep into the lungs with less effort. More air sacs are lower down in your lungs, so you get oxygenated more easily and with less effort. This form of breathing also massages your internal organs (massage is always good!), and triggers the body's relaxation response. It's a win-win!

Chest breathing isn't "bad" in every situation — for example, when you exercise intensely or face danger, chest breathing helps you gulp air quickly. But when chest breathing becomes your *habit*, even at rest, it can keep your body in a slight state of stress without your even realizing it.

Habitual shallow breathing relies on what are known as *accessory breathing muscles* found in your neck, shoulders, and upper back. If you breathe this way most of the time, it can lead to muscle tension and discomfort in those areas. (Plus, constantly lifting your shoulders to inhale can make you look like you're perpetually shrugging, which is not a great long-term fashion statement!)

Nose versus mouth breathing

Check in on yourself right now: Is your mouth open or closed? Ideally, you should breathe through your nose most of the time, especially when resting or doing light activity. The nose filters, warms, and humidifies the air, preparing it nicely for the lungs.

Mouth breathing can contribute to dry mouth, snoring at night, and even feelings of anxiety. If you find you're a habitual mouth-breather (breathing through your mouth even when not exercising), it could be a sign of nasal congestion or just an ingrained habit. It's worth becoming aware of this habit and training yourself to favor the nose during everyday breathing.

Learn more about the importance of nose breathing in Chapter 6.

Unconscious breath holding

Have you ever suddenly gasped and realized you weren't breathing for a bit? You may be doing something dubbed *email apnea* — holding your breath while focused on your screen or phone. It's more common than you'd think. I've had corporate clients discover that whenever they concentrate hard (like reading intense emails or scrolling their phone), they unconsciously hold their breath. This habit deprives your brain of optimal oxygen and can increase tension.

If you suspect you do this, start paying attention during those focused moments and gently remind yourself to breathe. You can even put a little sticky note on your monitor that says, "Breathe!" No shame in that.

Avoiding common breathing mistakes

People often fall into dysfunctional breathing patterns (see the nearby sidebar, "Functional versus dysfunctional breathing"). Here are the big ones to watch out for:

>> **Shallow/chest breathing:** This is when you breathe mostly with your upper chest (see "Shallow versus deep breathing," earlier in this chapter). Your breaths tend to be quick and shallow, using only a portion of your lung capacity. It's like sipping air instead of drinking it in. Over time, habitual chest breathing can keep your body in a mild fight-or-flight mode. You may notice tension in your neck or shoulders (from all that up-and-down movement), and you may not feel as relaxed as you could.

>> **Paradoxical breathing:** Paradoxical breathing means your chest and belly are moving opposite of the way they should. For example, on an inhale, instead of your diaphragm expanding outward, it sucks inward; then it pushes out on the exhale. Basically, the diaphragm isn't working correctly, and other muscles are taking over in a weird tug-of-war. This can happen due to poor habits or certain respiratory issues. It's inefficient and can cause a feeling of not getting enough air. If you notice something like this happening when you breathe (your belly going in as you inhale), that's a sign to retrain your breathing pattern (for example, with the exercises found in this book).

>> **Over-breathing:** Over-breathing (technically *hyperventilation*) may make you picture someone breathing rapidly into a paper bag during a panic attack, but it's not always that dramatic. Many people over-breathe in subtle ways throughout the day — they breathe a bit too fast or too deeply for what the body actually needs at that moment. This can lead to blowing off too much carbon dioxide, which, in turn, can make you feel lightheaded, tingly, or anxious. (It's a bit of a tricky cycle, because anxiety can cause faster breathing, which can cause more weird sensations, which can cause more anxiety. Fun, right?) Signs of chronic over-breathing include frequent sighing or yawning, feeling short of breath for no obvious reason, or getting dizzy when you stand up quickly. If you suspect you're a chronic over-breather, learning to slow down and lighten your breathing can do wonders.

>> **Holding your breath (see "Unconscious breath holding," earlier in this chapter):** This is a common mistake where you intermittently hold your breath without realizing it, often when you're concentrating or lifting something, or even during emotional stress. Holding your breath can raise your blood pressure and stress response (your body thinks something intense must be happening if you suddenly stop breathing). The fix here is mostly awareness — catching yourself in the act and then deliberately taking a gentle breath.

In one of my workshops, a participant once quipped, "I only hold my breath when I'm awake." It got a good laugh, but it rang true for a lot of folks in the room who realized they do it, too. Strangely, breath holding only seems to be harmful when done unconsciously. When you do conscious breath holds, which you can learn more about in Chapter 9, they can be really good for your health.

>> **Mouth breathing (see "Nose versus mouth breathing," earlier in this chapter):** Breathing through the mouth is fine when you're exercising hard or if your nose is stuffed up with a cold. But doing it as a habit, day in and day out, can be a mistake. Mouth breathing, especially when it's chronic, can lead to a dry throat and dental issues; plus, it bypasses the nose's filtering system, so you end up with more dust, bacteria, and viruses in your lungs. It's also linked to snoring and poorer sleep quality. If you frequently wake up with a

dry mouth, that's a clue you may be mouth-breathing overnight. During the day, if you catch yourself mouth-breathing while resting, practice closing your mouth and switching to nasal breathing.

Mouth breathing can actually make nasal congestion worse, creating a bit of a vicious cycle. When your mouth hangs open, the tongue tends to sit low in the mouth, which can narrow your airway and lead to a forward head posture. This, in turn, may contribute to headaches and neck pain and even worsen sleep issues like sleep apnea. In children, chronic mouth breathing can also affect how the face develops, sometimes resulting in a narrower face, crowded teeth, and a higher palate. Simply put, breathing through your nose is not only more efficient, but better for your overall health and posture, too.

TIP

If nasal congestion is forcing you to mouth-breathe, try doing the nose clearing exercise in Chapter 6. If problems with nasal congestion are persistent, consider talking to a healthcare professional or trying simple remedies like saline nasal rinses. Breathing well sometimes starts with addressing the nose.

THE POSTURE CONNECTION

I can't talk about breathing habits without mentioning posture — the modern-day villain. Thanks to computers and smartphones, many of us are walking (or sitting) around with a hunched back and a head jutted forward. This slouching posture compresses your chest and abdomen. Imagine your rib cage and diaphragm are a big balloon. Now imagine trying to inflate that balloon while it's being squeezed. That's what bad posture does to your poor lungs and diaphragm. In fact, some studies have found that slouching can reduce lung capacity by up to 30 percent. (Yes, 30 percent less air just because of how you sit or stand!) No wonder you may feel short of breath after sitting crouched over a laptop for hours.

Take a moment to straighten up whenever you can. Roll your shoulders back, lift your chest slightly, and if you're sitting, try to have both feet on the floor and your back supported. Good posture creates more room for your diaphragm to move and your lungs to fill. Plus, you'll look more confident — and who doesn't want that side benefit?

The good news is that breathing functionally — using your diaphragm — naturally supports good posture. It's when you rely on shallow, upper-chest breathing that muscles in your neck, shoulders, and upper back have to take over. Over time, this can lead to poor posture and discomfort in those areas. Try taking a deep, full breath down into the base of your lungs — you'll likely feel your posture improve right away!

The next time your smartwatch alerts you to stand up, consider it a reminder to also check your spine and take a deep breath. Your lungs will thank you for it.

Breathing and Technology

You may be thinking, "Breathing is the most natural thing — do we really need *technology* for it?" In an ideal world, probably not. But technology can be a fantastic helper when used right — kind of like having a personal coach or biofeedback buddy with you. This section explores some gadgets and apps that can make your breathing practice more effective (and even fun!). Welcome to breathing in the 21st century — there's an app for that!

Using wearable devices for real-time feedback

One of the coolest developments in breathing tech involves heart-rate variability (HRV) biofeedback devices. HRV is a fancy term for the slight variations in time between your heartbeats. Why should you care about HRV? Because it's a proxy for how balanced your nervous system is — higher variability (in a certain healthy range) generally means a more relaxed, resilient state. When you breathe slowly and smoothly, your heart rate tends to sync up with that rhythm (speeding up a bit as you inhale, slowing as you exhale), which increases HRV. Biofeedback devices measure your HRV in real time, letting you know when you're hitting that sweet spot of calm, coherent breathing.

A pioneer in this field is HeartMath (www.heartmath.com). At the time of writing, they offer gadgets like the Inner Balance Coherence Plus sensor (which clips to your earlobe and connects to an app on your phone) and the emWave Pro device (a stand-alone handheld device with a screen that shows your heart rhythm in real time — no phone needed). These devices give you a live display of your heart's rhythms and a coherence score. *Coherence* is HeartMath's term for a harmonious state where your heart, mind, and breath are in sync. Basically, when you breathe at a calm, steady rate (around 5 seconds in, 5 seconds out for many people), the device's screen shows a smooth wave pattern, and your coherence score goes up. When you're tense or your breathing is erratic, the wave looks jagged and the score drops. It gamifies peace of mind — you can literally watch your body calm down!

I admit, the first time I used it, I got *too* excited watching the screen, which made my coherence drop. Oops! When I learned to just breathe and not obsess over the score, it went much better.

Using something like HeartMath can be a real eye-opener. It's one thing to *feel* calmer after breathing exercises; it's another to *see* a tangible reading that confirms it. That visual feedback can motivate you to practice regularly. It's like having a little coach saying, "Slow down, breathe deeper . . . yes, like that!" Over time, this training can help you internalize a healthier breathing rhythm even when you're not using the device.

HeartMath is popular, but it's not the only game in town. Other devices and apps offer HRV or breathing biofeedback. Some smartphone apps can use your phone's camera or a finger sensor to detect your pulse and give HRV readings. Elite HRV (https://elitehrv.com) is a popular and well-respected app for HRV tracking. You can find many other apps simply by searching "HRV" in the app store for your device. They can measure your HRV through the camera flash as you breathe (though results will be less responsive or accurate than dedicated sensors). There are also wearables like chest-strap heart rate monitors (from companies like Garmin and Polar), which are more reliable — plus, when paired with an app like Elite HRV, they can give you real-time biofeedback for breathing exercises.

By now, you may be wondering, "I have a smartwatch/fitness tracker — can't that just coach my breathing?" The answer is: To some extent. Devices like the Apple Watch, Oura Ring, and WHOOP strap have sensors that track heart rate; some also track blood oxygen and other metrics. They measure HRV as well, but there are some limitations in using them for real-time breath training:

>> **Apple Watch** (www.apple.com/watch): Apple has a built-in Breathe app that reminds you to take a minute to breathe deeply. It even gives a pleasing animation (a little blue flower-like circle) and haptic taps on your wrist to pace you. It's a nice feature for mindfulness. Although the Watch measures your heart rate and can record your HRV (accessible in the Health app), it doesn't display your HRV changes live during a breathing session. In other words, it won't show you a coherence score or a waveform as you breathe. It simply concludes the session and may show your heart rate or how many "mindful minutes" you earned. So, it's good for guided breathing breaks, but it's not a full biofeedback tool — at least not at the time of writing, but who knows, Apple may update the app to do more in the future.

>> **Oura Ring** (https://ouraring.com): The Oura Ring is a smart ring that tracks sleep and recovery. It calculates your nighttime HRV and gives you a readiness score each morning. It's awesome for seeing trends (like whether that late-night pizza affected your recovery), but it doesn't provide real-time feedback during the day. The Oura Ring doesn't have a screen, and though the app can show your current heart rate if you check, it's not meant for moment-to-moment coaching. Some users do breathing exercises, and then look at their HRV score the next morning to see if consistent practice raises their baseline — but that's more of a long-term view, not immediate feedback.

>> **WHOOP** (www.whoop.com): WHOOP is similar to Oura in that it focuses on recovery, strain, and sleep, aimed at athletes or anyone serious about optimizing health. It gives a daily HRV reading and lots of analysis. However, WHOOP doesn't have a display (data goes to your phone app), and it doesn't guide breathing exercises. Like Oura, it's more about background data. You

could manually use it by starting a "breathwork" activity on the app, which will record your heart rate; then, later, you can analyze how your heart rate changed, but it's not real-time on-screen guidance.

In short, popular wearables are great for measuring your overall patterns and progress, but as of now, they aren't as interactive for breath training. They won't beep at you *in the exact moment* you start hyperventilating during a stressful meeting (maybe one day!). They will, however, encourage you to take breathing breaks (Apple's reminders) or show you that your HRV is improving over weeks of practice (Oura/WHOOP trends). If you already have one, by all means use it as part of your breathing improvement plan — just know its limits. For example, you can use an Apple Watch or Fitbit to check your heart rate before and after a five-minute breathing exercise to see the difference. Or track your sleep and notice if breathing exercises during the day correlate with better sleep scores. These indirect measures are still super valuable.

I've used HeartMath's Inner Balance device, which I found very helpful to optimize my coherent breathing (see Chapter 8). After several months of using it, I no longer feel I need to use the device daily because I can sense the feeling of coherence within me.

I currently have an Apple Watch and occasionally use it to track my sleep and other data. Over time, I've learned not to overanalyze the numbers. Instead, I trust my intuition and check the data only when something feels off, helping me identify patterns when needed. Everyone's different, so find a balance that works for you when using technology to support your breathing.

Trying breathing apps for support

If dedicated gadgets aren't your thing, no worries — a smartphone can do a lot on its own. Breathing apps range from very simple timers to comprehensive breathwork coaches. Here's a roundup of some popular ones:

>> **Breathing Zone** (https://breathing.zone): This simple app can measure your current breathing rate using your phone's microphone and then guide you to slow it down using visual cues (like a pulsing shape) and soothing sounds. It gradually lengthens your exhale to bring your breath into a calmer rhythm. It's great for those who want gentle, no-fuss breath training — and it tracks your progress, too.

>> **Breathwrk** (www.breathwrk.com): This app is dedicated to breathing exercises and mini classes. With short, targeted exercises for anxiety, energy, focus, and sleep, it makes breathwork engaging and easy to stick with. It uses visuals, audio, and haptic feedback (vibrations) to guide your breathing in

real time. The interface is fun and beginner-friendly, with a wide library of techniques and a progress tracker to keep you motivated.

>> **Calm** (www.calm.com): Known for meditation and sleep, Calm also has a breathing tool. The app can guide your inhale and exhale at a pace you choose. You can select themes and pair your practice with soothing voices or ambient music. It's ideal for people who already use Calm and want a simple breathing feature.

>> **iBreathe** (www.jadelizardsoftware.com/ibreathe): This no-frills app is great for people who like simplicity. Set your own inhale, exhale, and hold durations, and the app will guide you with a clean visual interface. No guided meditations, no music — just a straightforward, customizable breathing timer that gets straight to the point. Perfect for personal breath routines like 4-7-8 or 6-6 Coherent Breathing.

>> **Oxygen Advantage** (https://oxygenadvantage.com): Based on Patrick McKeown's breathing method, this app is designed for those who want to improve health, endurance, and breathing efficiency. It includes exercises for slow breathing, light breathing, and advanced breath-hold practices to build carbon dioxide tolerance. It's ideal for athletes, people with asthma, or anyone looking to learn how to breathe better. It's currently free and comes with a structured daily plan.

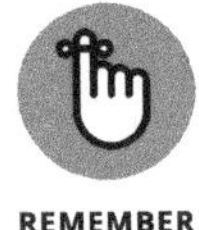

REMEMBER

Apps are great, but remember not to overthink or stress about "doing it right." The goal is to breathe better, not to get a high score or perfect streak. I once found myself getting stressed because my HRV biofeedback streak was about to break — oh, the humanity! Use these tools as gentle guides, not strict bosses. As I've gotten more experienced with breathwork, I've felt far less need to use these apps.

Opening up to the future of breathwork

Where is all this headed? The marriage of age-old breathing wisdom with modern tech is still relatively new, and it's evolving quickly. Here are a few things on the horizon or just starting to emerge:

>> **More advanced sensors:** We may soon see wearables that track breathing rate and even carbon dioxide levels. Imagine a smartwatch that notices you're breathing too fast and gently prompts you to slow down. Start-ups and researchers are already developing this tech.

>> **Continuous stress monitoring:** Building on HRV, companies are developing algorithms to detect stress in real time using heart rate and skin signals. Future devices may gently alert you when stress rises — like a coach reminding you to pause and breathe. This could be built into smartwatches or new wearables.

- » **Virtual reality (VR) and biofeedback games:** VR is now being used for meditation, with games that respond to your breath. Imagine a flower blooming as you exhale or a balloon rising with your inhale. Breathing becomes a fun, interactive challenge — perfect for kids and game-loving adults.

- » **Smart home integration:** Future smart homes may detect stress in your voice and suggest a short breathing exercise, dim the lights, and play calming music. With the data these devices collect, personalized wellness prompts are likely just around the corner.

- » **Breathing technique personalization:** Apps may soon track how your body responds to different techniques and guide you toward what works best — like recommending 4-7-8 Breathing if it calms you more than Box Breathing does. Think custom breathwork plans powered by artificial intelligence (AI).

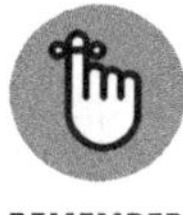

REMEMBER

The future is bright and breathing easy! But remember, you don't *need* high-tech gadgets to breathe better — they're just optional helpers. The core of breath training is you and your body. In fact, you're equipped with the original "breathing app" right now: your own awareness and conscious attention.

FRESH AIR AT HOME: WHAT WORKS

You may spend lots of time indoors and wonder, "Is this air actually healthy?" It may look clean, but indoor air often contains invisible pollutants — like dust, pollen, pet dander, cleaning product fumes, smoke, and even gases released from furniture.

If you have allergies, asthma, or lung issues, this can be a real problem. That's where air purifiers come in — but only the right kind. Look for ones with high-efficiency particulate air (HEPA) filters, which capture fine particles like PM2.5. If you're dealing with smoke or chemicals (VOCs), you'll also want an activated carbon filter.

Still, no air purifier can clean your whole home or eliminate all pollutants. They work best alongside good habits: regular cleaning, opening windows when you can, and avoiding indoor pollution (like smoking or using harsh sprays).

Also, don't underestimate indoor plants — they not only brighten a space but can help filter air naturally, especially when used with other strategies.

And of course, nothing beats real fresh air. Step outside often. A short walk in the park can clear your lungs and your mind.

2

Foundations of Healthy Breathing

This part provides the practical foundations you need to transform your breathing and enhance your health, emotional well-being, and quality of life. You begin by exploring mindful breathing, discovering how intentional breaths relieve tension, calm the mind, and soothe emotions, with simple ways to incorporate it into your everyday routine.

Next, you discover the transformative benefits of nasal breathing, including improved immunity and lung function. Essential exercises help you clear nasal blockages, while practical tips guide you away from mouth breathing.

Then you master diaphragmatic breathing, understanding how your diaphragm works, recognizing improper breathing patterns, and following step-by-step instructions to practice effectively. Through simple activities such as walking or yoga, you can seamlessly integrate this healthy breathing method into your daily life.

You find out about powerful techniques like coherent breathing, box breathing, and the 4-7-8 method — each proven to reduce stress, enhance focus, and improve sleep. Clear instructions and helpful tips ensure you can easily incorporate these practices into your routine.

Finally, you discover the subtle power of breathing less. Techniques such as the Buteyko Breathing Method gently reduce your breathing volume, improving oxygen efficiency, relaxation, and resilience, and offering practical ways to adopt breathing lightly as a lifelong habit.

Chapter **5**

Getting Started with Mindful Breathing

Breathing is central to life. However, you probably don't pay much attention to your breath. Mindful breathing offers a doorway to better physical health, emotional well-being, and mental clarity — which is surprising, because all you're doing is paying attention to your breath!

In this chapter, we dive into what mindful breathing is, why it matters, and how you can seamlessly integrate it into your daily life.

Discovering Mindful Breathing

Mindful breathing is simply bringing awareness to your breath. It's about shifting from unconscious, automatic breathing to conscious awareness as you inhale and exhale.

Modern life can pull you in many directions, leaving little room to connect with yourself — you're too busy paying attention to everything else. Mindful breathing helps create a meaningful way to connect back to yourself.

Think of your breath as an anchor — always there, always steady, ready to bring you back to the present moment when your mind wanders off. In this way, you can connect to that anchor and feel more grounded.

Whether you're feeling overwhelmed at work, stressed in traffic, or simply caught up in the hustle and bustle of everyday life, your breath is a tool you can use to regain control. The beauty of it? It's accessible to everyone, everywhere, at any time.

Mindful breathing is about noticing any experience associated with your breath. For example, you can notice the following:

» The sensation of your breath at your nostrils, back of your throat, chest, belly, or any other part of your body

» The speed at which you breathe

» How deep or shallow your breath is

» The sound of your breath

» Whether you're breathing through your nose or mouth (see Chapter 6 for more on nose breathing, which is best)

» The rhythm of your breath

» How your breath is changing from moment to moment

Whenever you *notice* your breathing, you're doing mindful breathing.

IF BEING CONSCIOUS OF YOUR BREATH MAKES YOU ANXIOUS

For some people, focusing on their breath can trigger feelings of anxiety rather than calm. This is more common than you may think, and it often happens because paying attention to the breath brings sensations to the surface that people may have ignored or suppressed. If you're not used to observing your body in this way, the act of tuning into your breathing may feel unfamiliar — even overwhelming at first. You may notice tightness in your chest, changes in your heart rate, or difficulty controlling your breath — and these sensations can be unsettling.

If this happens to you, know that it's completely okay, and you're not doing anything wrong. The key is to approach mindful breathing gently and with self-kindness. Start by practicing for just 10 to 15 seconds instead of several minutes, and gradually increase the length of time as you feel more comfortable. You can also try pairing breath awareness with something soothing, like listening to calming music, repeating a mantra (see "Tuning in during stressful moments," later in this chapter), or placing a hand on your chest for reassurance. Another option is to focus on external sensations, such as the feeling of your feet on the floor or the sounds in your environment, while keeping a light awareness of your breath in the background.

If focusing directly on the breath still feels too intense, try a related practice like walking meditation or mindful movement (see Chapter 7). These activities allow you to engage with your body and breath more indirectly, often easing any tension or anxiety. Over time, as you grow more familiar with these sensations, mindful breathing can become a helpful tool for navigating both calm and difficult moments.

Remember: Don't force yourself to do a breathing exercise if it doesn't feel right for you. Listen to your body.

Curious to learn more about other ways to practice mindfulness? Find out more in my book *Mindfulness For Dummies*, 3rd Edition (Wiley).

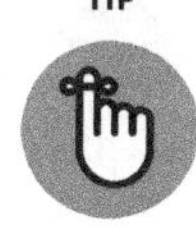

Mindful breathing is not about changing your breath. All the other breathing exercises in this book involve *breath control* (changing your breath in some way), but not mindful breathing. If, when you're practicing mindful breathing, you find that your breath changes in some way by itself, that's fine and to be expected. The key is *you're* not trying to change your breath — you're just passively observing your breath rather than actively controlling it.

Imagine your breath is a puppy. Mindful breathing is like having a puppy on a lead and taking it for a walk. You're paying attention and allowing the puppy to go wherever it wants. You're not pulling it this way or that. It's about following rather than directing — at least for this lucky puppy!

Mindful breathing involves simply cultivating an awareness of how you breathe, where your breath is going (into the chest, abdomen, or diaphragm), and how it feels in your body.

Mindful breathing is similar to meditation but goes beyond meditation. Meditation often involves sitting still and focusing for extended periods. Mindful breathing, on the other hand, can be practiced in the middle of your daily activities, no matter where you are.

You can take a simple step into mindful breathing right now. Just become aware of the sensation of three breaths. That's it — you've already made a start. It really is that easy. And starting small, with just a few breaths like this, is one of the best ways to ensure you enjoy the experience and keep going.

IF YOU FEEL LIKE YOUR MIND IS TOO BUSY TO FOCUS ON BREATHING

It's completely normal to find it difficult to focus on your breathing when your mind feels like it's racing in a hundred directions. Mindful breathing isn't about forcing your mind to be quiet — it's about gently guiding your attention back to the breath, no matter how often it wanders. If this feels like a challenge, try these three tips:

- **Anchor your focus with touch.** Place a hand on your chest or belly and notice the gentle rise and fall as you breathe. This physical sensation can make it easier to stay present.

- **Count your breaths.** Inhale and silently count "one"; then exhale and count "two." Continue up to ten, and then start over. If your mind wanders, simply return to the count without criticizing yourself.

- **Try shorter sessions.** Begin with just one mindful breath. When this feels manageable, gradually extend the time.

Remember: The goal isn't perfection — it's practice. Even if your mind feels busy, every moment of awareness is a step toward greater calm and focus.

Exploring the Benefits of Mindful Breathing

I first discovered mindful breathing when I was in my early 20s. It's an experience that changed my life. At the time, I was going through all sorts of stress at university, and my mind was often racing. By learning and practicing mindful breathing, I was given a powerful tool for life. Anytime, anywhere, I could turn my attention to my breath to center and ground myself — and no one could take that away from me. It was, and is, so empowering!

The benefits of mindful breathing go far beyond simply "feeling good." When practiced consistently, it can transform your body, mind, and emotions in profound ways. These findings have been backed up by research studies all over the world. Breathing mindfully positively changes almost all aspects of your life. You might even say the research is breathtaking (#dadjoke).

Releasing tension in your body

Tension can build up in your body, often without your realizing it. It manifests as tight shoulders, clenched jaws, or a feeling of restlessness in the limbs. One of the most accessible ways to release this built-up tension is simply becoming conscious of your breath.

Breath awareness works because the act of paying attention to your breathing brings you into the present moment. The body often holds onto stress as a result of unprocessed thoughts and emotions. When you're caught up in the swirl of mental activity, your body unconsciously reflects this situation with tension. However, when you direct your attention to your breath, you interrupt that cycle of reactivity. It's as if the act of noticing your breath reminds your body that it's safe to let go.

When you're consciously aware of your breath, you're not trying to change it or control it — you're simply observing it as it is, with a friendly awareness if you can. This observation brings a sense of neutrality and calm. For example, when you notice your breath moving naturally in and out of your nostrils, you may also notice your chest gently rising or your belly softly expanding. By observing these sensations, your body's stress response — the fight-or-flight mechanism — begins to downshift, and tension naturally starts to dissipate.

Being mindful of your breath also creates a feedback loop with your nervous system. When you pay attention to your breathing, your brain receives signals that you're engaging in a calm, restful activity. This, in turn, helps regulate your nervous system, promoting a state of relaxation. You may even notice that areas of tension, like your neck or hands, begin to soften without your actively trying to release them.

Here's an example: Let's say you've had a stressful meeting, and your shoulders are tight. Instead of immediately trying to fix the tension by stretching or deep breathing, simply pause and observe your breath. If just being conscious of your breath isn't engaging enough, ask yourself the following questions:

>> Where do I feel my breath most clearly?

>> Can I feel it in my nostrils, throat, chest, or belly?

>> Is it smooth or uneven, fast or slow?

>> What does it feel like to feel my breathing?

By tuning into your breath, you're directing your focus away from the source of stress and giving your body permission to reset. Often, you'll find that the simple act of observing the breath causes your muscles to soften and your posture to realign without conscious effort.

This process is powerful because it doesn't require any manipulation of the breath. Just by being aware of this natural rhythm, you anchor yourself in the present and allow tension to melt away. Over time, regular practice of breath awareness can create a habit of noticing tension as it arises, giving you a tool to address it before it builds up.

This simple but powerful exercise, called mindful breathing, will help you tune into your breath and possibly experience its tension-relieving effects. I say "possibly" because mindfulness is about accepting whatever your present-moment experience is, even if it's uncomfortable tension. That's the skill of mindfulness to develop over time. It's a simple idea, but not easy. Even 1 percent more acceptance makes a difference, so start with baby steps. You don't need any special tools or a quiet room (though you may want to play Track 9) — just yourself and a few moments of focus:

1. **Find a comfortable position.**

   Sit or stand in a position where you feel stable and at ease. You can do this lying down, if you prefer. Let your hands rest naturally on your lap or at your sides. Keep your back comfortably straight but not rigid — allow your body to feel supported. Be comfortable.

2. **Bring your attention to your breath.**

   Close your eyes if it feels comfortable, or soften your gaze. Notice your breath exactly as it is right now. Don't try to change it — just observe. If it changes by itself, that's fine. Where do you feel your breath most clearly? It may be at your nostrils, in the rise and fall of your chest, in the gentle movement of your belly, or perhaps in your lower back.

3. **Stay curious.**

   Focus on the sensation of the air entering and leaving your body. Is it cool or warm? Does it flow evenly? Notice the rhythm of your breath. Is it slow or fast, smooth or uneven? ***Remember:*** There's no right or wrong — your job is simply to observe.

4. **Manage distractions gently.**

   Your mind is bound to wander off to other thoughts. When you notice that has happened, just say to yourself, "Thank you, mind," and bring your attention back to your breath. If you notice tension, don't force it to release. Simply bring your attention back to your breath, allowing any tightness to soften naturally.

5. Wrap it up.

Stay with your breath for two to three minutes, or longer if you feel comfortable. When you're ready, gently shift your attention outward, noticing the room around you. Take one final moment to notice how your body feels now compared to when you started. Do you feel more aware or grounded?

Although at its simplest, mindfulness is about awareness, there is another important key part to mindfulness: acceptance. By *acceptance*, I mean an openness to however you're feeling. Acceptance is the opposite of resistance. So, when you feel physically tense, and you find that mindful breathing doesn't relieve the tension, just let the tension be there. Fighting, resisting, denying, or suppressing the tension can make it worse. Allowing the tension to be there isn't easy, but it's a skill you can learn. With practice, you'll get better at both mindful breathing and accepting any tension you feel.

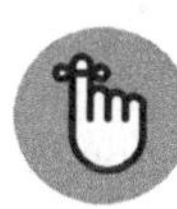

What you resist, persists. What you accept, transforms.

You can do this exercise anytime you feel tense — before a big meeting, while waiting in line, or as part of your morning or evening routine. The key is not to force or change anything but to let the simple act of observing your breath do the work for you. Over time, this practice will become second nature, helping you navigate stress and tension with ease. The more regularly you practice this exercise, the more beneficial you'll find it.

Calming your mind

The mind is a busy place. Thoughts come and go, often uninvited, creating a whirlwind of mental chatter. Worries can leave you feeling overwhelmed or unfocused.

Mindful breathing offers a simple yet profound way to bring stillness and clarity to your mind. By anchoring your attention to the breath, you create space between yourself and the constant stream of thoughts, allowing your mind to calm naturally.

Why mindful breathing calms the mind

Your mind and breath are deeply interconnected. When your mind is agitated — whether by stress, anxiety, or overthinking — your breath often mirrors this state, becoming shallow, rapid, or irregular. Similarly, when you focus on your breath, you send signals to your brain that you are safe and can be calm, creative, and focused.

Mindful breathing works by interrupting the mind's tendency to fixate on worries or distractions. When you deliberately pay attention to your breath, you shift your focus away from thoughts and into the here and now. This simple act of awareness quiets the mental noise and helps your mind find its natural rhythm.

Another reason mindful breathing calms the mind is its soothing effect on your stress response. By focusing on your breath, you're telling your brain that you can relax. Subsequently, your brain has less need to fill itself with worries. As you engage your relaxation response, you promote peace of mind.

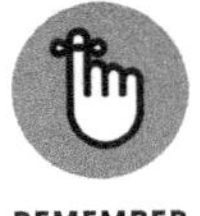

Regrets pull you into the past. Worries drag you into the future. Mindful breathing helps bring you into the peace of the present moment.

How to use mindful breathing to calm the mind

The beauty of mindful breathing is that you don't need to do anything complicated. The act of observing your breath as it flows naturally can be enough to step back from your thoughts and soothe your mental state.

Start by noticing the sensations of your breath. Perhaps you feel the air entering your nostrils, cool on the in breath and warmer on the out breath. Maybe you feel the gentle rise and fall of your chest or the subtle expansion of your belly. By directing your attention to these sensations, you give your mind something steady and neutral to focus on, which helps ease the mental clutter.

You'll find that your thoughts don't disappear — and that's normal.

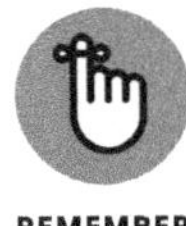

The goal isn't to stop thinking. The goal is to kindly and curiously notice your breathing as best you can and gently and almost effortlessly refocus each time your mind gets distracted.

Think of your thoughts like clouds passing through the sky, or like watching people walk past a café as you sip your favorite drink. By anchoring yourself to your breath, you remain grounded, allowing the thoughts to float by without pulling you along as much as they normally do.

THE SCIENCE BEHIND MINDFUL BREATHING

Research shows that mindful breathing reduces levels of *cortisol* (the stress hormone), enhances focus, and improves emotional regulation. It also activates the *vagus nerve*, which originates at the brain and travels through the neck, chest, and abdomen.

Activating the vagus nerve calms your nervous system, and increases serotonin, which promotes well-being. Regular practice boosts clarity, decision-making, creativity, and encourages the production of *gamma-aminobutyric acid* (GABA), a neurotransmitter that naturally reduces anxiety and fosters calmness — even after just a minute of practice.

By using your breath as a tool, you create a physiological shift that aligns your body and mind toward a state of balance. Over time, practicing mindful breathing strengthens your emotional resilience, making it easier to face challenges with clarity and calmness. See Chapter 2 for more on the science of breathing.

Tuning in during stressful moments

When I prepare for a big presentation, my mind sometimes races with thoughts like, "What if I forget what to say?" or "What if they don't like my ideas?" These thoughts can create a loop of anxiety, making it difficult for me to focus. By shifting attention to my breath, I can break the cycle.

Here's how I do it: I take a moment to pause and observe my natural breath. I notice its rhythm and how it feels in my body. At this time, my breathing may be a little faster than normal, and I may be able to notice my heart racing. Without trying to change it, I simply follow the flow of my inhalation and exhalation. As I stay with my breath, the intensity of my anxious thoughts begins to soften, and my mind becomes clearer. I may also notice my breathing rate begin to slow down naturally.

You can also break the cycle of unwelcome thoughts with these tips:

>> **Start small.** Begin with a few mindful breaths when you're feeling scattered or overwhelmed. Over time, you can extend this to a minute, a few minutes, and even ten minutes or more as you get comfortable with the practice. Little and often works well. For example, one minute of mindful breathing, five times a day.

>> **Use reminders.** Set a gentle alarm on your watch, phone, or computer, or use sticky notes with the word *Breathe* to remind yourself to pause throughout the day.

>> **Expect your mind to wander.** It's perfectly natural to find it difficult to focus on your breath for more than a few seconds. It's a bit like learning to walk. You're bound to fall again and again, and that's all part of the learning process. The same is true for mindful breathing for most people.

>> **Combine it with other activities.** Practice mindful breathing while doing something simple, like walking, washing dishes, or waiting in line. This makes it easier to integrate into your daily routine.

Calming the mind through mindful breathing is a skill that grows with practice. The more you tune into your breath, the more you'll notice a sense of calm becoming second nature. Eventually, you'll find it easier to access this sense of calm even in challenging situations, giving you a powerful tool to navigate life's ups and downs.

Mantras are simple words, phrases, or sounds that you can repeat silently or softly to help focus your mind. When paired with your breath, they create a rhythm that makes it easier to stay present and calm. This exercise, paired with Track 10, will guide you through using mantras with your breath and help you find one that resonates with you:

1. **Choose a comfortable position.**

   Sit in a chair or on a cushion with your back supported and your shoulders relaxed; if you prefer, lie down. Rest your hands gently on your lap or at your sides.

2. **Select a mantra.**

   Choose a simple word or phrase that feels calming or meaningful to you. Here are some suggestions:

   - *Peace:* Exhale and silently say, "Peace," and repeat.

   - *Let go:* Inhale as you think "Let," and exhale as you think "Go."

   - *Calm:* Inhale and then exhale and say, "Calm," and repeat.

   - *I am here:* Inhale and think, "I am," and exhale and think, "Here."

   - *So hum:* Inhale as you say, "So," and exhale as you say, "Hum." (This is a traditional Sanskrit mantra that means "I am that.")

   Alternatively, you can create your own mantra or *affirmation* (a positive statement that you find inspiring). Think of a word or phrase that reflects what you want to feel, such as *Steady, Ease,* or *I am enough.* Let the mantra feel natural and supportive — it doesn't have to be perfect. It can even be a neutral word like *One* or *Now.*

3. **Synchronize the mantra with your breath.**

   Close your eyes if it feels comfortable, or soften your gaze. Begin by noticing your natural breath without trying to change it. As you inhale, silently think or softly say the first part of your mantra (for example, "Let"). As you exhale, complete the mantra (for example, "Go").

Let the mantra flow naturally with your breathing. Don't rush or force it — let it follow your natural rhythm. Repeat the mantra in a way that works for you.

4. **Focus on the connection.**

   Keep your attention on the pairing of the mantra and your breath. Notice how the sound or thought of the mantra anchors your mind and creates a steady rhythm.

   If your thoughts wander (and they probably will!), gently bring your focus back to the mantra and your breath with kindness rather than judgment.

5. **Experiment and reflect.**

   Practice this exercise for one to five minutes at first, and gradually extend the time as you feel more comfortable.

   After the practice, take a moment to notice how you feel. Did the mantra help you stay focused? Did it evoke a particular feeling, such as calmness or clarity?

TIP

Here are some tips for finding your mantra:

>> **Reflect on your needs.** Ask yourself what you're looking for in this moment. Do you need calm, focus, strength, or reassurance? Choose a word or phrase that reflects this need.

>> **Experiment.** Try different mantras during your practice, and see which ones feel most effective.

>> **Keep it simple.** Short, clear words or phrases work best. Avoid anything too complex or intellectual.

>> **Focus on your breath, too.** Put part of your attention on the mantra, and part of your attention on your breath. Don't just focus on the mantra and forget about your breath.

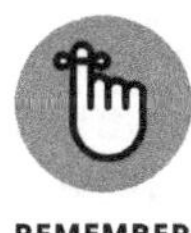

REMEMBER

Using a mantra with your breath can help, whether you're preparing for a stressful event, taking a moment to reset during the day, or winding down before sleep. Over time, this practice can become a trusted tool to center yourself in any situation.

Soothing and regulating your emotions

Emotions are a natural part of being human. But sometimes they can feel overwhelming, especially during moments of stress, sadness, or anger. Mindful breathing provides a gentle and accessible way to soothe your emotions, helping you navigate them with greater ease and understanding.

Over time, as mindful awareness of your emotions grows, you're better able to regulate your emotions. This means your feelings are less likely to highjack you. You're better able to respond to your emotional experiences in a healthy way instead of impulsively reacting.

Seeing how breath and emotions are connected

Your breath and emotions are deeply intertwined. Think about how your breathing changes when you experience strong feelings. When you're angry, your breath may become short and sharp. When you're anxious, your breath may feel shallow or rapid. And when you're calm and content, your breathing is likely steady and even.

This connection goes back to how your breath is closely tied to your nervous system. Understanding how stress impacts your breath helps you better regulate how you feel. Emotional states activate the fight-or-flight response, triggering physiological changes, including a faster heart rate and altered breathing patterns. By becoming aware of your breath and consciously observing it, you can shift your nervous system out of this heightened state and into one of calm and balance.

When I'm feeling irritable or stressed, I know even just one mindful breath will help me. If I can, I close my eyes and focus on feeling just one breath around my belly (lower abdomen). I like focusing there because it's away from my busy mind. I start with just one mindful breath because when I'm not feeling great, that's all I'm motivated enough to do. But the good news is, after just one conscious breath, it usually feels so good, I want to do more! A few breaths later, I'm feeling more refreshed and my emotions are a little more soothed. If you're like me and you find lengthy exercises challenging when you're not feeling good, start with just one mindful breath and do more only if you feel like it.

Discovering the role of mindful breathing in emotional regulation

Mindful breathing doesn't force emotions away. Instead, it allows you to create space around them. When you focus on your breath, you anchor yourself in the present moment. This reduces the tendency to get swept away by emotional waves. This practice helps you observe your feelings without being consumed by them. Just by observing emotions, you may start to notice a difference. Here are a couple examples:

>> **When feeling anxious,** observing your breath can interrupt the spiral of worry, giving your mind and body a chance to reset.

>> **During anger or frustration,** focusing on your breath can provide a pause, creating a moment to respond thoughtfully instead of reacting impulsively.

The process is simple but powerful. Here's how to start:

1. **Pause and notice.**

   When you feel an emotion rising, take a moment to pause. Instead of reacting, gently direct your attention to your breath. Notice where you feel your breath most strongly — at your nostrils, your chest, or your belly, for example.

2. **Anchor yourself in observation.**

   Simply observe your breath as it is. **Remember:** This exercise isn't about changing your breath. You may notice that it feels tight or irregular. That's okay. Just the simple act of observing itself can begin to calm your nervous system.

3. **Allow the emotion to be.**

   Emotions are like waves — they rise, peak, and eventually subside. By staying with your breath, you give yourself a stable anchor, allowing the emotion to flow without resistance. This practice helps you respond to feelings with openness rather than self-judgment or resisting the feeling.

Using techniques to help soothe your emotions

To soothe your emotions in various situations, try the following:

» If you're anxious: If your thoughts are racing and your chest feels tight, try silently saying "Breathing in, I'm aware I am breathing in" on the inhale and "Breathing out, I'm aware I am breathing out" on the exhale. These simple phrases keep your mind engaged with the present, easing anxious energy.

» If you're angry or frustrated: Focus on the sensation of your breath at the tip of your nose. Feel the air entering and leaving. Count each exhale up to ten; then start over. This practice creates a pause, allowing your anger to dissipate before it drives your actions.

» If you're sad: Rest your hands gently on your belly and observe the natural rise and fall with each breath. This tactile connection to your body fosters a sense of grounding and safety, helping you feel more supported.

The following exercise is designed to help you navigate intense emotions by combining mindful breathing with a mindset of friendly acceptance. It helps you create space around your feelings, allowing them to soften naturally. You may want to play Track 11 as you follow these steps:

1. **Find a comfortable position.**

   Sit, stand, or lie down in a position where you feel supported. Let your body be at ease as best you can. Rest your hands on your lap, your belly, or wherever feels natural.

2. **Tune into your breath.**

   Close your eyes if it feels comfortable, or soften your gaze. Without trying to change anything, notice your breath. Observe its natural rhythm — whether it's slow or fast, deep or shallow. Let it be as it is.

3. **Name the emotion.**

   Bring your awareness to how you're feeling. What emotion are you experiencing? Is it anxiety, sadness, frustration, or something else? Silently name it in your mind — for example, "I feel anxious" or "This is frustration." Acknowledging the emotion helps you approach it with awareness rather than resistance.

4. **Pair the emotion with your breath.**

   As you inhale, silently say to yourself, "Breathing in, I feel . . ." and fill in the emotion (for example, "Breathing in, I feel sadness"). As you exhale, say, "Breathing out, I allow it to be here." Repeat this for several breaths, staying present with both the emotion and your breathing.

5. **Create space around the feeling.**

   Imagine your breath creating more room inside your body for the emotion. With each inhale, feel that space gently expanding. With each exhale, feel tension softening.

   If the emotion feels intense, remind yourself that it's okay to feel this way. Your breath is your steady anchor, helping you ride the wave of emotion.

6. **Finish with a grounding breath.**

   After a few minutes, gently shift your focus back to your breath alone. Take three slow, steady breaths, inhaling through your nose and exhaling fully through your mouth. Open your eyes, stretch if you need to, and take a moment to notice how you feel now compared to when you started.

By naming the emotion and pairing it with your breath, you acknowledge its presence without resistance or judgment. This practice helps you respond to your feelings with kindness and curiosity, creating a pathway for them to dissipate naturally. Over time, this exercise can become a reliable tool for soothing emotions in any situation.

What you resist, persists. What you accept, transforms.

Practicing Mindful Breathing in Everyday Life

One of the things I love most about mindful breathing is its flexibility. You don't need to carve out loads of time or even find a quiet space to practice. You can integrate it seamlessly into your daily activities, turning ordinary moments into opportunities for mindfulness and calm.

This section offers practical ways to bring mindful breathing into different parts of your day.

Morning: Setting the tone for the day

Your mornings can shape how the rest of your day unfolds. Instead of rushing to check your email or social media, take a moment to ground yourself with mindful breathing as soon as you wake up.

This exercise is a simple yet powerful way to get your day off to a mindful start:

1. Sit up in bed, on the edge of your bed, or in a comfortable chair.

2. Close your eyes or soften your gaze and take a few moments to notice your natural breath.

3. Pair your breathing with a simple mantra or affirmation, such as "I am calm" on the inhale and "I am ready" on the exhale.

   Use words that are meaningful for you.

4. Spend one to five minutes breathing consciously, allowing yourself to feel centered and present before starting your day.

This short practice helps you transition from sleep to wakefulness with a sense of calm and intention.

Traveling: Finding calm amidst chaos

Travel — whether it's your daily commute, a long road trip, or a crowded airport — can be a source of stress. Mindful breathing can transform these moments of chaos into pockets of peace.

Here's how to do mindful breathing when on the move:

1. **On a train, bus, or plane, sit back and close your eyes if possible.**

2. **Observe your breath flowing in and out.**

   Focus on the sensation of the air entering your nostrils or the gentle movement of your body as you breathe.

3. **Try counting your breaths: When you get to five, start again from one.**

   Repeat this for a few minutes, or even your entire journey.

If you're driving, practice by focusing on the rhythm of your breath without altering it, especially during stops at traffic lights. Obviously, keep your eyes fully open when driving, and only do this exercise if you feel it's helping you to pay attention to the road when driving. Safety first!

This practice can help you stay grounded and patient, no matter what travel challenges arise.

Working: Boosting focus and reducing stress

Work often brings long hours, tight deadlines, and high levels of stress. Mindful breathing is a quick and effective tool to reset your mind and body, improving productivity and focus.

You can practice mindful breathing in two ways when you're at work: Either stop your work and be fully conscious of your breath from as little as one breath to as much as you have time for, or practice mindful breathing *while* you work. Combining mindful breathing with your work is easiest when you're doing repetitive work that doesn't require your full attention.

Schedule short breathing breaks throughout the day, setting an alarm or reminder. Even a few conscious breaths every hour can make a difference. These small moments of awareness can help you feel less reactive and more in control during a busy workday.

Try this if you feel your current task is repetitive and you can do it while being conscious of your breath:

1. **As you're doing your work, notice how your breath feels.**

2. **Be aware of your breath as you're doing your work.**

3. **Notice what effect this is having on your experience.**

   Whatever the impact, be curious and notice. That's what mindfulness is about.

4. **If your work is slowing down, notice if the quality of your work is increasing.**

With others: Enhancing connection and calm

Interactions with others — whether they're colleagues, friends, or family — can sometimes feel overwhelming, especially in challenging conversations. Mindful breathing can help you stay present and responsive rather than reactive.

Try this when you're expecting a difficult conversation:

1. **Before entering a meeting, social gathering, or conversation, pause for a moment and take three conscious breaths.**

2. **While talking with someone, bring your attention to your breath, especially if you feel tension rising.**

   Simply guiding your attention to your breath can prevent you from getting swept up in strong emotions.

3. **If the conversation is causing your emotions to overwhelm you, take a moment to step away; practice mindful breathing until you feel more grounded, and then return to the conversation if you need to.**

By staying aware of your breath, you can approach interactions with a sense of calm and compassion.

For sleep: Unwinding and letting go

Struggling to fall asleep? A busy, racing mind could be preventing you from falling asleep. Or maybe you find yourself wide awake in the middle of the night, and you just can't fall back asleep, no matter how much you know you need to.

If this happens, try mindful breathing. Mindful breathing can help quiet the mind and rest the body, creating the perfect environment for peaceful sleep.

Give this exercise a go to help you sleep:

1. **While lying in bed, place one hand on your chest and the other on your belly, or if this is uncomfortable, place your hands wherever you want.**

2. **Notice the natural rise and fall of your breath without trying to change it.**

3. **Feel your breathing with a sense of care and affection.**

   If you want, take a moment to be grateful that you are alive and able to comfortably breathe.

4. **Remind yourself that even if you don't immediately fall asleep, just being conscious of your breathing in this way has a beneficial effect.**

   If your mind wanders, gently bring your focus back to the sensation of your breath.

5. **Keep going until you fall asleep.**

   Good night!

This practice signals to your body that it's time to relax, helping you drift off more easily and improving the quality of your sleep.

Chapter **6**

The Amazing Power of Nose Breathing

Your nose isn't just for smelling roses or holding up your glasses — it's a sophisticated breathing apparatus designed to keep you healthy and functioning at your best. Yet many people completely bypass this amazing organ and breathe through their mouths instead.

In this chapter, you see why nasal breathing is a game-changer for your health and how to make the switch if you've always been a mouth breather. By the time you finish this chapter, you'll have a new appreciation for that prominent feature in the middle of your face!

Understanding Why Nasal Breathing Is a Game-Changer

Your nose is specifically designed to be your primary breathing pathway, while your mouth is built for eating, drinking, and telling bad jokes at dinner parties. When you bypass your nose and breathe through your mouth, you're missing out on several crucial physiological processes that keep you healthy and optimize your bodily functions.

Think of your nose as a sophisticated air-processing system that prepares every breath before it enters your lungs. Your mouth, in contrast, is more like the emergency backup system — useful when you're congested or doing very intense exercise, but detrimental when used regularly to breathe.

In the following sections, I explain some of the benefits of nasal breathing, in case you aren't convinced.

Feeling the joy of nitric oxide

One of the most remarkable benefits of nasal breathing comes from a molecule called nitric oxide.

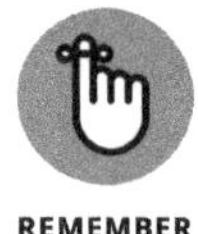

REMEMBER

Don't confuse nitric oxide with nitrous oxide, the laughing gas at the dentist's office. Nitric oxide is something your body produces naturally in your sinuses, and it's pretty amazing stuff.

When you breathe through your nose, your nasal passages and sinuses release nitric oxide, which is carried into your lungs with each breath. This powerhouse molecule performs several vital functions that can significantly improve your health:

>> **Nitric oxide is a *vasodilator*, which means it helps widen your blood vessels, improving circulation and lowering blood pressure.** This improved blood flow benefits your entire body, from your brain to your toes.

>> **Nitric oxide enhances oxygen uptake in the blood.** Studies have shown that nasal breathing can increase oxygen uptake by up to 20 percent compared to mouth breathing — like getting a free oxygen bonus just for using your nose! It accomplishes this partly by optimizing blood flow within your lungs and directing blood to the areas that are receiving the most air, which maximizes the efficiency of oxygen transfer.

>> **Nitric oxide is a potent antimicrobial agent.** It has antiviral, antibacterial, antifungal, and antiparasitic properties, actively helping your immune system fight off infections before they can take hold. This protective function is especially important during cold and flu season or when you're exposed to other respiratory pathogens.

The concentration of nitric oxide in healthy sinuses can be remarkably high — sometimes more than 20 parts per million. When you breathe through your nose, this nitric oxide gets swept into your respiratory system, providing continuous benefits to your lungs and overall health. It's like having a built-in medicine factory right in the middle of your face!

Conditioning the air for your lungs

Your nose acts as a built-in air conditioner, preparing each breath before it reaches your lungs. The nose:

>> **Filters air:** Nasal hairs trap dust, allergens, and pathogens, preventing them from entering your lungs — something mouth breathing bypasses.

>> **Humidifies air:** Your nasal passages add moisture, preventing dryness and irritation that can increase infection risk.

>> **Warms air:** Cold air can trigger respiratory issues, but your nose warms it to body temperature for smoother lung function.

These functions work together to optimize your breathing efficiency.

WARNING

Mouth breathing can actually trigger asthma in some people. This is because mouth breathing delivers cold, dry, unfiltered air to the lungs. This, in turn, causes *bronchospasm*, which is a sudden tightening of the muscles that line the *bronchi* (airways) in your lungs. Your airways then narrow, making it difficult to breathe.

Pressuring the air for your lungs

Nasal breathing creates slight resistance, helping your lungs inflate fully and promoting diaphragmatic breathing. This improves oxygen uptake and strengthens core muscles, supporting posture and reducing back pain.

Nasal breathing strengthens the respiratory muscles, enhancing lung capacity and efficiency during both rest and activity.

Exploring other benefits of nasal breathing

The benefits of nasal breathing are extensive. Here are some additional benefits that make nasal breathing a game-changer for your overall health and well-being:

>> **Improved sleep quality:** This is one significant benefit of nasal breathing. When you breathe through your nose during sleep, you're less likely to snore or experience sleep apnea, both of which can severely disrupt sleep quality.

>> **Dental health:** Mouth breathing dries the mouth, raising the risk of tooth decay, gum disease, and bad breath. Nasal breathing keeps saliva levels balanced, helping protect teeth and gums by neutralizing acids and removing bacteria.

- **>> Improved posture:** Chronic mouth breathing often leads to forward head posture as people extend their heads to open the airway. Nasal breathing encourages proper head and neck alignment, which can alleviate these issues and improve overall posture.

- **>> Reduced stress:** Nasal breathing activates the calming parasympathetic nervous system, helping you stay relaxed and focused — even during times of stress.

- **>> Improved brain functioning:** Nasal breathing leads to clearer thinking and energy levels. This is due to the increased oxygen getting into your brain cells and body.

- **>> Enhanced athletic performance:** Many athletes are discovering the benefits of nasal breathing during training and competition. It can improve endurance, reduce exercise-induced asthma, and help with recovery.

- **>> Proper development of the face, jaw, and airway:** Mouth breathing in childhood can affect facial development, causing issues like crooked teeth and narrow airways. Nasal breathing supports healthier growth and may reduce the need for orthodontics later on.

- **>> Deeper breathing:** Nasal breathers activate their diaphragm when they breathe, improving oxygen intake and easing stress and anxiety. Mouth breathing often results in shallow chest breathing.

With all these benefits, it's clear that something as simple as breathing through your nose can have profound effects on your health and well-being. It's one of those rare health interventions that costs nothing, requires no special equipment, and can be done anywhere, anytime.

Doing Nose Unblocking Exercises

Now that you understand why nasal breathing is so beneficial, you may be wondering, "But what if my nose is stuffy or congested?" It's a fair question — many people breathe through their mouths because they feel like they can't get enough air through their noses. The good news is that there are effective techniques to clear your nose and make nasal breathing possible, even if you've struggled with nasal congestion in the past.

Understanding why noses get blocked

Before diving into nose-clearing techniques, it helps to understand why your nose gets blocked in the first place. Common causes of nasal congestion include

>> **Allergies:** Pollen, dust, pet dander, and other allergens can cause nasal inflammation and excess mucus production, leading to that stuffy feeling that makes nasal breathing difficult.

>> **Infections:** Colds, the flu, and sinus infections often cause nasal congestion as your body fights the infection.

>> **Environmental irritants:** Smoke, pollution, strong odors, and changes in temperature or humidity can irritate your nasal passages and trigger congestion.

>> **Structural issues:** A *deviated septum* (where the wall between your nasal passages is off-center), *nasal polyps* (small growths in the nasal passages), or enlarged *turbinates* (structures inside your nose) can physically obstruct airflow and make nasal breathing difficult.

>> **Over-breathing (chronic hyperventilation):** This is one reason why mouth breathing can actually make nasal congestion worse over time — it creates a vicious cycle.

>> **Some medications:** Certain blood pressure drugs and other medications can cause nasal congestion as a side effect. If you notice increased nasal congestion after starting a new medication, consult your healthcare provider about possible alternatives.

>> **Hormonal changes:** Hormonal changes during pregnancy, menstruation, or due to thyroid issues can sometimes cause nasal congestion. Pregnancy rhinitis, for example, affects many women during pregnancy and typically resolves after delivery.

Understanding what's blocking your nose can help you address the root cause, but the exercises I cover next can provide immediate relief in many situations, regardless of the underlying cause.

Clearing your nose

The following nose-clearing exercise comes from the Buteyko breathing method, developed by Ukrainian doctor Konstantin Buteyko in the 1950s (see Chapter 9). This exercise is particularly effective because it temporarily increases carbon dioxide levels in your blood, which helps dilate your nasal passages and reduce inflammation.

When I first discovered this technique, I was amazed that I didn't know about it beforehand. I use it whenever my nose is blocked. If I ever get symptoms of hay fever, I find it to be really effective, too.

This nose unblocking exercise, while effective for many people, is not suitable for everyone. It should not be performed by pregnant women, individuals over 60 years old, or those with serious medical conditions. People with high blood pressure, epilepsy, panic attacks, migraines, or heart issues should also avoid this exercise. Additionally, those experiencing strong anxiety or any other serious health concerns should consult with a healthcare professional before attempting the exercise.

Here's how to do the nose-unblocking exercise, or listen to Track 12:

1. **Sit comfortably with your back straight and your shoulders relaxed.**

   Let the tip of your tongue gently rest on the roof of your mouth, just behind your front teeth.

2. **Take a small, silent breath in through your nose if possible, lasting about two seconds.**

   If your nose is completely blocked, take a tiny breath through the corner of your mouth instead.

3. **Exhale gently through your nose for about three seconds.**

4. **Pinch your nose with your fingers to hold your breath.**

   Keep your mouth closed during this step — remember, you're trying to transition away from mouth breathing, not encourage it.

   While holding your breath, gently nod your head or sway your body until you feel a moderate *air hunger* (the need to breathe). This should be a little challenging but certainly not extremely uncomfortable. At first, just start with two or three head nods as you hold your breath and build up gradually according to your comfort levels. The nodding is mostly a form of distraction. Experiment over time, with and without it, to see if you need to do it.

5. **When you feel a relatively strong need for air (but before it becomes too uncomfortable), release your nose and breathe *gently* through your nose.**

   If you're a beginner, start gently and don't push yourself too much on the breath hold. It's crucial to keep your mouth closed during this step. Focus on calming your breathing immediately after releasing your nose. Try to suppress the urge to take a big breath and instead keep your breathing gentle and controlled. You may find it helpful to repeat to yourself, "Relax and breathe less."

6. **Wait about 30 to 60 seconds, and repeat the exercise.**

Continue for three to five repetitions or until your nose clears. For many people, this exercise can clear the nose in just a few minutes. The key is to practice it regularly, especially when you notice your nose starting to get stuffy.

In the Buteyko Breathing Method, it's recommended to aim for a breath hold of at least 30 seconds to be effective, but you may not be able to do that. Just do what you comfortably can, and you'll be able to judge for yourself if it's working for you. Everyone is different.

It's quite common for the nose to become blocked again shortly after doing this exercise. However, with regular practice, your body will adjust to these higher, more normal levels of carbon dioxide, and your nose will remain clearer for longer periods.

Here's a fun fact that might surprise you: Humming can significantly increase the production of nitric oxide in your nasal passages and help clear your sinuses. In fact, humming can increase nitric oxide production in the nasal passages by up to 15 times compared to quiet breathing!

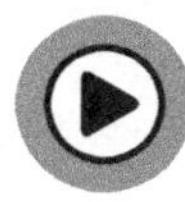

Here's a simple humming exercise for nasal clearing, also available in Track 13:

1. **Start by getting into a comfortable, relaxed posture for you.**

Let the tip of your tongue rest on the roof of your mouth, just behind your front teeth.

2. **Take a normal breath in through your nose, and as you exhale through your nose, make a "hmmmm" sound, keeping your lips closed.**

If you prefer, you can try humming a favorite tune.

You should feel a pleasant vibration in your nasal passages and sinuses.

3. **Continue this pattern for 10 to 15 breaths, humming on each exhale.**

Many people find that combining this humming technique with the nose-clearing exercise described earlier gives even better results.

Beyond clearing congestion, humming's ability to boost nitric oxide production may provide additional benefits. Because nitric oxide is a natural *bronchodilator* (it opens up the airways in your lungs), the increased nitric oxide levels from humming could potentially help people with asthma by relaxing the airways. The gentle vibration of humming also stimulates the vagus nerve, helping to activate the parasympathetic nervous system (the body's "rest-and-digest" state). More research is needed in this area, but it's an intriguing possibility that highlights the far-reaching effects of this simple practice.

Avoiding common mistakes

When practicing nose-clearing exercises, be careful to avoid these common mistakes that can reduce their effectiveness or cause discomfort:

>> **Forcing the breath hold:** Don't try to hold your breath for too long during the nose-clearing exercise in the preceding section. If you feel extremely uncomfortable, dizzy, or panicky, release your nose immediately. The exercise should be a little challenging but not distressing. ***Remember:*** You're aiming for a medium to strong air shortage, without overdoing it.

>> **Gasping after releasing the breath hold:** After you release your nose, breathe gently and calmly through your nose. Taking a huge gasping breath can undo the benefits of the exercise by causing your breathing to become erratic and heavier than usual. This indicates that you've held your breath for too long.

>> **Inconsistent practice:** Nose-clearing exercises work best when done regularly. Don't just do them when your nose is completely blocked; practice preventively when you notice the first signs of congestion. Like any skill, nasal breathing improves with regular practice.

>> **Ignoring underlying causes:** If you have persistent nasal congestion, it's important to identify and address the root cause. These exercises can help manage symptoms, but issues like structural problems, chronic allergies, or sinus infections may require medical attention.

>> **Breathing too deeply:** During and after these exercises, keep your breathing light and gentle. Deep breathing can actually worsen nasal congestion over time by reducing carbon dioxide levels, which can constrict nasal blood vessels.

>> **Mouth breathing:** After successfully clearing your nose, make a conscious effort to continue breathing through your nose. It's easy to slip back into mouth breathing out of habit, but maintaining nasal breathing helps reinforce this healthier pattern.

The goal isn't just to clear your nose once — it's to maintain nasal breathing as your default breathing pattern. Be patient with yourself as you work to establish this new habit, and celebrate small victories along the way.

THE NASAL BIOME: YOUR NOSE'S HELPFUL MICROBES

Just like the gut, the nose hosts a community of helpful microbes called the *nasal biome*. This mix of bacteria and fungi helps protect against harmful germs, supports your immune system, and keeps your nasal passages healthy.

New research shows that people with a diverse nasal biome are less likely to get sinus infections or chronic nasal issues. Some bacteria help block dangerous microbes. Interestingly, a healthy nasal biome may also be linked to better brain health in later life.

Here's how to support a healthy nasal biome:

- Breathe through your nose as much as possible.

- Use antibiotics wisely, only when prescribed.

- Stay hydrated to keep nasal passages moist.

- Eat a balanced diet, including plant foods and fermented foods.

- Avoid smoking and harsh environmental chemicals.

Identifying the Problems with Mouth Breathing

Now that you understand the benefits of nasal breathing and how to clear your nose, let's explore why mouth breathing can be problematic. Mouth breathing may seem harmless — after all, you're still getting oxygen, right? But breathing through your mouth regularly can lead to a surprising number of health issues, both in the short and long term.

Understanding why people mouth breathe

People breathe through their mouths for various reasons:

>> **Nasal obstruction:** Physical blockages like a deviated septum, nasal polyps, enlarged turbinates, or chronic congestion can make nasal breathing difficult or seemingly impossible.

>> **Allergies:** Whether seasonal or perennial, allergies often cause nasal congestion that leads to mouth breathing.

>> **Habit:** Mouth breathing often begins in childhood and continues into adulthood simply because it has become a habit.

>> **Sleep disorders:** When the airway becomes partially blocked during sleep, as occurs in sleep apnea, people often resort to mouth breathing in an unconscious attempt to get more air. This can create a vicious cycle. Turn to Chapter 13 to find ways you can improve your breathing while sleeping.

>> **Anatomical factors:** A narrow nasal passage, high palate, or other structural features can make nasal breathing more difficult, leading to a preference for mouth breathing.

>> **Stress and anxiety:** During periods of stress or anxiety, breathing typically becomes faster and shallower, and many people shift to mouth breathing as part of the "fight-or-flight" response. This stress-related mouth breathing can itself increase stress, creating another unhelpful cycle.

>> **Intense physical activity:** Many people switch to mouth breathing to get more air quickly when they're engaged in intense physical activity. This may be necessary during very high-intensity exercise, but many people resort to mouth breathing even during moderate activity when nasal breathing would be sufficient and more beneficial.

Understanding why you mouth breathe is the first step toward making a change.

Reducing mouth breathing

If you're a chronic mouth breather, you can try some strategies to reduce this habit:

>> **Bring awareness to your breath.** Many people don't even realize they're breathing through their mouths. Start by simply noticing your breathing pattern throughout the day. Is your mouth open or closed? Are you breathing through your nose or your mouth? This increased awareness alone can help you begin to shift your breathing pattern.

>> **Clear your nose regularly using the techniques in the "Clearing your nose" section, earlier in this chapter.** The Buteyko nose-clearing exercise and humming can help maintain clear nasal passages, making nasal breathing possible even if you're prone to congestion.

>> **Address allergies if they're contributing to your nasal congestion.** Talk to your doctor about appropriate treatments, which may include antihistamines, nasal sprays, or immunotherapy. Managing allergies effectively can make a significant difference in your ability to breathe through your nose.

>> **Stay properly hydrated throughout the day.** Proper hydration helps keep nasal mucus thin and flowing, reducing congestion and making nasal breathing easier. The exact amount you need varies widely depending on activity levels, weather, and health. If you're feeling thirsty and your urine is dark yellow, your fluid intake is probably inadequate.

>> **Use saline nasal sprays or rinses to keep your nasal passages clear and moisturized.** These products can help wash away irritants and thin mucus, making nasal breathing more comfortable. They're particularly helpful after exposure to allergens or irritants.

>> **Consider nasal strips or nasal dilators for nighttime use, especially if you have trouble breathing through your nose while sleeping.** These external strips can help open nasal passages and make nasal breathing easier during sleep. They don't address the root cause of nasal congestion, but they can be helpful as a temporary solution.

>> **Practice nasal breathing during exercise, starting with lower-intensity activities.** Begin by walking or light jogging while focusing on nasal breathing; then gradually increase the intensity of your activity while still breathing through your nose. This progressive approach allows your body to adapt to nasal breathing during physical activity.

>> **Seek medical attention for structural issues.** If you suspect a deviated septum or other structural issue is preventing nasal breathing, an ear, nose, and throat specialist can evaluate your nasal passages and recommend appropriate treatments.

These strategies can help reduce mouth breathing, but for a complete transition, you'll need the more comprehensive approach in the next section.

Transitioning away from mouth breathing

Transitioning from mouth breathing to nasal breathing requires patience and consistent practice. It's essentially retraining a habit that may have been with you for years or even decades. The following sections explore effective strategies to make this transition successfully.

Use it or lose it: Breathing using your nose

The more you breathe through your nose, the easier it becomes. This is partly because regular nasal breathing strengthens the muscles involved in keeping your nasal passages open, increases nitric oxide production (which helps dilate the airways), reduces nasal inflammation over time, and improves the overall function of your nasal passages.

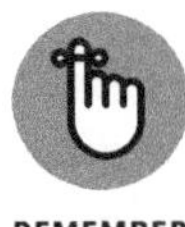

Think of nasal breathing as a skill that improves with practice, similar to learning a musical instrument or a new sport. Even if it feels difficult or uncomfortable at first, especially during physical activity or sleep, it gets easier with consistent practice. Your respiratory system actually adapts to nasal breathing, becoming more efficient over time.

Start with conscious nasal breathing during rest and light activities. Throughout the day, remind yourself to check your breathing pattern and switch to nasal breathing if you catch yourself mouth breathing. Setting regular reminders on your phone or placing sticky notes in strategic locations can help develop this awareness.

As nasal breathing becomes more comfortable at rest, gradually extend it to more challenging situations, such as during exercise or sleep. This progressive approach allows your body to adapt and helps make nasal breathing your default mode. Don't be discouraged if you can't immediately maintain nasal breathing during intense exercise — this is normal and will improve with practice.

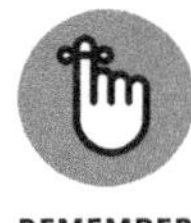

Your breathing pattern at night often reflects your daytime habits. If you consistently breathe through your nose during the day, you're more likely to maintain nasal breathing during sleep. This is why developing a solid daytime nasal breathing habit is crucial for addressing nighttime mouth breathing.

Mouth taping during the day

Mouth taping may sound extreme or uncomfortable at first, but it's actually a gentle and effective technique for transitioning to nasal breathing. By physically encouraging your lips to stay closed, mouth taping serves as a constant reminder to breathe through your nose.

For daytime practice, you can start with a small piece of 3M Micropore Surgical Tape placed vertically in the center of your lips. This serves as a physical reminder to keep your mouth closed. It's a great way of testing to see if you automatically have the urge to mouth breathe without knowing it.

Here are some mouth-taping tips:

>> **Start with short periods of just 15 to 30 minutes while engaged in a quiet activity like reading or watching TV.** This allows you to get comfortable with the sensation without feeling restricted or anxious. As you get more comfortable, you can gradually increase the duration.

>> **Use appropriate tape for this purpose.** Paper medical tape, like 3M Micropore Surgical Tape or specialized mouth tape, like MyoTape are good

options. Never use nonporous or strongly adhesive tapes like duct tape or electrical tape — these tapes can irritate your skin and are difficult to remove.

>> **When you use a piece of tape on your mouth, stick the tape on the back of your hand and remove it a few times.** This helps to ensure it's not too sticky when you put it on your mouth, so it doesn't hurt when you remove it.

>> **If your lips are dry, apply a small amount of lip balm before applying the tape to prevent irritation when removing it.** This tip is especially important if you have sensitive skin or if you're using mouth tape for extended periods.

>> **For daytime use, place the tape vertically from just above your upper lip to just below your lower lip.** This allows you to open your mouth if necessary but serves as a reminder to keep it closed. Some people prefer to use a strip placed across the whole mouth.

>> **As you become more comfortable with short periods of mouth taping, gradually increase the time you spend with mouth tape during the day.** Many people eventually work up to wearing mouth tape for several hours while at home or even during light exercise.

Many people report that even short periods of mouth taping help them become more aware of their breathing habits and make it easier to maintain nasal breathing throughout the day. It can also be done at night with more precautions (see Chapter 13). The physical reminder of the tape helps break the unconscious habit of mouth breathing and reinforces the new habit of nasal breathing.

Setting a timer and checking in

Changing your breathing pattern requires consistent awareness. Because breathing is mostly automatic, setting reminders can help make nasal breathing a habit:

>> **Use timers or cues.** Set phone alerts or place small notes in visible spots like your mirror or computer to remind yourself to check your breathing.

>> **Link check-ins to daily activities.** Check your breathing when looking at your phone, eating, or walking through a doorway. Associating it with routine tasks makes it easier to remember.

>> **Track patterns and set goals.** Keep a brief journal to identify when you tend to mouth breathe, such as during stressful times or when you're concentrating really hard. Set simple goals like maintaining nasal breathing during a commute or workout.

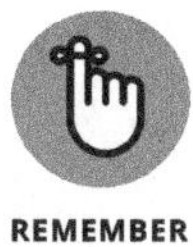

If you catch yourself mouth breathing, gently switch to nasal breathing — each correction reinforces the habit. Progress takes time, so focus on consistency rather than perfection.

REMEMBER

Improving your posture to encourage nasal breathing

Your posture and breathing are deeply interconnected. Poor posture makes nasal breathing harder, while proper posture supports it. Head position is key — forward head posture strains neck muscles and encourages mouth breathing. Keep your head aligned with your spine, with your ears over your shoulders, to promote nasal breathing.

Shoulder and spine alignment also impact breathing. Rolled shoulders compress the chest, restricting airflow, while a slumped spine limits diaphragm movement, leading to shallow breathing. Practicing good posture — relaxed shoulders and a long, neutral spine — creates space for deeper nasal breathing.

Here's a simple reset: Stand against a wall with your heels, buttocks, shoulders, and head touching the wall for 30 seconds; then try to maintain that alignment throughout the day.

Ergonomics and movement further support good posture. Adjust your screen to eye level, use a supportive chair, and take breaks to stretch. Mind-body practices like yoga, Pilates, and tai chi reinforce alignment and breathing. Because posture and breathing work in a feedback loop, improving one naturally enhances the other, making nasal breathing easier and more natural over time.

Optimizing your tongue posture

Believe it or not, one of the biggest helpers in healthy breathing is already in your mouth: your tongue! When you place your tongue in the right position, it not only helps keep your airway open but also naturally encourages nose breathing, even when you're not thinking about it.

Here's why your tongue's resting position matters:

>> **It keeps your airway clear.** When your tongue gently rests on the roof of your mouth (instead of sagging down), it acts like a built-in support beam to help keep your airway open.

>> **It supports nasal breathing.** With your tongue in the right spot, your lips are more likely to stay closed, which encourages you to breathe through your nose instead of your mouth.

>> **It shapes your face (really!).** In kids, good tongue posture can help the upper jaw grow properly. In adults, it helps maintain that shape, keeping your nasal passages more spacious.

Here's what good tongue posture looks like:

>> **Tongue on the roof of your mouth:** Gently press the broad, flat part of your tongue against the top of your mouth. The tip should be just behind your front teeth (but not touching them), and the rest of the tongue should make light contact with the hard palate.

>> **Lips together, teeth slightly apart:** Keep your lips closed softly — no tension in your jaw or face. Your teeth should have a tiny gap between them, about the width of a fingernail.

>> **Nose breathing only:** With your tongue in place, simply breathe through your nose. Easy does it.

This small change in how your tongue rests can make a surprisingly big difference to your breathing — day and night. Give it a go and see how it feels. It may feel strange at first, but you'll get used to it over time.

Chewing for nasal strength

Chewing plays a key role in nasal breathing and airway development. Modern soft diets require minimal chewing, leading to underdeveloped jaw muscles and narrower airways, which can make nasal breathing harder. In contrast, our ancestors' diets of tough foods promoted strong jaws and better nasal airflow. Proper chewing stimulates jaw and facial bone growth, supporting nasal breathing throughout life.

To strengthen your jaw, eat whole, unprocessed foods like crunchy vegetables, nuts, and seeds. Chew thoroughly — aim for 20 to 30 chews per bite — to aid digestion and exercise jaw muscles.

Sugar-free gum can also help. Chewing gum sweetened with xylitol not only avoids the blood sugar spikes of sugar but also starves cavity-causing bacteria, reducing both plaque and acid production. Research shows it can cut harmful mouth bacteria by up to 90 percent and significantly lower the risk of decay.

For children, chewing tougher foods encourages proper jaw development and lifelong nasal breathing habits. Results take time, but consistently choosing firmer foods can improve airway space and overall breathing efficiency.

Chapter **7**

Diaphragmatic Breathing: The Key to Healthy Breathing

magine this: You're feeling stressed, tired, or a bit overwhelmed. You pause, take a few deep breaths — and instead of feeling relaxed, you actually end up feeling a bit more tense or even dizzy! Sound familiar? Don't worry, you're not alone.

Many people think *deep breathing* means taking a big breath and inflating their chest and shoulders, without realizing they're missing the most important muscle involved in healthy breathing: the diaphragm.

In this chapter, I take you on an easy-to-follow journey into the world of diaphragmatic breathing. Here, you discover exactly what your diaphragm is (it's not just a fancy medical term!), how it can transform your breathing, and why simply breathing into your chest doesn't cut it.

I walk you step-by-step through simple exercises that'll get your diaphragm moving freely, help you spot common mistakes, and give you practical tips for integrating diaphragmatic breathing into everyday life — whether you're walking, doing yoga, or just relaxing on the sofa.

Exploring Diaphragmatic Breathing

Diaphragmatic breathing (also known as belly breathing or abdominal breathing) is your body's natural way of breathing, using your diaphragm — the powerhouse muscle beneath your lungs — to pull air deep into your lungs effortlessly. Let's get curious about your breathing habits and discover a healthier way to breathe.

Diaphragmatic breathing is a fancy term for a very natural way of breathing — using your diaphragm muscle to draw air deep into your lungs.

The diaphragm is a large, dome-shaped muscle that sits right under your lungs (at the bottom of your rib cage). Think of it as a movable floor between your chest and abdomen.

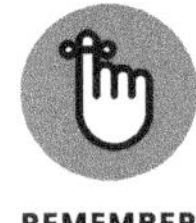

The term *belly breathing* is often used to describe diaphragmatic breathing, but they're not exactly the same. Diaphragmatic breathing uses the diaphragm to pull air deep into the lungs, which naturally makes the belly rise. Simply pushing your belly out isn't enough — it's the diaphragm doing the work that really matters. Just pushing your belly out doesn't mean you're using your diaphragm properly.

Understanding the diaphragm and how it works

When you take a proper diaphragmatic breath, this muscle contracts and moves downward, giving your lungs room to expand fully. On the exhale, the diaphragm relaxes and moves back upward, helping push air out of your lungs. You can see a diagram of the diaphragm in Figure 2-2 in Chapter 2.

In simple terms, when you inhale, the belly goes out and the lower ribs move outward slightly; when you exhale, the belly goes in and the lower ribs move in slightly. Your belly visibly expands because the diaphragm's downward movement makes your abdomen push forward. This is the key to healthy, efficient breathing — letting the belly lead instead of the upper chest.

Many people don't use their diaphragms effectively all the time. In fact, a lot of people breathe in a way that is essentially backward.

You can push your belly in and out without using your diaphragm. So, in "Figuring out if you're breathing correctly," later in this chapter, I show you a better test to find out if you're doing diaphragmatic breathing.

Seeing the signs of paradoxical breathing

Paradoxical breathing is like the opposite of diaphragmatic breathing. It happens when your body breathes in a way that works against itself. Instead of your belly expanding on the inhale, it pulls in, while your chest and shoulders lift up. Then, on the exhale, your stomach moves outward. This is the opposite of how healthy breathing should function.

Many people don't even realize they're doing it because it can feel normal, especially if they've been breathing this way for years. The good news? With awareness and practice, you can retrain your body to breathe in a way that is smoother, more natural, and better for your health.

Try this simple test to see if you're breathing backward:

1. **Sit or stand comfortably and place one hand on your belly and the other on your chest.**

2. **Take a deep breath in.**

3. **Watch what happens. Does your belly expand outward, or does it pull inward while your chest rises?**

4. **Now, exhale slowly. Does your belly fall naturally, or does it push outward at the end?**

If your stomach moves inward when you inhale and outward when you exhale, you're likely engaging in paradoxical breathing. This habit can make breathing feel more effortful than it needs to be, leading to increased tension and even mild dizziness or fatigue over time.

Understanding the causes of paradoxical breathing

Paradoxical breathing is often caused by habitual tension, stress, or posture issues. Here are the most common reasons:

>> **Holding in your stomach all day:** If you frequently suck in your stomach (to appear slimmer or as a habit), you may be restricting your diaphragm's movement. This forces you to rely more on chest breathing. Over time, this becomes your default way of breathing, even when you're relaxed.

>> **Stress and anxiety:** When you're stressed or anxious, your body often shifts into "fight-or-flight" mode, which naturally leads to shallower, more rapid chest breathing. Over time, your body adapts to this as a "normal" way to breathe, making diaphragmatic breathing feel unnatural.

- **»** **Poor posture and prolonged sitting:** Sitting for long periods, especially hunched over a desk, can compress your diaphragm and make it harder to breathe deeply. Slouching also restricts the rib cage, leading to more upper-chest breathing.

- **»** **Overusing the neck and shoulder muscles:** Some people compensate for weak diaphragm function by using their upper-chest and neck muscles to pull air in. This can lead to tension in the shoulders, neck, and even jaw, making breathing feel more effortful.

- **»** **High-altitude exposure:** If you've ever been to a high-altitude location where the air is thinner, you may have noticed your breathing felt different. Sometimes, the body adjusts by altering its breathing pattern, and paradoxical breathing can result.

- **»** **Underlying medical conditions:** In some cases, paradoxical breathing may be linked to medical conditions such as asthma, chronic obstructive pulmonary disease (COPD), sleep apnea, or neurological disorders. If you frequently struggle with breathlessness or extreme fatigue, it's worth speaking with a healthcare professional to rule out any underlying causes.

The good news? You can retrain your body to breathe properly! It takes practice, but with small adjustments, you can restore diaphragmatic breathing as your natural way to breathe. Doing the exercises in this chapter will help.

Reaping the benefits of diaphragmatic breathing

So, why should you care about switching to diaphragmatic breathing? The benefits are huge — for both your mind and your body. Here are some of the big perks experts attribute to good deep breathing:

- **»** **Triggers relaxation:** Breathing with your diaphragm activates your body's natural relaxation response (the parasympathetic nervous system). This empowers many systems in your body, including your immune system. You're less likely to get sick. It helps reduce stress hormones and can quickly calm you down. Many meditation and yoga techniques center on diaphragmatic breathing for this very reason.

- **»** **More energy and reduced brain fog:** Deep diaphragmatic breaths encourage full oxygen exchange — more fresh oxygen in and the right amount of carbon dioxide out. You may feel more energized and have greater clarity, because your brain works better with the right amount of oxygen. This also makes each breath more effective at nourishing your body. You may notice that you don't get winded as easily when you breathe this way, because you're using your lungs to their full capacity.

» **Lower heart rate and blood pressure:** Slow, deep breathing slows your heartbeat and can even lower or stabilize blood pressure. It's like a built-in blood pressure medication (without the pills!). If you've ever had a doctor or nurse tell you to "take a deep breath" during a stressful moment, this is why — diaphragmatic breathing signals your system to chill out. *Remember:* Don't stop taking any medication without speaking to your doctor.

» **More efficient workouts and movement:** When your diaphragm does the work, your other breathing muscles (neck, chest, shoulders) don't have to. This can improve muscle function during exercise and prevent those tense neck and shoulder feelings that come with stressful chest breathing. It also means less effort and energy spent on breathing, so you can use that energy for other activities. This also leads to improved athletic performance and reduced recovery time.

» **Improved core stability and digestion:** The diaphragm is part of your core muscle group. Engaging it can gently massage your internal organs, which has benefits like potentially easing abdominal bloating and improving digestion. Some breathing therapists even use it to help with constipation or irritable bowel syndrome (IBS) due to that gentle internal massage. A happy diaphragm can mean a happier tummy!

» **Lymphatic drainage and flow:** Your lymphatic system is a group of organs, tissues, and vessels that protect you from infection and keep the right balance of fluids in your body. By consciously using your diaphragm, you create a pumping action that moves and drains the fluid in an effective way. This helps to remove waste products and toxins from your body.

Figuring out if you're breathing correctly

TRY THIS

It's possible to push your belly in and out without actually using your diaphragm. That's like a trick — not belly breathing! So, to assess whether you're practicing diaphragmatic breathing correctly, do this test, which also doubles up as a deep breathing exercise:

1. **Stand upright with a relaxed posture, ensuring that your shoulders are down and your knees are slightly bent.**

2. **Place your hands on the sides of your lower rib cage, with your thumbs wrapped around your back and fingers resting on your sides.**

   This positioning allows you to feel the movement of your rib cage during breathing.

3. **Breathe in deeply through your nose, directing the air toward your lower ribs.**

   As you inhale, you should feel your lower rib cage expand slightly outward against your hands if you're doing diaphragmatic breathing.

4. **Exhale slowly through your nose.**

   You should notice your lower rib cage contract inward slightly as air leaves your lungs.

5. **Repeat this process for several breaths.**

   If you feel your lower rib cage expanding and contracting with each breath, you're effectively engaging in diaphragmatic breathing. If not, keep reading this chapter to learn how to do diaphragmatic breathing effectively.

Avoiding common mistakes

With all these benefits, diaphragmatic breathing sounds like a no-brainer. But when first learning it, people often run into a few common mistakes. Being aware of these can help you avoid them:

- **Chest breathing or "shrugging":** A very common mistake is using the upper chest and shoulder muscles, instead of the diaphragm, to inhale. If you notice your shoulders going up toward your ears with each breath, that's a sign. Breathing mainly with lifted shoulders and upper chest is inefficient and often linked to feeling anxious or panicky. It can also lead to tight neck and shoulder muscles. So, if you're practicing and your neck is getting sore, check in. You may be defaulting to chest breaths. The fix: Relax your shoulders down and focus on the belly moving first.

- **Pulling your belly in on the inhale:** This is paradoxical breathing — essentially holding your stomach tight. People sometimes do this without realizing, especially if they're used to holding in their abs all day. The result is very shallow air intake (because the diaphragm can't descend properly against tight abs). If you catch yourself doing this, don't beat yourself up — it's common. Just consciously allow your belly to *expand* when you breathe in. You may even say to yourself, "Soft belly," as a reminder. The exercises later in this chapter can help you fix this issue.

- **Breathing too fast or forcefully:** One of the top errors beginners make is rushed breathing — taking quick, big gulps of air in an effort to "breathe deeper." Ironically, this can make you lightheaded or dizzy (from blowing off too much carbon dioxide too fast). Deep breathing should be slow and steady, not a hyperventilation exercise. If you start to feel lightheaded or anxious while practicing, pause and breathe normally for a bit. Then resume at a slower pace (for instance, inhale for a count of 4, exhale for a count of 6, breathing as quietly and gently as you can). There's no prize for the largest and most breaths per minute — in fact, fewer is usually better.

>> **Pushing the belly out mechanically:** Some people hear "belly out" and then *only* move their bellies, without actually taking in much air. They kind of fake the motion. ***Remember:*** The belly should be moving because the lungs are filling with air and pushing the diaphragm down, not just because you're sticking your stomach out. Don't force your stomach forward unnaturally; instead, focus on the air flowing deep into your abdomen. The movement of your abdomen will happen naturally as a result.

>> **Expecting it to feel perfect immediately:** Diaphragmatic breathing is natural (babies do it!), but years of bad habits mean it can feel odd at first. It's normal to feel a little awkward or even tired when you start retraining your breathing. You may take a few good breaths and then suddenly gasp or feel yourself "lose it" — that's okay. Be patient with yourself and don't give up because it feels strange. With practice, it will become more automatic and comfortable.

Sarah, a client under constant stress, often felt short of breath at work. To relax, she took "deep breaths," but her version involved lifting her chest and pulling in her stomach — in other words, doing the opposite of diaphragmatic breathing. Instead of relief, she felt more tension in her neck and shoulders.

During a session, I noticed her pattern and guided her to lie down, place a hand on her belly, and breathe into it. At first, she struggled to relax her abs, because she was used to holding them in all day. But after a few tries, she felt an immediate shift — her breathing became easier and more calming.

With just a few minutes of practice each day, Sarah saw real changes. Her stress levels dropped, she felt less anxious, and even her shoulder tension improved. It was an eye-opening moment — something as simple as breathing the right way made a dramatic difference.

By now, you should have a good idea of what diaphragmatic breathing is (and isn't). The diaphragm is the star of the show, and the goal is to breathe in a way that lets it do its job — moving down on inhales to pull air in and up on exhales to push air out. No more chest-heaving or belly-sucking-in shenanigans.

Following a Step-by-Step Guide to Diaphragmatic Breathing

Before you dive into practicing diaphragmatic breathing, let's take some time to loosen up the diaphragm.

Loosening up the diaphragm

As you integrate diaphragmatic breathing into daily activities, you may also consider some techniques to keep your diaphragm and breathing muscles loose and free-moving. Just like any muscle, the diaphragm can become a bit tight or restricted if you've been chronically breathing shallowly.

Here are a couple of bonus tricks to loosen the diaphragm and surrounding muscles, making deep breathing even easier:

>> **Stretch it out.** One effective stretch for the diaphragm is a simple side stretch. Stand up and reach your left arm overhead, leaning your torso gently to the right side as you exhale. This increases the space on your left side where the diaphragm attaches (between your lower ribs and spine) and gives it a nice stretch. Inhale as you come back to center; then switch sides (right arm up, lean left on exhale). Do this a few times on each side. You'll stretch not only the diaphragm but also the intercostal muscles between your ribs. Afterward, you may notice that it feels even easier to get a deep breath, as if there's more room in your rib cage — because there is! This technique is actually used by singers and athletes to increase diaphragmatic flexibility.

>> **Try humming or singing.** Believe it or not, humming can help release tension in your breathing muscles. When you hum (especially a long, continuous hum on an exhale), your vocal cords vibrate and you naturally engage your diaphragm and core. This can improve the movement of your rib cage and diaphragm synergy. It also stimulates your vagus nerve, engaging relaxation and thereby making you feel good. So, next time you're alone, take a big belly inhale, and then hum as you exhale. Feel the buzz in your chest and belly. It's like a mini internal massage. Plus, it's hard to be stressed when you're humming your favorite tune! Singing works similarly — it forces you to use your breath support. No wonder singing in the shower feels so therapeutic. And if anyone complains about your singing, you can tell them you're activating your diaphragm, thank you very much!

>> **Do a belly massage.** You can also gently massage your upper abdominal area (just below your sternum, along the rib margins) with your fingers while breathing, to encourage the diaphragm to relax. Some people do this lying

down — placing their fingertips under the lower rib cage and massaging in small circles. If you find tender spots, be gentle, but a little massage can increase blood flow and remind those muscles to loosen up. Always be gentle — this shouldn't be painful, just a light, encouraging rub.

» **Practice good posture.** Lastly, consider your posture during the day. Slouching (like hunching over a desk) can compress your diaphragm. Every so often, sit up or stand up and do a big belly breath with arms stretched overhead to "reset" your torso. This literally gives your diaphragm space. If you spend a lot of time at a computer, ergonomics matter for breathing, too — keep your monitor at eye level, shoulders relaxed, and perhaps use a small, rolled towel behind your lower back to support the natural curve. This alignment allows your diaphragm to move without obstruction.

Practicing with a book on the floor

Now that you know the theory and you've loosened up a bit, let's put diaphragmatic breathing into practice. The best way to begin training your diaphragm is by practicing while lying down, which allows your belly to move freely without fighting gravity. Here's an exercise recommended by breathing expert Patrick McKeown.

TRY THIS

Grab a small book (nothing too heavy, a paperback or thin hardcover works well) and follow these steps:

1. **Lie down on your back on a flat surface (like a bed or a yoga mat on the floor), and bend your knees with your feet flat on the floor (to help take strain off your lower back).**

   You can put a pillow under your head and even under your knees if that's more comfy for you.

2. **Place the book on your belly, just below your rib cage (around the area of your navel), and place one hand on your chest.**

   If you don't have a book handy, you can simply rest one of your hands there instead, but a book gives a nice visual cue.

3. **Relax your shoulders and chest.**

   Take a moment to loosen up. Wiggle your shoulders away from your ears and let your neck relax. This ensures that tension isn't creeping into your upper body. You're aiming to keep your upper chest and shoulders at rest.

4. **Inhale gently through your nose and direct the breath toward your abdomen, as if you're filling your belly with air.**

   You should feel (and see) the book rise up as your stomach expands. The hand on your chest should stay relatively still — almost all the movement should be in your belly region. Don't force it — let the air naturally push the belly up instead of using your abdominal muscles.

5. **Slowly exhale through your nose.**

   As you exhale, feel your stomach fall and watch the book lower back down. You can imagine your belly button drawing in toward your spine, which means your diaphragm is moving back up, pushing the air out. Try to make your exhale long and steady — ideally a bit longer than your inhale. This not only expels more air but also further engages the relaxation response.

6. **Repeat for several breaths.**

   Continue this slow in-and-out breathing, focusing on the book rising on inhales and falling on exhales. Aim for about five to ten minutes of practice, if you can, or about ten breaths to start, if that feels like a lot. Go at a pace that's comfortable; for example, you might inhale for a count of four and then exhale for a count of six or eight. The exact count isn't critical as long as it's unforced and you're not getting lightheaded.

As you practice, remember the goal: Belly moves more than chest. If the book on your tummy is barely budging but the hand on your chest is bobbing up and down, refocus on sending the air lower. It may help to imagine your lungs filling from the bottom like a glass of water: First, the belly (bottom) expands, and then the chest (top) only if needed at the very end of the inhale. In the beginning, it may feel like you're not getting "enough air" when breathing this way — that's normal as your body adjusts to a new pattern. But rest assured, if the book on your belly is rising, you're getting plenty of air deep into your lungs, even if it feels different from the usual chest breathing.

When you get comfortable, you can increase the challenge slightly by using a slightly heavier book or object on your abdomen. This provides gentle resistance and helps strengthen your diaphragm muscle, like adding a tiny weight to a workout. Don't overdo it, though — a heavy textbook isn't necessary! Even a small hardcover is enough to give you feedback.

After you've practiced deep breathing lying down (with the trusty book), you'll likely start to get the hang of what it *feels* like to use your diaphragm. The next step is to try the same type of breathing in a seated position, because, of course, we spend a lot of time sitting or standing in daily life. Transitioning to sitting can be a bit more challenging (gravity isn't helping as much, and posture comes into play), but it's an important progression.

Practicing in a chair or sofa or standing

When you feel comfortable practicing diaphragmatic breathing lying down, try it while sitting or standing. You may sit on a chair, sofa, or even the edge of your bed — anywhere you can stay relaxed but upright. Or simply stand tall with soft knees and a relaxed posture. The key is to stay at ease and let the breath do the work.

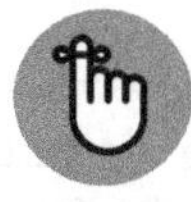

You can push your belly in and out without your diaphragm moving, but the next exercise is a good one to ensure you're doing it right.

Follow these steps to practice diaphragmatic breathing, or listen to Track 14:

1. **Find a comfortable position—either seated or standing.**

   If seated, rest your feet flat on the floor with your knees about hip-width apart. You can lean back for support if needed. If standing, soften your knees slightly so you're not locking them, and stand tall but relaxed. Either way, let your shoulders drop and your face soften, and imagine a gentle thread lifting the crown of your head to lengthen your spine.

2. **Place your hands on the sides of your lower ribs (minus the book now, unless you want odd looks in the office!).**

   Wrap your fingers around the sides of your rib cage — thumbs toward your back, fingers around the front. This hand placement helps you feel the natural movement of your diaphragm more accurately than placing a hand on your belly.

3. **Breathe in slowly through your nose and feel your ribs expand outward. Keep your shoulders down and relaxed.**

   As you inhale, gently direct the breath down and wide. Your ribs should press into your hands — sideways rather than upward into the chest. Keep your shoulders relaxed and still.

4. **Exhale slowly through your nose and feel your ribs soften inward.**

   Let the breath flow out smoothly, noticing your ribs return gently to center. If it feels comfortable, try extending the length of your exhale slightly longer than your inhale.

5. **Keep a relaxed rhythm and continue for a few minutes.**

   Whether seated or standing, allow your posture to support ease — not too slouched, not too stiff. Diaphragmatic breathing works best when your body is relaxed and your attention is gentle. Let the breath guide the movement instead of forcing anything.

As you practice in a chair, you may notice it takes a bit more awareness than when you were lying on the floor. That's completely normal. When seated, you have to maintain your posture and balance, so there are a few more muscle groups active. The key is to keep those other muscles (neck, shoulders, chest) as *inactive* as possible in the breathing process. They can hang out and relax while your diaphragm does the work.

Your diaphragm is three-dimensional. Imagine it as a jellyfish floating inside your torso. With each inhale, it gently lowers, expanding and drawing air into your lungs like a jellyfish spreading itself. Then, as you exhale, it rises and softens, like the jellyfish contracting to float upward again. So, when it moves downward as you inhale, it doesn't just push your belly out — it also expands the sides of your body and even your lower back. Try visualizing your breath as spreading in all directions — front, sides, and back. This fuller awareness can make the experience more enjoyable, effective, and natural.

If you find it challenging, you can alternate: Do a few minutes lying down (to remind yourself of the feeling), and then sit up and try to re-create that feeling. Over time, it will get easier and more natural to breathe diaphragmatically, whether you're lying, sitting, or even standing.

Troubleshooting

Now let's address some troubleshooting tips for diaphragmatic breathing. Not everyone gets it on the first try, and you may encounter some of these common issues:

- >> **Feeling like you can't get your belly to move:** If you're having trouble feeling your belly expand, you may be unconsciously holding tension in your abdominal muscles. First, make sure you're practicing at a time and place you can truly relax (not when you're in a rush or anxious about something else). Try placing a warm hand or a book on your belly as feedback and imagine your breath is filling up that area. Also, double-check that you're inhaling through your nose, not your mouth. Breathing in through the nose can naturally encourage the diaphragm to engage, whereas big gulps through the mouth may prompt more chest involvement. Think of the air "going to the bottom of your lungs." It may sound silly, but sometimes visualizing your breath like a wave filling your belly can help. Or try placing your hands on your ribs instead of your belly — some people find that helps. If all else fails, go back to lying down for a while — it's easier in that position, and with practice, you can gradually sit up more and more.

» **Feeling dizzy or lightheaded:** This is not uncommon when you start doing deep breathing exercises, especially if you're a little anxious. Usually, it's because you're breathing a bit too fast or too much (over-breathing can lower carbon dioxide in your blood and cause that dizzy feeling, which is what you're trying to avoid). If this happens, pause. Return to your normal breathing for a minute. You can also try shortening your inhales/exhales slightly or not breathing quite as deeply until your body adjusts. *Remember:* Quality over quantity. A comfortable breath is better than an exaggerated one. It's also a good idea, if you've been lying down practicing, to sit for a moment before standing up. Give yourself a second to get your bearings; standing up too quickly after a long breathing session may make you dizzy.

» **Feeling like your chest keeps taking over:** This is a very common frustration. You inhale and, *boom,* your chest lifts or your shoulders tense up out of habit. One trick is to intentionally soften your belly as you breathe. It's hard to tense your chest when your belly is jelly. You can also try breathing "against resistance" — for example, place a hand on your chest and gently hold it there, as if telling it, "Stay put," while you breathe into your lower hand. Another method: Practice in front of a mirror. Watch your shoulders — if they're moving up and down a lot, slow down and reset. Shrug them up, and then let them drop completely before your next inhale. Over time, you'll train yourself to isolate the diaphragm movement more.

» **Wearing tight clothing or having a full stomach:** If you're wearing very tight pants/trousers, a snug belt, or a restrictive waistband, it may physically prevent your belly from expanding comfortably. Try loosening your belt or practicing in loose clothing or pajamas. Similarly, attempting deep breathing right after a big meal can be uncomfortable because your stomach is physically full and pushing up on your diaphragm. (Anyone who's ever tried to take a deep breath after a big festive dinner knows the struggle!) In fact, eating a large meal can limit the diaphragm's movement. So, you may want to practice before meals or at least an hour after eating. If you must practice after eating, do it gently and stop if it feels like it's making you reflux.

» **Getting discouraged:** Don't be too hard on yourself if this takes time. It's like learning any new skill; at first, you have to consciously think about it, which can feel awkward. The good news is that with consistent practice, your body will start doing it more automatically. *Remember:* You used to breathe this way as a baby, so in a sense you're reactivating an old natural habit. Studies and experts note that at first it may take more effort and you may even get tired using your diaphragm consciously, but keep at it, and it will become automatic again. One day, you'll realize that you're diaphragmatically breathing without even thinking about it, and that's the goal!

By troubleshooting and adjusting, you'll overcome most initial challenges with diaphragmatic breathing. If you ever feel discomfort (beyond mild dizziness) or have a medical condition that affects breathing, of course check with a healthcare provider. But for the vast majority of people, these exercises are safe, gentle, and incredibly beneficial.

Integrating Diaphragmatic Breathing into Daily Activities

Diaphragmatic breathing isn't meant to be confined to your practice sessions on the yoga mat or the five minutes before bed (though those are great!). The real magic happens when you start incorporating this healthy breathing style into your everyday activities. The more you can make diaphragmatic breathing your "default" mode, the more you'll reap its benefits throughout the day.

In the following sections, I show you a few practical ways to blend deep breathing into daily life: while walking, during yoga or other mindful movement, and by building simple habits that remind you to breathe deeply regularly.

Breathing while walking

Walking is a great opportunity to practice diaphragmatic breathing in a natural, rhythmic way. By syncing your breath with your steps, you can make breathing more efficient, reduce tension in your body, and turn an ordinary walk into a calming, moving meditation. This technique can also improve endurance and help you breathe better during more intense activities like jogging or cycling.

Here are some tips for breathing while walking:

>> **When you start walking, notice if you're hunching your shoulders or tensing your neck.** Relax your upper body and let your abdomen do most of the work.

>> **Inhale and exhale through your nose whenever possible.** If you catch yourself mouth breathing, slow your pace and return to nasal breathing.

>> **Sync your breath with your steps.** Get into a rhythm that feels good for you. For example, inhale over two or three steps. Exhale over four steps (making your exhale slightly longer). Adjust the count so it feels natural — don't force it. This is a great way of combining breathing exercises while walking.

>> **Engage your diaphragm.** Focus on your belly and lower ribs expanding with each inhale and gently contracting with each exhale. If you're in a comfortable setting, place a hand on your lower ribs to feel the movement.

>> **Let your breathing set the rhythm for your walk.** If your mind wanders, gently bring your attention back to the rise and fall of your belly with each step. Enjoy the calming effect as you breathe smoothly and evenly.

I often enjoy adding a tiny smile during breathing exercises — just when it comes to mind. Smiling gently activates the relaxation response and makes the practice feel lighter and more enjoyable. Give it a try and see how it feels for you. No pressure to smile, of course — it's just a gentle invitation, not a requirement!

Yoga and mindful movement

If you practice yoga, Pilates, tai chi, or any form of mindful movement, diaphragmatic breathing is one of the best ways to enhance your experience. These activities already emphasize deep, smooth breathing, often linking breath with movement. By actively engaging your diaphragm, you improve oxygen flow, reduce tension, and move with greater ease and awareness.

Breathing deeply while moving also trains you to maintain diaphragmatic breathing in different positions — twisting, bending, stretching — helping you stay relaxed and present. Whether you're in a yoga pose, flowing through tai chi, or even just stretching at home, using your breath effectively can make movements feel more fluid, efficient, and enjoyable.

Some yoga instructors encourage mouth breathing or loud, forceful breaths, but I'd approach this with caution. It can lead to shallow, upper-chest breathing, which may trigger unnecessary stress. You also miss out on the many benefits of calm, diaphragmatic breathing — like deeper relaxation, better oxygen exchange, and nervous system balance. A little bit of mouth breathing won't do any harm, but ideally, you're mostly doing nasal, slow, quiet breathing in class.

Here are some tips for getting the most out of this practice:

>> **Sync your breath with your movement.** Inhale during expansion or opening movements (for example, lifting your arms or stretching up). Exhale during effort or contraction (for example, bending forward, twisting, or engaging your core). Let your breath guide your movements instead of holding or forcing it.

>> **Practice deep breathing in different positions.** In yoga, try deep diaphragmatic breathing in resting poses like Child's Pose or Savasana. In Pilates or tai chi, focus on "breathing into your back" or expanding your lower ribs. Experiment with conscious deep breathing while twisting, stretching, or balancing.

>> **Use the diaphragm fully.** Inhale slowly, allowing your belly to expand first, then your ribs. Exhale fully, sighing out tension and letting your abdomen gently contract. Avoid shallow chest breathing — keep your breath deep and steady.

>> **Apply deep breathing beyond structured practices.** When doing household chores, inhale as you reach or extend, and exhale as you bend or lift. Try deep breathing while walking or stretching before bed. Use breath awareness to stay relaxed and mindful in everyday movements.

The more you practice diaphragmatic breathing during movement, the more automatic it becomes. Over time, it will help you feel more energized, less fatigued, and more connected to your body — whether you're on the yoga mat or simply going about your day.

Building a daily deep-breathing habit

The ultimate goal is to make diaphragmatic breathing your go-to way of breathing, even when you're not thinking about it. To get there, it helps to set up some daily habits and reminders until it becomes automatic.

Here are a few strategies to weave deep breathing into your routine:

>> **Set aside dedicated time for it.** Consistency is key in forming any habit. Try to practice your diaphragmatic breathing exercises at least once or twice a day, especially in the beginning. Doing it at the same times each day can reinforce the habit. For example, you might do five to ten minutes of deep breathing every morning when you wake up and again at night before you go to sleep. These are naturally peaceful times and can bookend your day with relaxation. Find a peaceful, quiet spot if possible (it helps you focus). Over a few weeks, you'll start to notice you don't have to *force* yourself — you may even look forward to these little breathing sessions as a way to destress.

>> **Attach it to existing habits.** Tie your breathing practice to something you already do daily. For instance, each time you take a work break or during your lunch hour, take two minutes to breathe deeply. Or every time you get into bed, make the first few minutes about deep breathing. Some people tape a little note to their computer screen or set an alarm on their phone that simply

says "Breathe." That cue can snap you out of whatever you were caught up in and remind you to check in with your breath. In the car — perhaps at every red light — you take a couple of nice diaphragmatic breaths (eyes open, of course!). This turns mundane moments into opportunities for relaxation.

>> **Use technology or tools.** There are many breathing apps and even smart-watch reminders nowadays that can guide you through a short breathing exercise. These can be helpful if you like structured guidance.

>> **Incorporate breathing into stress management.** When you notice yourself feeling stressed, anxious, or angry during the day, *deliberately* switch to diaphragmatic breathing. It can help to close your eyes (if appropriate for the situation) and take three slow, deep breaths. This technique can be incredibly effective in moments of tension — it's like pressing a reset button on your mood. The more you do this, the more you'll start automatically taking a deep breath whenever something stressful happens, instead of a shallow gasp or holding your breath. It's a healthy reflex to develop.

>> **Be patient and trust the process.** Don't worry If some days you completely forget to breathe deeply, or if you catch yourself chest breathing when life gets hectic. It's all part of the process. The fact that you're aware of your breathing at all is a big step forward! Over time, as your diaphragm strength-ens and the habit forms, you'll find yourself doing it without consciously choosing to. Many people report that after a few weeks of practice, they suddenly realize while watching TV or walking that "Hey, I'm breathing deeply right now!" — and that's a great feeling.

By regularly stretching and relaxing the areas involved in breathing, you ensure that your diaphragm can move freely. It's similar to how a runner may stretch their legs to run more easily — you're just stretching your breathing apparatus for easier, deeper breaths.

Putting it all together

At this point, you may be thinking, "Breathing is breathing — do I really need to think about it this much?" Consider this: You take tens of thousands of breaths per day. By making those breaths a little deeper and calmer, you're essentially practicing mini relaxation sessions all day long. It can transform your baseline mood and energy levels.

Remember my client, Sarah, whose story I tell earlier in this chapter? When she learned to breathe with her diaphragm, she started integrating it into her daily routine — a few breaths before her stressful team meetings, deep breathing while commuting in traffic, and so on. She found that not only was she less stressed, but she also had more stamina and felt less fatigued in the afternoons. That's the real payoff of diaphragmatic breathing: It's not just an exercise, it's a lifestyle change for healthier breathing.

TIP

Take a moment now as you're reading to notice your breath. Are you breathing through your nose or mouth? Is your belly moving? If not, here's your gentle nudge: Put one hand on your abdomen, relax your shoulders, and take a nice, slow inhale. Let your belly expand, and then exhale slowly, feeling any tension melt away. Feels good, right? Keep that up, and soon, diaphragmatic breathing will be as natural to you as it was when you were a baby.

Chapter **8**

Slow Breathing for Stress Relief

S low breathing is a powerful, portable tool for stress relief, focus, and even heart health that you carry with you everywhere. In this chapter, I share how techniques like Coherent Breathing (my personal go-to for finding calm), Box Breathing (great for staying sharp and cool under pressure), and the 4-7-8 Breathing technique (a handy trick for dozing off to sleep) can help you out.

These exercises are simple and effective, and they can even be fun to practice! By the end of this chapter, you'll see why mastering slower breathing is one of the best ways to keep stress in check and your mind and body in balance.

The Science of Coherent Breathing

Let's start with my favorite breathing exercise of them all: Coherent Breathing. This technique is so powerful that many researchers consider it the "ultimate breath." If there's one breathing exercise that covers all the keys to a healthier, happier, and perhaps even longer life, my recommendation is Coherent Breathing.

Defining Coherent Breathing

The word *coherent* means forming a unified whole. The reason this technique is called Coherent Breathing is because it creates a synchronicity between your lungs, heart, and brain.

Coherent Breathing is all about breathing slowly and steadily at a rhythm your body loves. In practice, it usually means taking around five breaths per minute — much slower than normal breathing. This slow, consistent pace gently nudges your body into a state of balance. Your heart, lungs, and nervous system start to sync up, switching off the "fight-or-flight" alarm and turning on the relaxed "rest-and-digest" mode. In simple terms, Coherent Breathing is like telling your body, "It's okay to chill now," and everything from your heartbeat to your brain waves begins to calm down and cooperate. It's a bit like all the notes from a piece of music come together in harmony.

Coherent Breathing is also called resonance frequency breathing, heart-rate variability (HRV) biofeedback breathing, cardiac coherence breathing, or paced breathing at resonance frequency.

THE AMAZING DISCOVERY OF COHERENT BREATHING

In the early 2000s, Stephen Elliott, an engineer and life scientist, observed that breathing at a rate of approximately five breaths per minute — with equal durations of inhalation and exhalation — could harmonize the autonomic nervous system (see Chapter 2), leading to a state of balance and calm. This breathing pattern, termed *Coherent Breathing,* was detailed in his 2005 publication, *The New Science of Breath,* 2nd Edition (Coherence Publishing). Elliott's work emphasized the role of the diaphragm in promoting optimal circulation and brain function through rhythmic breathing.

Concurrently, Dr. Richard Gevirtz, a clinical psychologist, was exploring heart rate variability (HRV) *biofeedback* (a way of using technology to learn how to control your body's functions, like your heart rate or breathing, by giving you real-time information about what's happening inside).

He found that slow, paced breathing could enhance HRV, indicating improved autonomic balance. Gevirtz's research supported the idea that breathing at a resonant frequency — around five to six breaths per minute — could optimize physiological coherence. This state of physiological coherence means your heart, breath, and nervous system are all working smoothly together, like a well-conducted orchestra. This leads to greater calm, clarity, and resilience.

Interestingly, this optimal breathing rate wasn't a novel discovery. Ancient traditions incorporated similar rhythms into their practices. Studies have shown that Gregorian chants (which were part of the Roman Catholic tradition) and the Ave Maria prayer (a traditional prayer, most often associated with the Catholic Church) naturally induce a breathing rate of approximately six breaths per minute, promoting a meditative state and physiological relaxation. Similarly, yogic practices like pranayama and Bhramari (humming bee breath) often involve slow, rhythmic breathing that aligns with this coherent frequency.

These findings suggest that ancient cultures intuitively recognized the benefits of slow, rhythmic breathing, embedding them into spiritual and meditative practices. The convergence of modern scientific research and ancient wisdom underscores the universality and timelessness of Coherent Breathing patterns.

Adding to this, Dr. Patricia Gerbarg and Dr. Richard Brown, psychiatrists based in New York with whom I have trained, have extensively researched and promoted the therapeutic benefits of breathing techniques. They developed the BREATH-BODY-MIND program (www.breath-body-mind.com), integrating breathwork with movement and meditation to address stress, anxiety, and trauma. Their work emphasizes the power of breath to regulate the nervous system and enhance mental health. Their research has demonstrated that breathing practices can reduce symptoms of stress, anxiety, insomnia, post-traumatic stress disorder (PTSD), and depression. Notably, a study involving Australian Vietnam War veterans found that a breathing-based meditation intervention significantly decreased PTSD symptoms and anxiety with benefits maintained at a six-month follow-up.

Exploring the benefits of Coherent Breathing

Coherent Breathing offers numerous benefits for both physical and mental well-being. Here are seven key benefits, each explained in brief:

» **Reduced stress and anxiety:** Coherent Breathing activates the parasympathetic nervous system (see Chapter 2), moving the body out of the "fight-or-flight" response. This helps quiet the amygdala, which is responsible for emotional responses like fear, promoting a sense of calm and relaxation.

» **Improved cardiovascular function:** This breathing technique has been shown to lower heart rate and blood pressure while increasing HRV. Higher HRV is associated with better cardiovascular health and increased resilience to stress

>> **Enhanced respiratory function:** Coherent Breathing engages the diaphragm, improving overall breathing efficiency and gas exchange. This leads to better oxygenation of the body and can be particularly beneficial for those with respiratory issues.

>> **Improved cognitive function:** By increasing blood flow to the brain, Coherent Breathing can improve focus, clarity, and overall cognitive performance. It helps clear mental fog and enhances attention control.

>> **Reduced symptoms of depression:** Studies have shown that regular practice of Coherent Breathing can lower levels of depression. It helps regulate emotions and creates a greater sense of overall well-being.

>> **Improved sleep quality:** The relaxation response induced by Coherent Breathing can help reduce insomnia and improve overall sleep patterns. It calms racing thoughts that often interfere with both falling asleep and staying asleep.

>> **Increased emotional regulation:** By grounding practitioners in the present moment, Coherent Breathing helps manage challenging emotions. It reduces reactivity and improves the ability to navigate difficult feelings.

Discovering your optimal breathing rate

Your optimal breathing rate is the frequency at which your heart rate and breath synchronize most effectively, maximizing the benefits of Coherent Breathing. At your optimal breathing rate, you'll likely experience the greatest increase in HRV and the most pronounced calming effect.

Everyone has a slightly different "sweet spot" for Coherent Breathing because everyone's body is slightly different. The optimal rate is typically between four and a half to seven breaths per minute for most adults, but this can vary based on factors such as age, height, fitness level, and overall health.

Here's how to find out the right Coherent Breathing rate for you:

1. **Try breathing in for five seconds and out for five seconds (about six breaths per minute).**

   This is a common starting pace for Coherent Breathing.

2. **Notice how this rate feels.**

   If five-second breaths feel *too slow* (causing discomfort or dizziness), shorten your inhale and exhale to four seconds each. If five-second breaths feel *too fast* (you think you could breathe even more slowly comfortably), lengthen each breath to six seconds.

3. **Adjust the inhale/exhale length up or down by a second until the breathing feels *calming and unforced.***

    The goal is a pace where you're breathing deeply and slowly without straining. When you find a rhythm that makes you feel relaxed and centered (usually around four to six breaths per minute for most people), you've found your optimal rate.

Beginners often find a faster breathing rate easier. And over time, as they get used to it, it tends to slow down. So, don't force yourself too much — that'll just make you more stressed rather than calm. Over time, your breathing rate will slow to around five breaths a minute.

Using technology to track progress

If you're into gadgets, there are apps and devices that can help you monitor your breathing progress. Many smartphone apps provide a visual or audio guide (for example, a little circle expanding and contracting to coach your inhale and exhale), and some even give you a "calm score" based on your heart rate or HRV.

There are also HRV trackers and smartwatches that show how your heart rate steadies or your HRV improves as you practice Coherent Breathing. These tools can be fun and motivating, but they're totally optional — the real proof lies in how calm and focused you feel after a good breathing session.

A basic smartphone app to start with is Paced Breathing (`https://paced breathing.app`) or Breathing Zone (`https://breathing.zone`). These apps are quite easy to use, and you can set a specific breathing rate and see how it feels; then adjust accordingly.

Practicing Coherent Breathing

That's enough talk about Coherent Breathing. It's time to have a go! Follow these steps to do it effectively, or listen to Track 15:

1. **Sit in a comfortable position; relax your shoulders and unclench your jaw.**

    You can close your eyes if that helps you focus. Rest your tongue on the roof of your mouth, just behind your front teeth.

2. **Breathe in gently through your nose for about five seconds (count slowly in your head or use an app).**

Let your belly expand as you inhale, drawing air deep into your lungs. Gentle is the key — no need to draw a big breath in. Keep your shoulders down as you breathe in.

3. **Breathe out through your nose for about five seconds.**

   Feel your belly fall as the air leaves. Try to make your exhale just as smooth and steady as your inhale.

4. **Continue to inhale and exhale at this slow, even pace (about five seconds in, five seconds out).**

   Don't pause between breaths — one breath flows right into the next. If five seconds is your optimal count (or whatever count you found works best for you), stick to that timing consistently.

5. **Pay attention to the sensation of breathing — the feeling of air entering your nose, and your belly rising and falling.**

   If your mind starts to wander (and it might), gently bring your focus back to your breath and counting.

6. **Do this Coherent Breathing for up to five minutes to start with.**

   Within a few minutes, you should start to feel your body relax and your mind calm down. You can practice this a couple of times a day or whenever you need to quickly shift into a more relaxed state.

If you're just starting out, a five-second inhale and five-second exhale may feel a bit too slow — and that's totally normal. Instead, begin with two or three seconds in, and the same out. Keep it easy and comfortable. As your body and breath get used to it, you can gently build up to the five-second rhythm over time.

When doing Coherent Breathing, I like to imagine a sine wave, which is a smooth wave going up and down, like in Figure 8-1. The vertical axis represents the expansion and contraction of the lungs as you breathe in and out. The horizontal axis represents time passing. When I breathe in, I imagine smoothly breathing up to the top of the wave, and when breathing out, I imagine breathing out smoothly to the bottom of the wave. This makes your breath smooth and enhances the effect. Also, there's no need to take big breaths — just gentle nasal breaths in and out is the key.

Consistency helps — the more you practice Coherent Breathing, the quicker your body will respond to it. Over time, you'll notice you can enter a calm, focused state on demand just by controlling your breath.

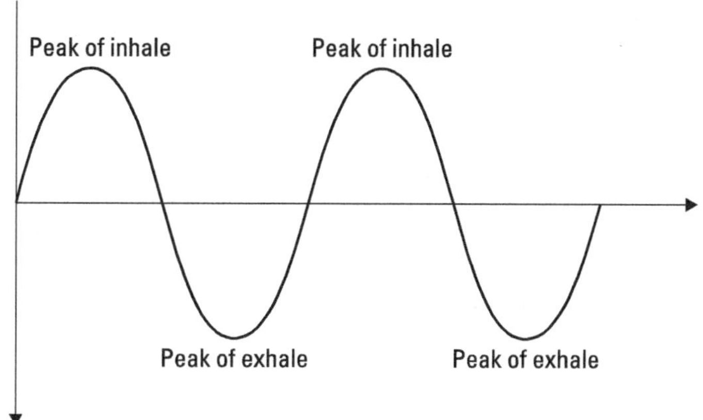

FIGURE 8-1: Imagine Coherent Breathing like a smooth sine wave.

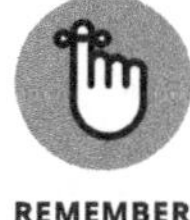

REMEMBER

You can practice Coherent Breathing anytime, anywhere. On the bus, on the train, standing in line, or between sips of tea or coffee. For maximum benefit, practice up to 20 minutes twice a day. Some people find Coherent Breathing to be a life-changing discipline in their life. But if 20 minutes isn't manageable, even 5 minutes a day will start to make a noticeable difference after a couple of weeks.

Using Box Breathing for Calm and Focus

They say it's good to think outside the box. Well, when it comes to breathing, you may want to try breathing *in* the box. In this section, I introduce the Box Breathing technique.

Defining Box Breathing

Box Breathing is a quick, go-anywhere technique that can bring you back to center when stress strikes. It's called Box Breathing because it has four equal parts (like the four sides of a square; see Figure 8-2). The pattern is simple: Inhale for a count of four, hold your breath for a count of four, exhale for four, and hold again for four. This creates a steady, rhythmic breathing cycle that helps reset your body and mind.

By making your breath slow and even, Box Breathing sends a signal to your nervous system that it's time to calm down. At the same time, focusing on the consistent count (1-2-3-4 for each part) clears your head of distractions.

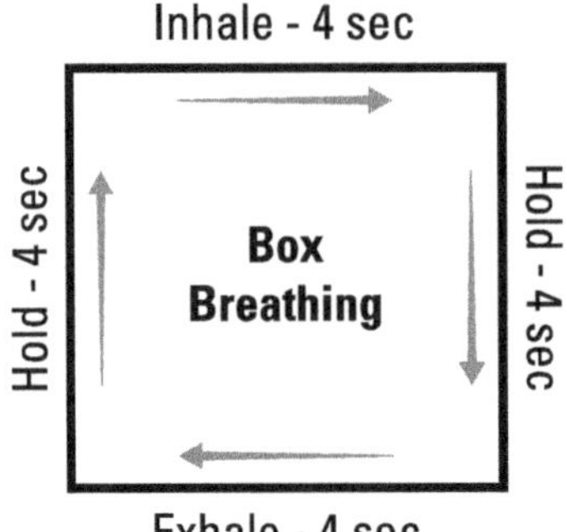

FIGURE 8-2: Box Breathing.

Box Breathing is so effective that people in high-pressure jobs — even Navy SEALs — use Box Breathing to stay calm and alert in tense situations. The good news is that it's extremely easy to learn, so you can use it anytime, anywhere to find a pocket of calm and focus.

Following a step-by-step guide to Box Breathing

PLAY THIS

Give Box Breathing a try with these simple steps or listen to Track 16. If a count of four for each side of the box doesn't feel comfortable, feel free to adjust it. You can make it less or more — whatever feels good is a good sign you're on the right track for you.

1. **Sit up comfortably with your back straight (or stand if you prefer), and relax your shoulders.**

   Soften any tension in the face and jaw if you can. Rest the tip of your tongue gently on the roof of your mouth, just behind your front teeth.

2. **Take a normal exhale to start, emptying your lungs gently.**

3. **Breathe in slowly through your nose while counting to four in your mind.**

   Feel your lungs filling up. Breathe deeply and slowly, using your diaphragm. Your shoulders should stay down, and your upper chest shouldn't need to move.

4. **Keep your lungs full and hold your breath for a count of four.**

   Try to stay relaxed during the hold. Avoid tensing your shoulders or face.

5. **Breathe out slowly through your nose for a count of four.**

   Let the air out in a controlled, steady stream.

6. **With your lungs now empty, hold your breath for another count of four.**

7. **Repeat the cycle.**

Continue this pattern for a few minutes or until you feel calmer and more focused. Even doing it for one minute (about four or five rounds) can make a difference.

Another variation of this exercise is to breathe out with pursed lips rather than your nose. A little reminder: *Pursed lips* mean breathing through your mouth as if breathing through a straw. Either way is good for you.

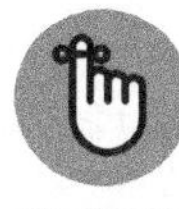

Note, I say a count of four, which is not necessarily four seconds for you. If four seconds for each side of the box feels uncomfortable, adjust to three or two seconds for each side. Start with what feels good, and you'll feel some benefits. If you feel good, you'll make rapid progress and feel better and better as you do more of the breathwork exercises — a positive spiral of well-being.

It may help to visualize moving along the four sides of a square as you breathe — imagine drawing a line for four seconds as you inhale, turning a corner as you hold, drawing the next side as you exhale, and so on (refer to Figure 8-2).

Appreciating the benefits of Box Breathing

Box Breathing packs a lot of benefits into a short exercise. Here are a few perks, delivered in just a minute or two of practice:

>> **It calms your nerves quickly.** The slow, deliberate breathing pattern activates your body's relaxation response. Your heart rate can slow down and blood pressure can drop within a few cycles, melting away feelings of stress or panic.

>> **It improves focus and clarity.** By concentrating on the counting and the rhythm of your breath, you push aside distractions and racing thoughts. This leaves you feeling clearheaded and centered, ready to tackle whatever is in front of you.

>> **It provides on-the-spot stress relief.** Box Breathing is easy to do anytime, even in the middle of a busy day. Whether you're in a meeting, stuck in traffic, or about to give a presentation, a minute of Box Breathing can steady your nerves without anyone noticing you're doing an exercise.

Avoiding common pitfalls

Although Box Breathing is simple, a few common mistakes can trip you up. Here are some pitfalls to watch out for and how to fix them:

>> **Overdoing the breath (too fast or too deep):** Breathing too quickly or taking giant gulps of air can make you lightheaded. Slow down your count and take normal, gentle breaths. The goal is a *comfortable* four count, not a race or a huge inhale.

>> **Struggling with the hold:** If holding your breath for four seconds makes you anxious or uncomfortable, you're not alone. Try a shorter hold (start with two or three seconds) and gradually increase it as you get more used to the feeling. Also, remember to stay relaxed during the hold — no need to clamp down or tighten up.

>> **Tensing up your body:** Sometimes people inadvertently raise their shoulders, clench their jaw, or tense their muscles while focusing on the breathing. Check in with your body. Make a conscious effort to relax your shoulders and jaw. You want to be calm and loose, not stiff, as you breathe.

>> **Losing count or concentration:** It's easy for the mind to wander, and suddenly you forget where you are in the cycle. If you lose track, no worries — just start the next inhale at one and continue. You can also visualize a box or square in your mind and "trace" its sides with each phase to help you keep the pattern.

If you prefer, use an app to help you time the four counts.

Adapting Box Breathing for various needs

One great thing about Box Breathing is its versatility. Everywhere you go, you can tweak or apply it in different ways depending on what you need in the moment:

>> **For better sleep:** Use Box Breathing as a wind-down exercise at bedtime. Do it while lying in bed, with your eyes closed. Slow down the four count a little and keep the breathing gentle. After a few cycles, you may find your whole body relaxing and your mind ready to drift into sleep. (See Chapter 13 for more tips on sleep and breathing.)

>> **For sports or exercise:** Before a big game or race, or even during a break in your workout, Box Breathing can help control jitters and center your focus. It steadies your breathing and heart rate so you stay calm yet alert. Athletes sometimes do a quick one or two minutes of Box Breathing to get in the zone and reduce tension. (See Chapter 16 for more tips for breathing in sports.)

>> **For high-stress moments:** Whenever you feel panic, anger, or overwhelm rising (say, during a heated meeting or after receiving bad news), excuse yourself for a minute and practice Box Breathing. It will help interrupt the stress response, giving you a moment to reset. After a minute of breathing, you'll likely find you can think more clearly and respond more calmly to the situation. (See Chapter 8 for more tips on breathing for stress relief.)

REMEMBER

You can adjust the basic timing however you want. The key is the controlled rhythm. Whether you use Box Breathing to fall asleep, pump the brakes on anxiety, or prepare for a big moment, it's a reliable all-purpose tool for finding calm and focus on demand.

Breathing Like a Calm Sea: Ocean Breath (Ujjayi Breath)

Ocean Breath, or Ujjayi (which means "victorious" in yoga) is a slow, steady nasal breath with a slight constriction in the throat, creating a soft whispering or ocean-like sound as you breathe. The key point is, it's not a loud gasp or wheeze. You'll feel the breath gently brushing the back of your throat, and the sound gives your mind something soothing to focus on. Ocean Breath is often used in yoga and meditation, but you don't need a mat to try it — just a moment and a bit of curiosity. Ocean Breath is another one of my favorites — I'm doing it right now in a cafe. No weird looks so far . . . apart from the usual ones when I order a decaf oat milk latte with extra mindfulness.

TRY THIS

The tricky part for most people is constricting the throat in the right way. Here's an easy way to learn how to gently constrict your throat to create that soft ocean-like sound:

1. **With your mouth open, take a long, slow breath *out* through your mouth as if you're trying to fog up a mirror — "Haaaah."**

    This should make a soft whispering sound in the back of your throat. That's the feeling you're aiming for.

2. **Still with your mouth open, breathe in as if you're *sucking fog* back in from the mirror.**

    Again, feel that slight constriction in the throat. It should create a soft, breathy sound without strain.

3. **Repeat Steps 1 and 2 a few times till you feel you've got the hang of it.**

4. **Now, gently close your mouth and breathe in and out through your nose, keeping the same feeling of slight throat constriction.**

    You should still hear a soft, wave-like sound — like a seashell held to your ear.

    Keep it light and steady. The sound should be gentle and consistent on both the inhale and exhale. If it feels rough or forced, relax your throat a little. It's a whisper, not a wheeze. Others around you shouldn't be able to hear you.

Now that you know how to constrict your throat in the right way, you can do Ocean Breath. Follow these steps or listen to Track 17:

1. **Sit comfortably and close your eyes or lower your gaze. Relax your jaw and shoulders. Rest the tip of your tongue on the roof of your mouth, behind the front teeth.**

2. **Breathe in slowly through your nose, slightly constricting the back of your throat.**

    You'll hear a faint whispering sound. Keep your shoulders down as you breathe in. Breathe gently down into your belly.

3. **Breathe out through your nose, keeping the same gentle constriction in your throat.**

    Let the exhale be steady, slow, and smooth — again, with that gentle ocean wave sound.

4. **Continue breathing like this for a few minutes.**

    Keep your attention on the sound and sensation of your breath. If your mind wanders, just return to the rhythm, like returning to the shore.

The soft, audible breath acts like a mini metronome for your mind, especially useful when you're feeling distracted or anxious. It's also incredibly soothing for the nervous system.

Like Coherent Breathing, Ocean Breath naturally slows down your breath rate, often to five or six breaths per minute, helping you tap into the parasympathetic nervous system (your relaxation mode). And because it gently engages your throat muscles, it's thought to stimulate the vagus nerve, which helps calm your heart and mind.

I find Ocean Breath especially helpful when I want to combine breathing with gentle movement (like walking or stretching) or when I want to calm my mind but feel too fidgety to sit completely still. It's subtle, it's simple, and you can do it without drawing any attention in public — unless you start sounding like Darth Vader. Keep it soft!

Mastering the 4-7-8 Breathing Technique for Sleep

Don't worry, 4-7-8 isn't your locker combination — it's a breathing technique. And this is one of the most popular breathing exercises you'll find. It's simple and easy to remember, and it has its roots in ancient yoga practice, popularized by Dr. Andrew Weil.

Defining 4-7-8 Breathing

The numbers stand for the counts: Inhale for four seconds, hold for seven seconds, exhale for eight seconds. This pattern may feel a bit exaggerated, but it's basically a recipe for deep relaxation. In fact, 4-7-8 Breathing is often touted as a "natural tranquilizer" for your nervous system because it can mellow you out quickly. Many people use it as a go-to method for falling asleep faster or calming intense anxiety. In short, it's a simple trick that can tell your body it's time to power down when you're wide-eyed and stressed.

Seeing how 4-7-8 Breathing can help you sleep

How does 4-7-8 Breathing send you off to dreamland? The magic is in the way it influences your physiology. By dramatically slowing down your breathing, this technique prompts your nervous system to switch into chill-out mode. The seven-second breath hold and especially the long eight-second exhale work together to stimulate your *vagus nerve* (a major nerve that tells your body to relax). This causes your heart rate to drop and your blood pressure to go down, basically signaling to your body that it's safe to relax.

Meanwhile, because you're busy counting 4-7-8 in your head, your mind has less room to spiral into anxious or busy thoughts. Altogether, it's a one-two combination of physical *and* mental calm. After a few cycles, you may feel your whole system slowing down, making you drowsy and ready for sleep.

Practicing 4-7-8 Breathing

Here's a quick guide to performing the 4-7-8 Breathing technique correctly. Follow these steps or listen to Track 18:

1. **Sit up with your back straight or lie down if you're doing this in bed; relax your shoulders and let your hands rest at your sides or in your lap.**

2. **Start by exhaling through your mouth, pushing all the air out with a gentle "whoosh."**

   This resets your lungs and prepares you to start the 4-7-8 cycle.

3. **Close your mouth and inhale quietly through your nose for a count of four.**

   Try to fill your belly, rather than your chest, with air. Remember to keep your shoulders down.

4. **Hold your breath for a count of seven.**

   Keep your face and jaw relaxed as you hold. Avoid clenching or tightening up.

5. **Open your mouth and exhale for a count of eight.**

   Make this exhale slow and steady. Imagine you're blowing out through a small straw or trying to make a candle flame flicker, not extinguish. By the end of the eight count, you should have emptied your lungs.

6. **Repeat the cycle.**

   Aim to do four cycles in total when you're just starting out. (Avoid doing many more than four breaths in one session when you're new to this technique — too many in a row may make you lightheaded.) After completing the cycles, return to breathing normally.

If you're using 4-7-8 Breathing to fall asleep, you can do your four cycles and then simply relax and allow yourself to drift off. If you're using it to calm down during the day, four cycles should be enough to noticeably reduce tension. With practice, you can increase to eight cycles or more if needed, but it's usually not necessary to do a lot of repetitions — the calming effect kicks in quickly.

Getting the most out of 4-7-8 Breathing

To get the most out of the 4-7-8 Breathing technique, keep these tips in mind:

>> **Start small.** In the beginning, limit yourself to two to four cycles at a time. It's normal to feel a little lightheaded when you first try extended breathing like this. By keeping the number of breaths low, you give your body a chance to

adjust. You can do another short round later if needed, but avoid turning it into a marathon in one go.

>> **Adjust the timing if needed.** When I say a count of 4-7-8, I mean counts, not necessarily seconds. If holding your breath for seven counts or exhaling for eight feels uncomfortable, try a gentler version like 3-5-6 or even 2-4-4 to begin with. What matters most is keeping the same pattern: Inhale, hold, and exhale, with the exhale being the longest. You can also speed up the counting if that helps. The key is to stay relaxed, not to push yourself. Over time, as your lung capacity and skill grow, you can work your way toward the classic 4-7-8 rhythm.

>> **Focus on a smooth exhale.** The long exhale is key to triggering the relaxation response. Make sure you're really emptying your lungs over the full eight count. You may purse your lips a bit to control the flow of air. Imagine blowing out very slowly to make a small flame flicker — slow and steady wins here. A complete, unhurried exhale helps maximize the calming effect. You can also breathe out of your nose if you prefer.

>> **Practice consistently.** Like any skill, 4-7-8 Breathing gets more effective with practice. Try doing it every night when you get into bed, even if you think you're relaxed. Over time, your body will recognize the 4-7-8 cue and start relaxing faster. You can also use it during the day if you feel stressed — regular practice will make it a reliable tool in your stress-relief toolkit.

>> **Make yourself comfortable.** For best results, do 4-7-8 Breathing in a comfortable, safe setting. If you're aiming to sleep, lying down in a dark, quiet room will enhance the effect. If you're at work or somewhere public and you need to calm down, even doing a few cycles with eyes closed at your desk or in a parked car can help. The more at ease you are, the more you'll get out of the exercise.

By following these tips, you'll master the 4-7-8 Breathing technique more quickly and get maximum benefit from it. Before you know it, you'll be using your breath like a natural tranquilizer to find calm or drift off to sleep whenever you need it. Sweet dreams and happy breathing!

Chapter **9**

Light Breathing for Better Health

Have you ever watched a sleeping baby breathe? Their tiny chests barely move — their breathing is so gentle you may need to look closely to see it at all. Compare that to many adults who heave their chests dramatically, sigh heavily throughout the day, or breathe loudly through their mouths. What if I told you that the baby's way of breathing is actually healthier and something we should all aspire to?

In this chapter, you explore the counterintuitive concept that breathing less can actually deliver more oxygen to your cells, calm your nervous system, and potentially transform your health. You learn practical techniques, including the Buteyko Breathing Method and other light breathing approaches, and discover how to integrate them seamlessly into your daily life for better health, energy, and well-being.

Introducing Breathing Light

The idea of "breathing light" often stops people in their tracks. "Wait a minute," they ask, "aren't we supposed to take deep breaths?" This common reaction highlights how deeply ingrained our misconceptions about breathing have become. But breathing light doesn't mean depriving yourself of oxygen — quite the opposite!

Understanding the concept of breathing light

Breathing light refers to a breathing pattern that:

>> Is gentle and quiet (no audible breathing)

>> Is primarily done through the nose

>> Is relaxed and effortless

>> Involves a smaller volume of air per breath

>> Is done at a comfortable, slower pace

TIP

Think of light breathing as quality over quantity. It's like savoring a small piece of high-quality dark chocolate instead of mindlessly consuming a giant candy bar. Both give you chocolate, but the experience and effects are completely different.

I first encountered the concept of light breathing during a particularly stressful period in my life. As a mindfulness teacher, I was ironically burning myself out while teaching others how to be peaceful! My breathing was rapid and shallow, I suffered from frequent headaches, and sleep didn't feel rejuvenating. A book by breathwork expert Patrick McKeown suggested I look into the Buteyko Breathing Method, and I was skeptical at first — how could breathing light help when I already felt starved for air?

Two weeks after beginning to practice light breathing techniques, my headaches disappeared, my sleep improved dramatically, and I found myself with a level of sustained energy I hadn't experienced for ages! This wasn't just a subjective improvement — my measured breath hold time (a key indicator of breathing efficiency that I explain later in this chapter) had markedly increased.

TRY THIS

Try this light breathing exercise for beginners:

1. Sit upright but relaxed; rest your hands loosely in your lap.

2. Close your mouth, let your tongue rest gently on the roof of your mouth, and breathe only through your nose.

3. Without changing anything, simply observe your breath for a few seconds.

4. **Gradually make each breath a little quieter and a little slower — almost like you're trying not to disturb a sleeping kitten on your lap.**

Breathe so lightly that if you placed a feather under your nose, it wouldn't move! That's the art of light breathing: soft, easy, and calming.

5. **Aim for a tiny feeling of wanting just a *little* more air, but stay completely relaxed.**

If you feel panicky or uncomfortable, you're trying too hard — ease off.

6. **Keep breathing softly and quietly for one minute, imagining your breath as a gentle whisper.**

Doing this one-minute exercise once or twice a day to begin with is a great way to ease yourself into light breathing.

Recognizing the signs that you may be over-breathing

Over-breathing, also known as *hyperventilation*, simply means breathing more air than your body actually needs. Contrary to popular belief, hyperventilation doesn't just mean rapid breathing during a panic attack. *Chronic* (ongoing), subtle hyperventilation can occur even when breathing appears normal but is slightly deeper or faster than physiologically optimal.

It may sound harmless, but consistently over-breathing can negatively impact your health and well-being. Here are some common signs that suggest you may be breathing too heavily or quickly:

>> **You're breathless at rest.** Oddly, breathing too much can make you feel short of breath.

>> **You feel dizzy or lightheaded.** Over-breathing messes with your oxygen and carbon dioxide balance.

>> **You have cold hands and feet.** Too much air narrows blood vessels, cooling your extremities.

>> **You feel more anxiety or panic.** Over-breathing triggers the fight-or-flight alarm.

>> **You're not sleeping well or snoring.** Excess breathing at night disrupts deep sleep.

>> **You frequently sigh or yawn.** This is your body's hint that you're overdoing it on air.

>> **You breathe through your mouth.** Mouth breathing pulls in too much air and dries out your mouth and throat.

>> **You engage in chest breathing.** Fast, shallow breathing feeds the over-breathing cycle.

If these signs sound familiar, don't worry — you're not alone. Many people unknowingly fall into the habit of over-breathing, especially during stressful periods. The good news is, by practicing the techniques in this chapter, you can restore your breathing patterns to a healthier rhythm.

Seeing why modern life leads to over-breathing

I remember teaching a mindfulness course to corporate executives in London. During our first session, in a short, one-minute meditation, I noticed that nearly everyone in the room was breathing primarily into their upper chests, taking rapid, shallow breaths even while sitting still. When I asked how many people were dealing with significant stress, every hand went up. Their breathing patterns were locked in a stress response, even when they were physically safe. By teaching them not only how to breathe more slowly, but also how to breathe lighter, they immediately began to reap the benefits. They now invite me to regularly run a live online breathwork session to help them stay calm, focused, resilient, and creative. By following the exercises in this chapter, you can reap these same benefits within weeks, if not sooner.

You may be thinking, "Our ancestors didn't need breathing classes. Why do many of us unconsciously fall into over-breathing today?" Several aspects of modern life contribute to this epidemic:

>> **Cultural advice:** "Take a deep breath!" can actually make breathing worse if done forcefully.

>> **Chronic stress:** Ongoing stress keeps people stuck in fast, shallow breathing mode.

>> **Ultra-processed foods:** A junky diet can mess with blood chemistry and breathing.

>> **Soft foods:** Eating mostly soft foods weakens the jaw, leading to mouth breathing.

>> **Sedentary lifestyle:** Lack of movement means less healthy, natural breathing.

>> **Poor indoor air:** Stale or polluted air indoors can mess with breathing patterns.

>> **Mouth breathing:** Breathing through your mouth skips the nose's natural filtration system and encourages over-breathing.

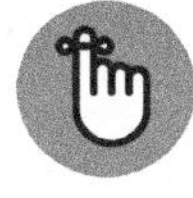

Deep breath doesn't mean *big* breath — it means to breathe using your diaphragm.

Many people today have developed a habit of chronically taking in more air than their bodies actually need, breathing through their mouths, using the upper-chest muscles rather than the diaphragm, and breathing faster than optimal for health.

Understanding the science behind light breathing and carbon dioxide tolerance

Most people think carbon dioxide is just waste we need to get rid of. But it's actually like a traffic controller for your oxygen delivery system.

Imagine oxygen molecules are passengers on a bus (your red blood cells). Carbon dioxide acts like the bus driver's signal to stop and let passengers off. Without enough carbon dioxide, the buses just keep driving — and the oxygen stays stuck, instead of getting into your brain, muscles, and organs where it's needed.

Carbon dioxide also does other important jobs:

>> It keeps your blood's pH in balance — too little can make you unwell.

>> It helps blood vessels stay open so oxygen-rich blood can flow freely.

>> It calms your nervous system and helps you feel relaxed and alert.

When you over-breathe, even a little, you blow away too much carbon dioxide, which causes a state called *hypocapnia* (low carbon dioxide), in which your blood may *look* full of oxygen but your cells are still waiting at the bus stop, feeling stranded!

By breathing lightly, you keep just the right amount of carbon dioxide in your system — so the oxygen buses can stop where they're supposed to, and your body and brain can thrive.

Dr. Konstantin Buteyko observed this paradox in his clinical work. While monitoring terminally ill patients, he noticed that their breathing became heavier as their condition worsened. This led him to question the relationship between breathing patterns and health.

The Control Pause test, a cornerstone of the Buteyko Breathing Method, is a simple way to assess your current carbon dioxide tolerance. Here's how to perform it:

1. **Sit comfortably with your back straight.**

2. **Take a minute or so to simply breathe at your natural pace, allowing your body to settle into a restful state**

3. **After a normal exhale (not forced), gently pinch your nose closed.**

4. **Time how many seconds you can comfortably hold your breath until you feel the first definite desire to breathe.**

   You may sense a slight movement of your diaphragm or an urge to swallow.

5. **Resume normal breathing immediately after the test — don't take a big breath.**

If, after holding your breath, you need to gasp for air, you held your breath for too long. You should be able to breathe at a normal pace after the breath hold. That is the length of the Control Pause. It's not an exact number, but it gives you a rough idea.

According to Buteyko practitioners, here's what the length of your Control Pause means:

Length	Indicates
Less than 15 seconds	Poor
15 to 20 seconds	Room for improvement
21 to 40 seconds	Good
More than 40 seconds	Great

If your score was less than 20 seconds, don't worry. That's very common for beginners. Over time and using the exercises in this chapter, your score will slowly improve.

According to the Buteyko Breathing Method, a Control Pause of less than 20 seconds suggests you're likely breathing from your upper chest, breathing too fast, and taking in more air than needed. This can lead to symptoms like a blocked nose, snoring, insomnia, fatigue, coughing, wheezing, breathlessness, and even exercise-induced asthma. If your Control Pause is above 20 seconds, most symptoms usually begin to improve. The good news? Every five-second increase in your Control Pause usually comes with noticeable improvements in how you feel.

This test measures your body's sensitivity to carbon dioxide buildup. The longer your comfortable breath hold, the better your carbon dioxide tolerance, which generally correlates with more efficient breathing and better health outcomes.

Light breathing techniques gradually and safely increase your body's tolerance to carbon dioxide, restoring a healthier breathing pattern and improving oxygen delivery throughout your body. It's not about forcing yourself to breathe less, but rather retraining your respiratory center in the brain to accept slightly higher carbon dioxide levels as normal.

Appreciating the Benefits of Breathing Less

One of the most counterintuitive benefits of breathing less is that it can actually improve oxygen delivery to your tissues. This seeming paradox is explained by a phenomenon known as the *Bohr effect*, named after the Danish physiologist, Christian Bohr, who discovered it in 1904.

Improving oxygen efficiency and delivery

Think of it like this: Hemoglobin is like a bus carrying oxygen (passengers), and carbon dioxide is like the signal that tells the bus to stop and let the passengers off. If there isn't enough carbon dioxide, the bus keeps driving, and the passengers (oxygen) stay stuck on board instead of getting to their destinations (tissues).

Even with normal oxygen saturation levels of 95 percent to 99 percent in your blood, if you're over-breathing and have low carbon dioxide levels, much of that oxygen remains bound to hemoglobin and isn't released to your tissues. This condition, where there's plenty of oxygen in the blood but not enough reaching the tissues, is called *tissue hypoxia despite normal blood oxygen levels.*

The benefits of improved oxygen delivery include the following:

>> Enhanced cellular energy production

>> Better brain function and mental clarity

>> Improved physical endurance and recovery

>> Support for all energy-dependent healing processes

>> Reduced fatigue and brain fog

When I first started practicing light breathing techniques, one of the first changes I noticed was a marked decrease in afternoon energy slumps and a better ability to stay calm and focused. I'd previously combated these energy slumps with coffee or mindfulness meditation. But with light breathing, my focus improved significantly, and I found myself thinking more clearly throughout the day.

Activating the relaxation response

When you practice light breathing properly, you'll start to notice several positive changes in your body — gentle signals that your system is shifting into a healthier, more balanced state.

Your hands and feet may begin to feel warmer as your blood circulation improves. You may notice an increase in saliva in your mouth, a classic sign that the parasympathetic ("rest-and-digest") branch of your autonomic nervous system is kicking in. Your eyes may become slightly more moist or watery — another indicator of relaxation. Most importantly, you'll likely feel calmer and more relaxed, and a sense of general well-being may gently fill you, like the warmth of sunlight through a window.

These changes can be subtle at first, so stay curious and patient. Keep an eye out for them as signs that you're on the right track.

This is all because your breathing pattern directly influences your nervous system state. Heavy, upper-chest breathing activates the sympathetic ("fight-or-flight") branch of your autonomic nervous system, while light, diaphragmatic breathing triggers the parasympathetic ("rest-and-digest") response.

When you breathe lightly, several calming mechanisms activate:

>> The vagus nerve (a key component of the parasympathetic nervous system) is stimulated.

>> Stress hormones like cortisol and adrenaline decrease.

>> Heart rate variability, or HRV (a measure of autonomic nervous system balance), improves.

>> Blood pressure tends to normalize.

>> Digestive function improves.

>> Immune system function is enhanced.

I observed this dramatically when working with a client who suffered from panic attacks. She had been taught traditional deep breathing techniques that actually

made her symptoms worse. When we switched to light breathing approaches —
focusing on gentle, slow exhalations through the nose — her panic attacks
decreased in both frequency and intensity within just a few weeks. We had to go
very gradually and slowly, but she noticed the benefits almost immediately.

If you ever feel anxious, resist the urge to take big breaths. Instead, focus on
extending your exhale and making your breathing gentler and quieter. This sends
powerful calming signals to your brain. Slow and steady is the key.

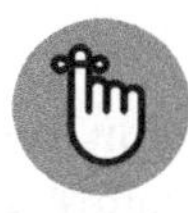

The relaxation benefits of light breathing extend beyond the immediate physiological effects. As you develop a habit of breathing lightly, you're essentially
retraining your nervous system to maintain a calmer baseline state, making you
more resilient to stress triggers and less prone to anxiety.

Boosting mental clarity, emotional calm, and physical endurance

The benefits of light breathing extend across all dimensions of human experience —
mental, emotional, and physical.

Mental benefits

Light breathing optimizes blood flow and oxygen delivery to the brain, supporting
cognitive function. Many practitioners report

>> Improved concentration and focus

>> Enhanced memory

>> Clearer thinking and decision-making

>> Reduced brain fog

>> Better creative problem-solving abilities

The connection between breathing and mental clarity makes perfect sense when
you consider that your brain, while comprising only about 2 percent of your body
weight, consumes roughly 20 percent of your body's oxygen supply.

Emotional benefits

Our breathing patterns and emotional states are intimately connected in a two-
way relationship. Just as emotions affect breathing (notice how your breathing
changes when you're angry versus content), breathing patterns influence emotions.

Light breathing helps

>> Reduce anxiety and stress responses

>> Improve emotional regulation

>> Decrease reactivity to triggers

>> Enhance overall mood and sense of well-being

>> Support sleep quality, which further stabilizes emotions

WARNING

Breathing techniques can significantly help with emotional regulation, but they are *not* a replacement for professional mental health treatment if you're dealing with clinical depression, severe anxiety disorders, or other serious mental health conditions. Breathing practices are a complementary approach to appropriate professional help.

Physical benefits

Athletes and fitness enthusiasts are increasingly turning to light breathing techniques to improve performance and recovery. Benefits include

>> Increased exercise endurance

>> More efficient oxygen utilization during activity

>> Quicker recovery between exercise sets or training sessions

>> Reduced exercise-induced asthma symptoms

>> Better sleep quality, supporting physical recovery

>> Enhanced overall energy levels

I was amazed at the impact on my own brisk walking ability after several months of consistent light breathing practice. Not only could I walk farther with less perceived effort, but the post-walk fatigue I used to experience virtually disappeared. The key was learning to maintain nasal breathing even during brisk walking, which initially required slowing down but ultimately led to better performance. I also had to take some tissues with me as I got a runny nose when I started to do nasal breathing while briskly walking. Keep practicing, and it'll get easier with time. The more you use your nose, the easier it'll get and the healthier you'll become.

Practicing Breathing Light

The Buteyko Breathing Method, developed by Dr. Konstantin Buteyko in the 1950s, offers a systematic approach to retraining your breathing pattern. At its core, the method involves a series of exercises designed to gradually reduce breathing volume while increasing carbon dioxide tolerance.

The Buteyko Breathing Method: Gentle breath reduction for health

The Buteyko Breathing Method is based on a simple but powerful idea: Many modern breathing habits — like breathing through the mouth, breathing heavily, and taking in more air than needed — can actually harm our health.

The method teaches you to breathe mainly through your nose, breathe lightly and quietly, and reduce the volume of each breath, creating a gentle feeling of air hunger.

This approach helps restore the natural levels of carbon dioxide in the body. Carbon dioxide is a key player in getting oxygen from your blood into your tissues, keeping your blood vessels open, and calming your nervous system.

The Buteyko Breathing Method first emerged in the 1950s and has since helped thousands of people around the world improve asthma symptoms, sleep quality, anxiety, blood pressure, and even exercise performance. Instead of focusing on big breaths, Buteyko breathing retrains your body to breathe in a way that's more efficient, more natural, and ultimately, more healing.

Today, Buteyko techniques are used by everyone from elite athletes to people simply wanting better everyday energy and resilience — all by learning to breathe just a little bit less.

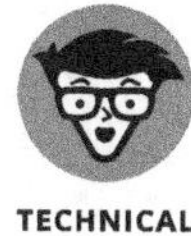

TECHNICAL STUFF

Studies suggest potential benefits of the method in asthma management, but it's important to note that the technique is considered a complementary approach. The medical community acknowledges the need for further high-quality, large-scale studies to conclusively determine its efficacy and understand the underlying mechanisms. Patients interested in the Buteyko Breathing Method should consult healthcare professionals to ensure it complements their existing treatment plans.

THE SURPRISING STORY BEHIND THE BUTEYKO BREATHING METHOD

In the 1950s, a young Ukrainian doctor named Konstantin Buteyko faced a terrifying diagnosis: severe high blood pressure and not much hope of improvement. Told he had only a short time to live, Buteyko did something unusual: He turned his attention inward and began observing his own breathing.

He noticed something strange: Whenever his symptoms worsened, his breathing became heavier and louder. Curious, he tried an experiment — he deliberately slowed and softened his breath. Almost immediately, he felt a little better.

Intrigued, Buteyko spent years studying patients in hospitals. Again and again, he found that people who were the sickest often breathed the heaviest. He came to a radical conclusion: Over-breathing — taking in more air than the body needs — was making people sicker, not healthier.

From this, the Buteyko Breathing Method was born:

- Breathe through your nose, not your mouth.

- Breathe less air, not more.

- Keep your breathing soft, slow, and silent.

By teaching people to retrain their breathing patterns, Buteyko helped thousands improve their health, from reducing asthma attacks to calming anxiety.

Although his ideas were controversial at the time, today the Buteyko Breathing Method is recognized around the world — and continues to change lives, one lighter breath at a time.

Even King Charles III turned to the Buteyko Breathing Method! In 1999, Dr. Buteyko and his wife, Ludmila, were invited to meet Charles. Then Prince Charles was struggling with severe allergies — especially to horses and ceremonial uniforms (not ideal when you're expected to attend parades!). By teaching Charles how to gently reduce his breathing volume, Dr. Buteyko was able to help ease his symptoms.

A basic Buteyko reduced-breathing exercise

This fundamental exercise trains your body to comfortably accept slightly higher carbon dioxide levels. Follow these steps to practice it, or listen to Track 19:

1. **Sit comfortably with your back straight but not rigid.**

2. **Observe your normal breathing for about a minute.**

3. **Gradually reduce the volume of each breath by approximately 20 percent to 30 percent.**

   Make your breathing quieter. Use less effort. Focus on relaxing your breathing muscles. Try to create a slight but comfortable level of air hunger.

4. **Maintain this reduced breathing for three to five minutes.**

   If you feel significant discomfort, ease back to a more comfortable level.

Practice two to three times per day, gradually increasing the duration or frequency as comfortable.

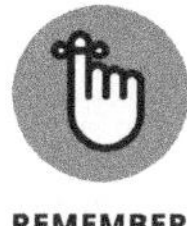

The goal is gentle reduction, not strain. You should feel a slight air hunger (like when you've climbed a flight of stairs), but never gasping or significant discomfort. If you overdo it, you'll stress yourself, reduce your progress, and feel uncomfortable. Take it easy, but ensure you have a slight sense of air hunger.

Light Slow Deep Breathing

This is one of my favorite breathing exercises. Light Slow Deep (LSD) Breathing is about breathing so gently and quietly that it's almost as if you're not breathing at all. You're helping your body relax, improving oxygen delivery, and restoring calm — without needing any fancy gadgets or apps.

LSD Breathing is a term first coined by Patrick McKeown, one of the world's leading teachers of the Buteyko Breathing Method.

Follow these steps to do Light Slow Deep Breathing or listen to Track 20:

1. **Sit comfortably and relax.**

   Find a quiet spot where you can sit upright yet relaxed — shoulders soft, face relaxed, and hands resting loosely in your lap. Imagine you're sitting on a beach chair, just watching the waves.

2. **Close your mouth gently and breathe only through your nose.**

   Nose breathing warms, filters, and humidifies the air, making it easier on your lungs and helping you breathe naturally slower and lighter.

3. **Gently soften your breathing.**

   Imagine you're breathing in just enough air to barely feel it. If someone placed a feather under your nose, it would hardly move. You may notice a slight feeling of wanting a little more air — that's okay. Stay comfortable. If you feel breathless or stressed, lighten even more.

4. **Allow your breath to naturally slow down.**

   Lengthen the pauses between breaths slightly — no forcing, no straining. Think of each breath as a slow tide coming in and out. If it helps, you can mentally count, breathing in for about five seconds, breathing out for about five seconds — but don't worry about getting it perfect. Breathing at this slower pace supports both your heart and lungs by encouraging *Coherent Breathing* (a rhythm that helps balance your nervous system and improves heart rate variability). (Turn to Chapter 8 for more.)

5. **Without pushing or forcing, encourage the breath to gently move lower into your body — toward your lower ribs or belly area.**

   Imagine your breathing is a gentle wave washing through your whole body, not just your chest. That's diaphragmatic breathing (see Chapter 7).

6. **Practice breathing light, slow, and deep for about five minutes.**

   You're aiming for a feeling of calmness, stillness, and quietness inside — like sitting under a big shady tree on a warm afternoon. You can do this for just 30 seconds, or feel free to extend for as long as it's comfortable for you.

7. **When you finish, allow your breathing to return to its natural rhythm.**

   Take a moment to notice how you feel before moving on with your day.

If you ever feel short of breath or stressed, stop and breathe normally. Think: Less is more. Lighter breathing often feels like you're not doing much — that's the magic.

You can combine this exercise with your daily activities. For example, I'm practicing it right now as I'm writing this sentence.

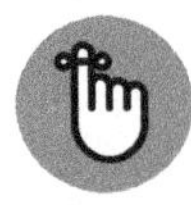

Nasal breathing is key. Keep your mouth closed throughout.

Mini breath holds: Gently training your body to need less air

When you've started breathing more lightly and slowly, the next gentle step is to add short breath holds — just a few seconds — to retrain your body to feel safe with slightly higher levels of carbon dioxide.

This may sound a bit odd at first, but here's the logic: Breath holds create a temporary rise in carbon dioxide, which helps improve your body's tolerance over time. And as your tolerance improves, your breathing naturally becomes lighter, calmer, and more efficient. It's like teaching your body that it doesn't need to overreact to a little air hunger.

Breath holds also help activate the vagus nerve, improve heart-rate variability (HRV), and reduce over-breathing — especially helpful if you experience coughing, wheezing, or anxiety.

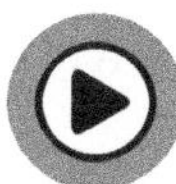

Follow these steps to do mini breath holds, which you can do anytime, or listen to on Track 21:

1. Sit or stand comfortably, with an upright posture and your mouth closed.

2. Breathe quietly through your nose for a few breaths, relaxing your body.

3. After a normal exhale (not a big breath out), gently pinch your nose and hold your breath.

4. Hold for three to five seconds, or until you feel the first small desire to breathe.

5. Release your nose and resume gentle nasal breathing, staying relaxed.

6. Wait about 10 to 15 seconds, and then repeat.

    Repeat three to five times, once or twice a day to start.

The good news is, mini breath holds are generally safe for most people when done correctly. The key is to keep them short and comfortable and always return to gentle nasal breathing straight after the hold.

You can also try this technique while walking. Take a normal breath in and out through your nose, pinch your nose and hold, walk five to ten steps, and then resume nasal breathing.

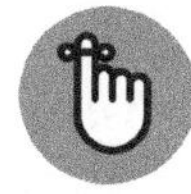

Mini breath holds are especially useful when you're feeling anxious or over-breathing, to reduce coughing or wheezing, or as a gentle warm-up before deeper light breathing exercises. They're also helpful during walking or light activity, and they can be a great quick reset between meetings or screen time. Many Buteyko breathing students use mini breath holds throughout the day, seamlessly integrating them into everyday moments.

Nasal breathing with slow exhales

The nose is designed to be the primary breathing organ for good reason. Nasal breathing has so many benefits (see Chapter 6).

Yet many people habitually breathe through their mouths, especially during sleep, exercise, or when feeling stressed. Retraining yourself to breathe through your nose is a fundamental aspect of light breathing. Your nostrils are much smaller than your mouth, so it makes light breathing much easier.

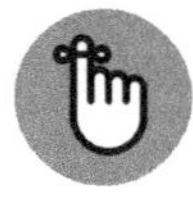

If your nose is blocked, use the nose-unblocking technique in Chapter 6 to unblock your nose.

A particularly effective way to enhance the benefits of nasal breathing is to slightly extend your exhale:

1. **Breathe in normally through your nose for a count of three.**

2. **Exhale slowly through your nose for a count of six.**

   Make the exhale relaxed and gentle (not forced).

3. **Practice for three to five minutes, several times daily.**

If 3-6 doesn't feel comfortable, try 2-4 or 4-8. The aim is to extend the exhale and breathe lightly instead of taking huge breaths in and out.

This extended exhale activates the parasympathetic nervous system even more effectively than equal-length breathing, promoting deeper relaxation and reducing stress hormones.

I discovered the power of this technique when helping a client with insomnia. After trying various approaches, the extended exhale practice — done for just ten minutes before bed — was what finally helped her fall asleep without medication for the first time in years.

If you find nasal breathing difficult due to chronic congestion or anatomical issues, consider consulting an ear, nose, and throat (ENT) specialist. Physical obstructions like a deviated septum or an issue with *turbinates* (small structures in your nose that clean, warm, and humidify the air) may need medical intervention before nasal breathing becomes comfortable. However, I recommend you check the advice given in the book *Breath: The New Science of a Lost Art* by James Nestor (Riverhead Books) before making any decisions around surgery. You want to make sure it'll make things better rather than worse, because you can't reverse surgery.

Silent breathing: Listening to the subtle rhythm of your breath

One of the simplest yet most powerful approaches to light breathing is making your breath completely silent. Audible breathing — whether it's loud inhales, sighing exhales, or the sound of breathing through an open mouth — is often a sign of over-breathing.

Here's how to do silent breathing:

1. **Find a quiet place where you can hear subtle sounds.**

2. **Close your mouth and breathe only through your nose.**

3. **Gradually reduce the volume of your breath until it becomes completely silent.**

   Even when placing your finger near your nostrils, you should feel minimal airflow. Your chest and abdomen should move very little.

4. **Maintain this silent breathing for three to five minutes.**

5. **Notice the calming effect this has on your mind and body.**

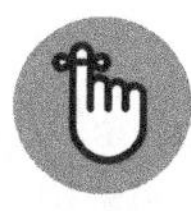

As with all the breathing exercises in this book, just practice for as long as you can manage. If three minutes feels like an eternity, start with three breaths. Baby steps!

Practice regularly throughout the day, especially during transitions between activities.

I often use this practice when traveling or before important presentations. Once, before giving a talk to more than 3,000 people, I found myself in the grips of stage fright. Five minutes of silent breathing in a quiet corner backstage gently shifted my state, allowing me to speak with calm confidence rather than nervous energy.

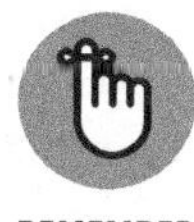

The goal isn't to reduce your breathing to an unhealthy level, but rather to find the natural, efficient rhythm your body actually needs — which is often far less air than we habitually breathe.

Counting breath holds: Training your body to breathe lightly

Controlled breath holds are a powerful way to systematically increase your carbon dioxide tolerance and train your body to breathe more lightly.

TRY THIS

Try the following basic breath retention exercise:

1. **Sit comfortably with good posture.**

2. **Breathe normally for a few moments.**

3. **After a normal exhale (not forced), gently pinch your nose closed.**

4. **Hold your breath until you feel the first distinct desire to breathe (not to your maximum capacity).**

5. **Release and breathe normally (not deeply) for about 30 seconds.**

6. **Repeat three to five times.**

Practice this exercise two or three times daily.

As your carbon dioxide tolerance improves, your comfortable breath hold time will naturally increase. This is a measurable sign of progress.

Box breathing (see Chapter 8) is also a good exercise in light breathing. The empty-lung breath hold (after exhale) is particularly effective for increasing carbon dioxide tolerance. If this is challenging at first, start with shorter holds and gradually extend as comfortable.

WARNING

Never practice breath retention exercises while driving or in situations requiring full attention. Some lightheadedness can occur as your body adjusts to higher carbon dioxide levels. Always practice in a safe environment, preferably seated or lying down.

Incorporating Light Breathing into Daily Life

The true power of light breathing comes when you integrate it into your daily life, not just during dedicated practice sessions.

Breathing light during everyday activities

Here are strategies for maintaining light breathing throughout your day.

Morning reset

Start your day with intentional light breathing:

1. **Upon waking, before getting out of bed, take a moment to notice your breathing.**

2. **If you're breathing through your mouth, gently close it and switch to nasal breathing.**

3. **Take ten gentle, quiet nasal breaths to set the pattern for your day.**

Throughout your morning routine, periodically check in with your breathing and reset to light, nasal breathing if needed.

Breathing checkpoints

Establish regular times to check and reset your breathing:

» Every time you check your phone

» Before meals

» When stopping at traffic lights

» Before entering meetings

» When washing your hands

» When feeling stressed or tired

At each checkpoint, ask yourself: "Am I breathing through my nose? Is my breathing quiet and gentle?" If not, take a moment to reset to light breathing.

I set reminders on my phone that simply say "Breathe light" at various points throughout the day. These mini-interventions take just seconds but help maintain awareness and prevent slipping into dysfunctional breathing patterns during busy or stressful periods.

Environmental cues

Place small reminders in your environment:

» A small sticker on your computer monitor or fridge

» A special bracelet or ring that reminds you of light breathing when you notice it

» A background image on your phone with a breathing reminder

Mealtimes

TRY THIS

Have you ever devoured a meal so quickly that you barely tasted it, only to regret it later with a bloated stomach? Light breathing transforms eating from a rushed necessity into a nourishing ritual. Start with a three-bite reset:

1. **Before your first bite, take three gentle nasal breaths to activate your parasympathetic ("rest-and-digest") mode.**

2. **Sync your chewing with slow exhales — try five chews per exhale.**

   This not only aids digestion but also prevents you from swallowing excess air, a common cause of post-meal discomfort.

3. **After swallowing, exhale fully through your nose before reaching for the next bite.**

   This simple pause prevents overeating and gives your body time to register fullness.

I once coached a client who also suffered from chronic indigestion. By practicing these steps during lunches, her "afternoon food coma" decreased and was replaced by steady energy. "It's like my gut finally learned to keep up with my schedule," she marveled.

TIP

Diaphragmatic breathing during meals massages the stomach and intestines, enhancing enzyme secretion and nutrient absorption. Imagine your breath as a gentle internal masseuse kneading away tension with every exhale! Learn more about diaphragmatic breathing in Chapter 7.

Walking

TRY THIS

Walking doesn't have to leave you huffing like a steam engine. Try the 4-4-4 stride sync:

1. **Inhale nasally for four steps.**

2. **Hold your breath gently for four steps.**

3. **Exhale nasally for four steps.**

Start with short distances — even a few steps counts! If 4-4-4 doesn't work for you, try 3-3-3 or any other similar combination. Starting with what works best for you is better than over-forcing yourself.

On uphill climbs, shorten your exhale ratio to 2:1 (inhale two steps, exhale one step). This maintains light breathing without triggering panic-like gasping.

Working at a desk

Modern workspaces are minefields for breath-holders and screen-starers. Combat this with micro-resets:

>> **Monitoring breath:** Each time you click Send on an email, take two silent nasal breaths.

>> **Chair yoga:** While seated, place your hands on your lower ribs. Inhale, expanding the ribs sideways; exhale, hugging them inward. This desk diaphragm drill combats slouched breathing.

>> **Zoom Zen:** During video calls, discreetly practice tongue-on-palate breathing (in which your tongue is pressed to the roof of your mouth and you take silent nasal breaths). It keeps you calm without audible sighs.

A tech CEO client reported that these techniques cut his afternoon caffeine cravings by half. "My brain fog lifted once I stopped treating my lungs like accordions," he joked.

Using light breathing to manage stress and improve sleep

When stress strikes, ditch the "take a deep breath" cliché. Instead, try Buteyko's Emergency Reset:

1. **Pinch your nose closed after a normal exhale.**

2. **Walk slowly until you feel moderate air hunger.**

3. **Release your nose, and breathe nasally for 30 seconds.**

4. **Repeat three times.**

This controlled *hypoxia* (under-breathing) triggers your body's innate calm response. Research shows that just 90 seconds of this practice lowers spikes of *cortisol* (the stress hormone).

For one of my community members, I suggested this technique while pacing hospital corridors. The rhythmic focus prevented panic from hijacking their decision-making.

If your mind tends to race at night or your body feels too wired to drift off, 7–11 Breathing can help. It's a simple way to activate your body's relaxation response — shifting you out of stress mode and into rest mode. It's easy, soothing, and surprisingly effective. Here's how to do it:

1. **Lie down or recline somewhere comfortable, ideally where you plan to sleep.**

2. **Close your eyes, and if it feels good, place one hand gently on your belly.**

3. **Inhale slowly and quietly through your nose for a count of seven.**

   Try to breathe into your belly so it gently rises.

4. **Exhale even more slowly through your nose or slightly parted lips for a count of 11, letting your body soften as you breathe out.**

5. **Repeat for five to ten rounds, or longer if you like.**

   Don't worry if your mind wanders. Just gently return to the counting and the rhythm of your breath.

Pair it with cool-down tactics:

>> Sleep with your lips lightly sealed, using a special tape if it's safe for you to do so (see Chapter 13 for more information).

>> Place a warm pack on your diaphragm to relax your breathing muscles.

One student reported, "After years of counting sheep, I now count exhales — and rarely reach ten before drifting off."

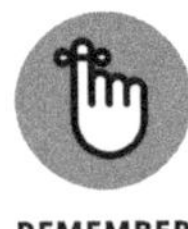

Slow exhales stimulate the vagus nerve, which lowers your heart rate and signals your brain to transition into *delta-wave sleep*, the deepest stage of sleep, marked by slow brain waves called *delta waves*. Delta-wave sleep is when your body repairs, your immune system strengthens, and your brain consolidates memories. Breathing and heart rate slow right down. It's the most restorative sleep you get.

Imagine each exhale as a lullaby for your overactive mind. By weaving light breathing into life's daily rhythms, you transform ordinary moments into opportunities for renewal — one gentle breath at a time.

Making breathing light a lifelong practice

Let's face it — adopting new habits is like trying to teach a cat to fetch. Even the most well-intentioned practitioners (myself included!) stumble when life gets chaotic.

Overcoming challenges and staying consistent

The key to making light breathing second nature lies not in perfection, but in compassionate persistence.

Here are the three big obstacles to light breathing (and how to overcome them):

>> **Forgetting:** This is the most common hurdle. Unlike brushing your teeth, breathing happens automatically, so conscious retraining requires gentle reminders. Early in my practice, I'd often realize mid-lecture that I'd reverted to mouth breathing. My solution? Strategic sticky notes. I placed them on my laptop ("Nose breathing!"), bathroom mirror ("Breathe light!"), and even inside my wallet. Over time, these cues rewired my habits without judgment.

>> **Discomfort:** Mild air hunger can feel unsettling at first. One client described it as "trying to drink a thick milkshake through a tiny straw." This discomfort often arises from years of over-breathing — your body isn't accustomed to optimal carbon dioxide levels.

Start with mini sessions. Even 30 seconds of conscious light breathing while waiting for coffee to brew counts. Try mini breath holds of three to five seconds whenever you remember. Gradually increase duration as your tolerance improves, much like building workout stamina. You'll make progress faster if you don't rush it and overexert yourself.

>> **Time:** Who has 20 minutes daily for breathing exercises? Sound familiar? Here's the secret: Integrate, don't add. Practice light breathing while:

- Walking to your car (nasal breathing with extended exhales; see Chapter 3 for how to do extended exhales)

- Scrolling emails (silent breath awareness; more in Chapter 5)

- Washing dishes (diaphragmatic breathing rhythm; more in Chapter 7)

I once coached a busy corporate leader who mastered light breathing during his taxi commute to work. He learned to fully focus on breathing less each morning and evening. Within weeks, his resting respiratory rate dropped from 18 to 12 breaths per minute according to his smartwatch — all without "finding time." He also found, as I do, that it was easier for him to stay focused on his breath when breathing light, compared to just doing mindfulness breathing.

Tracking progress and celebrating milestones

What gets measured gets mastered. But forget complex spreadsheets — effective tracking should feel rewarding, not burdensome.

Relapses are inevitable. After contracting COVID-19, my measured Control Pause plummeted from 25 to 15 seconds. Instead of berating myself, I applied this 3R framework:

- **Recognize** the lapse without judgment.

- **Reset** with one minute of nasal breathing.

- **Recommit** to the next actionable step.

This compassionate approach reduced my recovery time by half compared to previous setbacks. Before long, I started to increase my control pause and my COVID symptoms reduced, too. The secret was to listen to how my body was feeling and go gently instead of using too much force.

Try recording this information each day:

>> Date

>> Length of Control Pause in seconds

>> Which Buteyko exercise you did and how many times a day

A student of mine created a "breathing win" jar. Each time she noticed improved stress resilience, she dropped in a marble. Within six months, the jar overflowed, visually reinforcing her progress.

Combining breathing light with other mindfulness practices

Light breathing isn't a solo act — it's the rhythm section of your mindfulness orchestra. When harmonized with other practices, it amplifies their benefits exponentially. For example:

>> **Yoga:** During sun salutations, inhale nasally while reaching upward, and exhale slowly during forward folds.

>> **Meditation:** Settle into your favorite meditation posture. Perform three cycles of 2-4 Breathing (a two-count inhale, and a four-count exhale). Let your breath return to its natural light rhythm. Observe sensations without manipulation. This light breathing can become part of your meditation practice.

>> One corporate team using this method reduced its perceived stress scores in eight weeks.

>> **Mindful eating:** At your next meal, pause for three light breaths before the first bite. Chew rhythmically with nasal breathing. Exhale fully between bites.

Not only did this technique slow my rushed lunches, but my digestion improved markedly.

BREATH TRAINING DEVICES: SMALL TOOLS, BIG BENEFITS

If you want to breathe better, feel calmer, and boost your energy, breath training devices are worth a try. These small tools add gentle resistance to your breathing, helping you slow down, breathe deeper, and strengthen your diaphragm. They look a bit like a whistle. The idea is you breathe in lightly through your nose and breathe out through the device, which has some resistance to help slow down and lighten your breathing.

One popular option is the Relaxator, developed by breathwork expert Anders Olsson. I tried it out at a conference Olsson organized. You breathe out through it, adjusting the resistance to train relaxed, rhythmic breathing. He says just 15 minutes a day can help reduce stress, improve focus, cut cravings, and support fat burning. Some people love using the device and find it a great way to train themselves to breathe slowly and lightly. (You can check it out at www.consciousbreathing.com/products/relaxator.)

There are other devices like this on the market, too. These devices are like mini gyms for your lungs — easy to use, portable, and surprisingly effective.

3

Breathing for Physical and Mental Health

Here you explore how breathing can support both your physical and mental well-being. You start by finding out how breath helps you navigate stress, anxiety, and emotional challenges. Practical exercises guide you in using breath to manage panic attacks, anger, and even trauma, while enhancing emotional intelligence and relaxation.

Next, you discover how breathing improves physical health, from strengthening your lungs and boosting circulation to easing pain and aiding digestion. You discover specific techniques to manage conditions like asthma, high blood pressure, and long COVID, as well as how breath can support recovery and overall well-being.

This part also introduces dynamic breathing techniques for those looking to boost energy. You explore how to stay energized throughout the day while balancing stress and avoiding burnout, with practical guidance on safely practicing energizing breathwork.

Improving sleep is another key focus, with breathing exercises designed to help you fall asleep faster and stay asleep longer. You'll find out how to establish a presleep breathing routine, correct common breathing mistakes that disrupt rest, and use breathwork to manage sleep apnea and nighttime awakenings.

Finally, I introduce you to breathwork for children, making breathing fun and accessible for all ages. I offer simple exercises to help kids with focus, relaxation, and emotional regulation, along with creative ways to integrate breathwork into daily routines, from bedtime to school stress.

Chapter **10**

Stress, Anxiety, and Mental Health

n a world where stress seems to come with your morning coffee and anxiety comes with every deadline, your breath may just be your most underrated superpower. Before I dive into the transformative breathing techniques in this chapter, here's the good news: You already have everything you need. No fancy equipment required — just the breath that's been with you since day one.

This chapter explains how this natural, always-available tool can help you navigate emotional storms, manage anxiety and depression, heal trauma, build emotional intelligence, and create pockets of peace in your hectic day. The techniques here range from simple 30-second interventions to deeper practices, all designed to help you breathe your way to better mental well-being.

Breathing through Emotional Storms

I don't know how you deal with the stress of life, but for me, mindfulness and meditation have always been a great help. However, these practices work best for me when things are going okay. When things get really stressful, I've found mindfulness alone isn't as helpful as breathing exercises. In this section, I explore why that may be true for you, too.

Exploring why breathing matters in tough times

When emotions hit like a tidal wave, your breath becomes your lifeline. But why is breathing such a big deal when you're emotionally overwhelmed? Well, your breath isn't just keeping you alive (though that's a pretty neat trick, too) — it's intimately connected to your emotional state.

Picture this scenario: You're stuck in traffic, late for an important meeting, and your boss has already texted twice asking where you are. Notice what happens to your breathing in this moment. It likely becomes shallow and rapid, moving high into your chest rather than deep into your belly. This isn't just a coincidence — it's your body's automatic response to stress. When you're emotionally charged, your breathing changes. But, and here's the kicker, when you change your breathing, your emotions shift, too.

This two-way street between breath and emotions gives you a powerful tool. Unlike many aspects of your autonomic nervous system (see the next section), like your heartbeat or digestion, breathing is unique because you can control it consciously. This makes it your direct line to influencing how you feel. It's like having access to the control panel of your emotions — not to shut them down, but to turn down the volume when they're screaming too loudly.

Breathing is one of the few bodily functions that bridges both your voluntary and involuntary systems. You breathe automatically when you're not thinking about it (thank goodness!), but you can also choose to control your breathing patterns. This dual nature makes breath the perfect gateway to influencing your emotional state — a backdoor into systems that usually run on autopilot.

During tough times, your breathing pattern often reveals your emotional state before you've even consciously acknowledged what you're feeling. Anxiety typically leads to shallow, rapid breathing from the chest. Anger may cause you to hold your breath or breathe in sharp bursts. Sadness sometimes manifests as sighing or irregular breathing patterns. By noticing these patterns, you gain valuable insight into your emotional landscape — often before your thinking mind has caught up.

Calming your nervous system

Let's get a little nerdy for a moment (but just a little, I promise). Your autonomic nervous system has two main branches: the sympathetic ("fight-or-flight") and parasympathetic ("rest-and-digest") nervous systems. These two systems are constantly working to keep you in balance, like the world's most important seesaw.

When you're stressed, your sympathetic nervous system dominates, pumping stress hormones through your body and preparing you to either battle a woolly mammoth or run away screaming (neither of which is typically helpful in modern scenarios like work presentations or awkward family dinners). On the other hand, your parasympathetic nervous system promotes relaxation, proper digestion, and recovery — basically all the good stuff that keeps you healthy and happy in the long run.

Here's where breathing becomes your superpower: Certain breathing patterns can actually switch your body from sympathetic overdrive to parasympathetic calm. For example, lengthened exhalation — breathing in for a count of three and out for a count of five — stimulates the parasympathetic branch of your nervous system. This isn't just feel-good advice — it's based on solid physiology. When you extend your exhale, you activate the vagus nerve, a key component of your parasympathetic nervous system. This sends a signal throughout your body that it's safe to relax. Your heart rate slows, blood pressure decreases, and stress hormones reduce. All from simply adjusting how you breathe!

Interestingly, different breathing patterns can have opposite effects. If you're feeling lethargic or foggy, you may benefit from energizing breathing techniques. Lengthened inhalation — breathing in for a count of five and out for a count of three — stimulates the sympathetic branch of the nervous system, bringing energy into the body and reducing lethargy.

The beauty of breathing techniques is that they put you in the driver's seat of your nervous system, allowing you to shift gears depending on what you need in any given moment.

Discovering how breath impacts thoughts and emotions

Have you ever noticed how your thinking changes when you're stressed versus when you're relaxed? When your breathing is rapid and shallow, your thoughts often race accordingly. Conversely, when your breath is slow and deep, your mind tends to settle like a snow globe after the shaking stops.

This isn't coincidental. Your breathing pattern directly influences your brain chemistry and function. Studies have shown that controlled breathing practices can change brain-wave patterns, leading to enhanced mental clarity, improved focus, and emotional regulation. Our thoughts can directly change our breath pattern and subsequently affect our physiology and disease processes.

Breathing also connects to our emotional centers through our sense of smell. Every breath you take brings information about your environment to your brain, influencing your emotional response to what's around you. This explains why certain scents can trigger powerful memories and emotions — your breath is literally carrying emotional information to your brain with every inhale.

On a physiological level, mindful breathing increases heart rate variability (HRV), a key indicator of overall health and stress resilience. A higher HRV corresponds to greater emotional flexibility and better stress management. Think of it as having a wider emotional bandwidth to handle life's challenges without becoming overwhelmed.

Perhaps most important, conscious breathing creates a pause between stimulus and response — that crucial moment where you can choose how to react rather than being swept away by automatic emotional responses. As you develop awareness of your breath, you simultaneously develop awareness of your emotional landscape, creating space to respond thoughtfully rather than react impulsively to emotional triggers.

Managing Stress, Anxiety, and Depression with Breath

Do you ever feel overwhelmed by stress, anxiety, or depression? If so, the pathway to feeling better may be, at least partly, through healthier breathing. I explain how in this section.

Using breath to manage anxiety or panic attacks

When anxiety strikes, it often feels like you're trapped in a whirlwind with no way out. Your heart races, your breathing becomes shallow, and your thoughts spiral faster than a caffeinated squirrel. The good news? Your breath can be your path out of Anxiety Land.

During anxiety or panic attacks, your breathing pattern typically shifts to rapid, shallow chest breathing. This breathing pattern actually reinforces the physical symptoms of anxiety — creating a frustrating feedback loop that intensifies the experience. By consciously changing your breathing pattern, you can interrupt this cycle and signal to your body that you're not in danger.

This type of breathing reduces carbon dioxide levels in your blood, leading to symptoms like dizziness, tingling, and feelings of suffocation — all of which can intensify the panic.

One approach to address this is by focusing on slowing down your breath, increasing carbon dioxide levels, and activating your parasympathetic nervous system (the "rest-and-digest" mode). By doing so, you interrupt the feedback loop that perpetuates the panic attack and restore a sense of calm.

This technique, known as the Cupped-Hands Rescue Breath or simply SOS Breathing, can be your go-to exercise for stopping a panic attack in its tracks. Follow these steps or listen to Track 22:

1. **Sit upright or lie down if possible.**

   Keep your back comfortably straight to allow for optimal diaphragm movement.

2. **Cup your hands over your nose and mouth with minimal gaps between your fingers.**

   This creates a small pocket of air.

3. **Inhale gently through your nose for three seconds and exhale softly through your nose for three seconds.**

4. **As you inhale, focus on the gentle outward expansion of your lower ribs; as you exhale, feel your ribs contract inward.**

5. **Maintain this slow, steady rhythm while keeping your breathing light and quiet if possible, for two minutes.**

6. **If you feel *air hunger* (a slight need for more air), take a break by removing your hands for 30 seconds, before resuming.**

Wondering how this works? Cupping your hands helps retain carbon dioxide in the small air pocket you create, which stabilizes blood pH and improves oxygen delivery to your brain and body. This calms the central nervous system and reduces symptoms like dizziness or tingling.

If cupping isn't feasible or comfortable, try this alternative method to regulate your breathing:

1. **Sit or lie down comfortably.**

   Ensure your back is straight to allow for unrestricted airflow.

2. **Place your hands on your ribs.**

   This helps you focus on diaphragmatic (belly) breathing rather than shallow chest breathing.

3. **Inhale lightly through your nose for three seconds, allowing your lower ribs to expand outward.**

4. **Exhale softly through your nose for three seconds, feeling your ribs contract inward.**

5. **If it's comfortable, extend the exhale slightly longer than the inhale (for example, inhale for three seconds, and exhale for four to five seconds).**

6. **Continue until you feel calmer.**

Slow diaphragmatic breathing reduces *hyperventilation* (over-breathing) by encouraging light nasal breaths that balance oxygen and carbon dioxide levels. The extended exhale activates the *vagus nerve* (a long nerve that connects your brain to your heart, lungs, and digestive system, helping to regulate your body's restorative mode), signaling relaxation to your brain.

Another effective approach for anxiety is breath focus, where you combine deep breathing with visualization. Close your eyes if they're open. Take a few big, deep breaths. Breathe in and, as you do, imagine that the air is filled with a sense of peace and calm. Try to feel it throughout your body. Breathe out and, while you're doing so, imagine that the air is leaving with your stress and tension.

Several other breathing exercises in this book could work best for you. In particular, you could try:

>> Mini breath holds (see Chapter 9)

>> Deep diaphragmatic breathing (see Chapter 7)

>> Coherent Breathing (see Chapter 8)

>> Ocean Breath (see Chapter 8)

>> 4-7-8 Breathing (see Chapter 8)

These techniques require practice to be most effective. Don't wait until you're in the midst of severe anxiety to try them for the first time — just as you wouldn't want to start learning to swim when you're drowning. Instead, practice regularly when you're relatively calm so that the techniques become second nature and are readily available when you need them most.

Breathing for anger management

We all get angry sometimes — it's part of being human. But when anger threatens to hijack your better judgment or damage your relationships, breathwork can help you cool those flames before they burn everything down.

When anger surges, your breathing typically becomes rapid and forceful. You may even unconsciously hold your breath, building pressure like a pressure cooker. These breathing patterns actually fuel your anger response, making it harder to think clearly or respond appropriately. By intentionally shifting your breathing pattern, you can defuse anger's intensity and regain your emotional equilibrium.

The yogic breathing technique of Cooling Breath (Sitali Pranayama) is known for its cooling and calming effects, making it particularly useful when experiencing intense anger. Follow these steps:

1. **Sit upright in a comfortable chair or on the floor, ensuring your spine is straight.**

2. **Purse your lips to create a small O shape with your mouth.**

3. **Slowly inhale through your O-shaped mouth, as if sipping air through a straw. Focus on the cool sensation of the air entering.**

4. **After a full inhalation, close your mouth and exhale slowly through your nose.**

5. **Continue this pattern for several minutes, concentrating on the cooling sensation and the rhythm of your breath.**

This technique helps reduce the body's heat and calms the mind, aiding in defusing anger. It's a simple yet effective method to incorporate into your breathwork practice. You can also use it to help you cool down on a hot day, as I have been today, in the midst of a heat wave!

Straw Breathing is another effective method that involves exhaling through a straw to promote relaxation and reduce anger. Here's how to practice it:

1. **Sit upright in a comfortable chair or on the floor, ensuring your spine is straight.**

2. **Take a slow, deep breath in through your nose, filling your lungs completely.**

3. **Place a straw between your lips and exhale slowly and steadily through it.**

   The resistance created by the straw helps to control the exhalation and promotes a calming effect.

4. **Continue this breathing pattern for several minutes, focusing on the sensation of the breath and the calming effect it has on your body.**

This technique can be particularly useful in moments of heightened anger, because it encourages slower breathing and helps activate the body's relaxation response.

Other breathing exercises that will help you manage anger are:

>> Box Breathing (see Chapter 8)

>> 4-7-8 Breathing (see Chapter 8)

>> Deep diaphragmatic breathing (see Chapter 7)

>> Humming Breath (see Chapter 6)

For particularly intense anger, adding sound to your exhalations can provide additional release. Try making a *haaa* sound as you exhale forcefully through your mouth. This audible exhale helps discharge pent-up emotional energy while physically relaxing tension in your jaw and throat (areas where people often hold anger).

Breathing for easing sadness and depression

When sadness or depression settles in, it often feels like a heavy weight pressing down on your chest, making even breathing feel like an effort. Your breathing pattern typically becomes shallow and restricted, which unfortunately can deepen feelings of lethargy and emotional heaviness.

Breathing exercises won't cure clinical depression, but they can help lift some of the physiological patterns that maintain and deepen depressive states. They're a valuable complementary approach alongside appropriate professional treatment.

Energizing breath practices can be particularly helpful for depression's low-energy states.

Another approach is combining a breathing exercise with some mindful awareness. When you're feeling down, overwhelmed, or stuck in your head, the 5-4-3-2-1 Grounding Breath helps you gently return to the here and now using your breath and senses. It's a technique you can do almost anywhere — quietly, privately, and within a few minutes. Here's how to practice it step-by-step:

1. **Take a Deep Breath**

   Breathe in slowly through your nose, letting the air fill your lungs. Then exhale gently through your mouth. Let this breath be your signal to begin.

2. **Notice 5 Things You Can See**

   Look around you. Silently name five things you can see right now. These could be objects, colors, shapes, patterns, or movement.

Example: "The light on the wall, the cup on my desk, a shadow, the color blue, my hand."

Take another slow, steady breath.

3. **Silently name four things you can feel — on your skin, beneath your body, or in contact with your hands or feet.**

   For example, "I can feel the warmth of my sweater, my feet on the floor, the chair's back, and my hands on my lap."

4. **Take a gentle breath in and out.**

5. **Silently name three things you can hear right now, whether they're loud or quiet, inside or outside.**

   For example, "I can hear a car passing, a clock ticking, and the sound of my breath."

6. **Take another soft, calming breath.**

7. **Silently name two things you can smell.**

   If nothing stands out, simply notice the neutral scent of the air or your clothes. For example, "I can smell my tea and a hint of soap on my sleeve."

8. **Take a deep, grounding breath.**

9. **Silently name one thing you can taste.**

   This might be something you recently ate or just the natural taste in your mouth. For example, "I can taste the mint from my toothpaste" or "I taste nothing in particular."

This practice grounds you in the here and now by gently shifting your focus to your senses. It helps quiet the mental chatter and lifts you out of overthinking or rumination — a common part of depression. You're not trying to *fix* anything, just noticing, with kindness and curiosity.

The lion's breath technique can also be beneficial for depression. Lion's Breath (known as *Simhasana* in yoga) is a powerful, energizing breathing technique that can help lift a low mood and break through the heaviness often associated with depression. It's playful, physical, and a little silly — which makes it an antidote to the depression. Think of it as shaking off mental cobwebs with your breath and face. It's not for everyone, but give it a try once if you're willing!

TRY THIS

Here's how to do Lion's Breath:

1. **Kneel on the floor, sitting back on your heels, or sit upright in a chair if that's easier.**

2. **Place your hands on your knees and spread your fingers wide like lion claws.**

   Lean slightly forward to engage the posture more fully.

3. **Take a strong, deep breath in through your nose, filling your lungs.**

4. **Open your mouth wide, stick your tongue out as far as possible, pointing it toward your chin, and exhale, making a loud *haaa* sound, like a lion's roar (but with breath, not voice).**

5. **Look up as if you can see between your eyebrows or just gaze upward.**

   This facial stretch engages tension-holding muscles.

6. **After the exhale, return to normal breathing. You can repeat the practice three to five times.**

Another approach is breath visualization. While breathing deeply, imagine your inhales bringing in light, energy, and hope, while your exhales release heaviness, lethargy, and sadness. This combines the physiological benefits of deep breathing with the psychological power of visualization.

TIP

For persistent sadness or depression, establishing a regular breathwork routine can be more effective than isolated practices. Breathwork meditation may boost mood and reduce symptoms of anxiety and depression. Committing to even five to ten minutes of intentional breathing each morning can provide cumulative benefits for your emotional well-being.

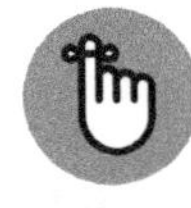

REMEMBER

If you don't feel motivated enough to do five minutes, even doing just one of these breathing exercises for ten seconds makes a difference. That's the beauty of breathing exercises — everyone can do them.

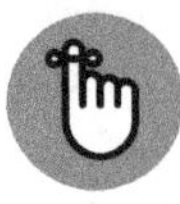

REMEMBER

Although breathing exercises can be helpful, they should complement rather than replace professional treatment for clinical depression. If you're experiencing persistent depression, reach out to a healthcare provider.

Managing Trauma

In recent years, there's been a greater realization of just how prevalent trauma is and what a challenge it can be for people to manage. Fortunately, breathwork can be a vital part of the package of strategies for managing trauma.

Understanding and identifying trauma

Before diving into how breathing can help with trauma, let's get clear on what trauma actually is. Despite what many people think, trauma isn't just about experiencing something terrible like war or natural disasters.

Trauma is a deeply distressing or disturbing experience that overwhelms an individual's capacity to cope, leading to difficulties in functioning. There are different types of trauma: "big T" events such as physical or sexual abuse, war, natural disasters, or significant losses such as the death of a loved one; and "small t" events like breakups, financial worries, or interpersonal conflict.

Trauma affects an estimated 70 percent to 75 percent of people at some point in their lives, with about 10 percent developing post-traumatic stress disorder (PTSD). That means trauma is incredibly common — you're certainly not alone if you've experienced it.

How do you know if you're carrying trauma? Your body often provides the clues. Trauma responses commonly include the following:

>> Hypervigilance (feeling constantly "on guard")

>> Being easily startled

>> Sleep disturbances

>> Unexplained physical pain

>> Emotional numbness

>> Strong emotional reactions that seem disproportionate to current situations

People can store psycho-emotional pain or traumas in the form of physical tension or pain in the body.

When it comes to breathing patterns, trauma often manifests as restricted, shallow breathing or holding your breath. Trauma and overwhelm freeze the breath entirely. This is because during traumatic experiences, we often unconsciously hold our breath or breathe very shallowly — and this pattern can persist long after the trauma itself has passed. It becomes a physical habit that reinforces the psychological impact of trauma.

Importantly, trauma isn't just psychological — it's physiological, too. Trauma literally changes how your nervous system functions, often leaving it stuck in either hyperarousal (fight or flight) or hypoarousal (freeze or disconnect). These states affect everything from your heart rate and digestion to your thinking patterns and, of course, your breathing.

Understanding that trauma lives in your body — not just your mind — is crucial because it points to how breathing exercises can help. Because breathing is both voluntary and involuntary, it provides a bridge between your conscious awareness and your body's automatic responses, making it an ideal tool for trauma recovery.

Appreciating how breathing exercises impact trauma

Now that you understand how trauma affects both mind and body, let's explore why breathwork can be particularly powerful for trauma recovery. Simply put, breathing exercises offer a direct path to reprogramming the nervous system patterns established during and after traumatic experiences.

The science behind this is fascinating. Studies indicate that breathwork can contribute to symptom reduction in individuals with trauma. Specific breathwork techniques such as Holotropic Breathwork (Chapter 17) may activate the somatic-cognitive cycle, helping release unresolved trauma.

Conscious breathing helps reset the dysregulation in your body by activating the parasympathetic nervous system — the "rest-and-digest" response that counterbalances stress activation. This explains why proper breathwork can help reduce many common trauma symptoms, including anxiety, hypervigilance, and emotional reactivity.

Beyond nervous system regulation, breathing practices create a safe way to reconnect with your body. Many trauma survivors unconsciously disconnect from bodily sensations as a protective mechanism. Gentle breathwork offers a nonthreatening way to rebuild body awareness, gradually increasing your capacity to feel sensations without being overwhelmed by them.

Breathing exercises also help establish a sense of agency and control — something that's often lost during traumatic experiences. Step-by-step, you can illuminate the way home. The simple act of consciously controlling your breath reminds your system that you are safe now and have choices about how to respond to triggers.

Additionally, breathwork helps process "stuck" emotional energy associated with trauma. During breathwork sessions, individuals may experience an emotional release, which can manifest as spontaneous tears, trembling, temperature changes, or emotional insights. This may sound intimidating, but these releases are actually signs of the body processing and integrating experiences that were too overwhelming to process fully when they occurred.

It's worth noting that although breathwork can be tremendously helpful for trauma recovery, it should be approached mindfully. Breathwork for trauma can be powerful but also emotionally intense. To navigate this process safely and effectively, working with a qualified breathwork facilitator and therapist is highly recommended. For severe trauma, breathwork is best used as a complement to professional trauma therapy rather than as a stand-alone treatment.

Discovering ways of healing your past traumas through breath

Specific breathing techniques can support trauma healing, but remember to approach these practices gently, honoring your own pace and boundaries.

One of the most accessible techniques for trauma recovery is coherent breathing, a simple practice of bringing your breath into a steady, rhythmic pattern. This balanced breathing pattern helps regulate your autonomic nervous system, bringing it back into equilibrium when trauma responses have disrupted its natural balance.

For moments when trauma triggers are activated, the extended exhale technique can be particularly helpful. Lengthened exhalation involves breathing in for the count of three and out for the count of five, for example. Making the exhalation longer than the inhalation stimulates the parasympathetic ("rest-and-digest") branch of the nervous system. This technique counteracts the "fight-or-flight" state often triggered by trauma reminders.

Alternate-Nostril Breathing (also known as *Nadi Shodhana*) offers another valuable approach. This technique involves gently closing one nostril with your finger while breathing through the other, and then switching sides. This practice is helpful for enhancing empathy. Beyond balancing your nervous system, Alternate-Nostril Breathing helps integrate the right and left hemispheres of your brain, which can support processing traumatic memories that are often stored in fragmented ways.

For deeper trauma release work, a technique called Breath of Fire (or *Kapalabhati*) can be effective, though it should be approached cautiously and ideally with guidance for trauma survivors. This involves a series of short, forceful exhales through the nose while allowing inhales to occur naturally. This energetic breathing helps release tension from the body while activating and moving stagnant emotional energy.

For sustainable trauma healing, consistency matters more than intensity. Establishing a daily practice of five to ten minutes of conscious breathing creates cumulative effects, gradually retraining your nervous system and building your capacity to stay present with sensations and emotions. The path requires patience, self-forgiveness, and trust in your body and mind to heal over time.

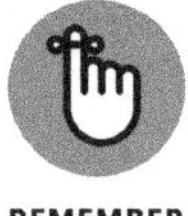

REMEMBER

Trauma recovery isn't linear, and breathwork should be approached as a complementary practice alongside appropriate professional support for significant trauma. Breathwork for trauma can be powerful but also emotionally intense. To navigate this process safely and effectively, working with a qualified breathwork facilitator who's trained to work with trauma is highly recommended. Your facilitator should be well-qualified, experienced, and compassionate toward you.

Developing Emotional Intelligence through Breath

Emotional intelligence isn't as complicated as it sounds. It's the skill of noticing and understanding your own feelings and the feelings of others. It also means managing emotions well, so you can stay calm, connect with people, and handle situations thoughtfully.

As your emotions and breath are so closely tied together, by getting more skillful at using breathing exercises, you can become more emotionally intelligent.

Tuning into your breath to navigate emotions

Emotional intelligence begins with awareness — the ability to recognize and name what you're feeling. Your breath serves as a remarkably accurate barometer of your emotional state, making it an excellent tool for developing emotional self-awareness.

Have you noticed how each emotion tends to create a characteristic breathing pattern? Anxiety typically manifests as shallow, rapid chest breathing. Anger often involves held breath or forceful breathing. Sadness may show up as sighing or irregular breathing. Joy frequently appears as full, expansive breathing. By tuning into your breath throughout the day, you gain valuable information about your emotional state, often before you've consciously registered what you're feeling.

And there's more good news! By consciously altering your breathing patterns, you can influence your emotional state and improve your emotional intelligence. This two-way relationship between breath and emotion means your breath not only reflects your feelings but can also help you understand and navigate them more effectively.

Try this simple practice: Several times throughout your day, pause to notice your breathing pattern. Is it fast or slow? Deep or shallow? Smooth or irregular? Centered in your chest or your belly? Without trying to change your breathing, simply observe it with curiosity. Then ask yourself: "What am I feeling right now?" You may be surprised at the insights this simple practice reveals.

Beyond identifying emotions, breath awareness helps you recognize emotional transitions as they're happening. That moment when irritation starts bubbling toward anger, or when mild concern begins escalating toward anxiety — these shifts usually register in your breathing before they fully capture your conscious awareness. This early-warning system gives you valuable moments to choose how to respond rather than being swept away by emotional reactivity.

Breathwork supports improved mental health, better communication skills, and enhanced personal relationships. These benefits stem largely from increased emotional awareness and the ability to recognize your own triggers and patterns. When you can identify what you're feeling and what triggered it, you gain freedom to respond thoughtfully rather than react automatically.

The beauty of using breath for emotional navigation is its accessibility — your breath is always with you, making this tool available anytime, anywhere. Whether you're in a challenging work meeting, in a difficult conversation with a loved one, or just feeling emotionally confused, your breath offers immediate insight into your internal landscape.

For example, I remember sitting in a cafe recently, feeling a bit off but not quite sure why. As I waited for my coffee, I took a moment to tune into my breath. It was shallow and tight, sitting high in my chest. I paused and asked myself, "What am I feeling right now?" That simple question, paired with my breath awareness, revealed that I was feeling overwhelmed — something I hadn't consciously noticed. Just naming it helped me feel a bit lighter. I took a few slow belly breaths, and almost instantly, my body softened. It reminded me how breath can be a quiet guide to emotional clarity.

Using breath as a tool for emotional resilience

Emotional resilience — the ability to adapt to challenging situations and recover from difficulties — isn't about avoiding emotional storms but rather about weathering them skillfully. Your breath can be a powerful anchor during these storms, helping you stay present and responsive rather than being swept away by intense feelings.

Adding attention and energy to breathing can help you manage your emotions and open you to a deeper level of understanding. The internal softening that occurs through breathwork connects you deeply with yourself. This internal connection forms the foundation of emotional resilience.

One key aspect of emotional resilience is the ability to tolerate uncomfortable feelings without immediately reacting to them or trying to escape them. Conscious breathing creates a safe container for experiencing difficult emotions. By anchoring your awareness on your breath while allowing emotions to flow, you develop greater emotional capacity — like strengthening a muscle through regular exercise.

Breathwork is a powerful tool for emotional healing, offering a path to greater self-awareness, emotional resilience, and inner peace. This occurs partly because conscious breathing activates your parasympathetic nervous system, creating a physiological state of safety that helps you process emotions without becoming overwhelmed by them.

TRY THIS

One approach is to practice what can be called "breathing through difficult emotions." When you notice an uncomfortable feeling arising, rather than resisting it or getting caught in its story, simply direct your attention to your breath. Here's how to do it:

1. **When you sense a wave of discomfort — maybe anxiety, anger, or sadness — see if you can gently label it.**

   For example, "Ah, this is anxiety" or "This is anger." This act of naming can bring awareness and a touch of distance from the feeling, so you're not completely caught up in it.

2. **Tune in to where you sense the feeling in your body.**

   Is it a tightness in your chest? A heaviness in your stomach? Tension in your jaw? By focusing on the physical sensation, you can ground yourself in the present moment instead of getting lost in the story your mind may be weaving.

3. **Direct your breath to that area.**

   Imagine your inhale gently expanding around the uncomfortable sensation, and your exhale softening any resistance. This doesn't mean you're trying to make the emotion vanish — instead, you're creating space around it.

4. **Stay present with what arises.**

   As you continue to breathe, you may notice thoughts popping in ("I can't handle this" or "I shouldn't feel this way"). Acknowledge them but let them pass, like clouds in the sky. Keep coming back to your breath and your body. *Remember:* It's okay to feel the way you do.

5. **As you breathe with the emotion, notice how it shifts and changes over time.**

   Remind yourself that all emotions — no matter how intense — are temporary. You're not defined by this feeling; it's simply a passing experience.

Another classic breathing exercise for challenging emotions is box breathing (see Chapter 8). This offers a particularly effective technique for building emotional resilience. This balanced breathing pattern helps calm your nervous system while creating mental space to process emotions.

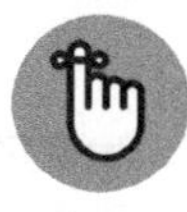

Regular breathwork practice builds emotional resilience much like regular exercise builds physical strength. Breathing exercises help cultivate emotional resilience, making you better equipped to navigate life's inevitable challenges with grace rather than reactivity.

Breathing to improve your emotional intelligence

These specific breathing techniques are carefully designed to help you develop greater emotional intelligence. By practicing regularly, you'll become better at recognizing, managing, and expressing your emotions clearly. Let's get breathing!

The following exercise, the Emotional Check-in Breath, develops emotional self-awareness by linking your breath directly with how you're feeling. Regular practice helps you notice emotions early, allowing you to respond consciously rather than automatically.

1. **Find a comfortable position, sitting upright but relaxed.**

   Close your eyes gently if comfortable.

2. **Breathe softly through your nose into your belly, inhaling slowly for four seconds.**

3. **Exhale gently and smoothly through your nose or mouth for around six seconds.**

4. **After a few calming breaths, ask yourself silently, "What am I feeling right now?"**

5. **Notice any emotions or sensations (like tightness, warmth, or tension).**

   Simply acknowledge them without judgment and continue breathing calmly.

TIP

If 4-6 feels uncomfortable, try 3-5 or 2-3.

TRY THIS

When emotions like anxiety, stress, or anger arise, your breathing typically becomes short or shallow. The Extended-Exhale Breath activates your body's natural relaxation response, helping you quickly return to emotional balance and clarity.

1. **Pause and notice your breathing whenever you feel strong emotions building.**

2. **Inhale gently through your nose, comfortably filling your lungs for however long feels good.**

3. **Exhale slowly through pursed lips, as if blowing gently through a straw, extending your exhale longer than your inhale.**

4. **Repeat this breathing pattern for at least five breaths, gradually helping you to feel calmer and more in control.**

5. **When you're calm, return to breathing naturally, and notice how your emotional state has shifted.**

TRY THIS

Expressing emotions clearly and appropriately can sometimes feel difficult. The following breathing exercise, the Vocal Release Breath, links your breath to sound, helping you comfortably express a range of emotions and become more confident in your emotional communication.

1. **Sit or stand in a relaxed position, and take a deep belly breath through your nose for about four seconds.**

2. **As you exhale slowly, make a vocal sound matching the emotion you want to express.**

   For example, a sigh — *ahhhh* — can release tension or stress.

3. **Experiment with different sounds.**

   Try a short *ha* sound to express confidence or assertiveness, or a gentle humming *mmm* to reflect contentment.

4. **Repeat several times, varying your vocal expressions according to how you feel or what you want to communicate.**

5. **After finishing, pause briefly to notice your emotional state.**

   Notice how connecting breath with sound can make emotional expression clearer and easier.

I taught some of these exercises to a business client who often struggled to manage his emotions during stressful interactions both at work and home. He found the emotional check-in breath particularly helpful. Whenever tension rose at home, he paused and quietly asked himself, "What am I feeling right now?" Through recognizing his emotions early, he found he could respond calmly rather than react impulsively. Within weeks, his family and staff noticed his increased patience and openness, transforming not just how he felt inside, but significantly improving his relationships, too.

This is an example of how something as simple as breath and a simple question you ask yourself can end up impacting emotional intelligence and relationships. Wow!

Relaxation and Recovery Practices

Imagine having your own personal relaxation coach everywhere you go! Well, in a way, you do. Your breath — that ever-present, ever-reliable companion — can act as your personal relaxation coach.

This section explores how to integrate breathing practices into your daily routine to unwind after stress and enhance rest. Whether you're looking for a quick reset or a deeper sense of calm, these techniques will help you create a sanctuary of stillness amidst the noise of life.

Creating a daily relaxation routine

Let's face it: Relaxation doesn't just *happen*. It requires intention and a bit of planning. Think of creating a daily relaxation routine as building a cozy little corner in your day where stress isn't allowed to enter. And the cornerstone of this sanctuary? Your breath.

The following sections walk you through exercises to try throughout your day. Here are some tips to make the most of the routine:

>> Start small. Just five minutes per session is enough to build a habit.

>> Gradually extend your practice or add additional sessions as your comfort increases.

>> Enhance relaxation by pairing breathwork with mindfulness meditation or gentle yoga stretches.

Creating a daily relaxation routine isn't about perfection; it's about progress. Even if you miss a session or two, simply returning to your practice when you can will yield long-term benefits. Over time, you'll find that these moments of intentional breathing become not just a part of your day but something you look forward to — a sacred pause amidst life's busyness.

Morning: Setting a calm and focused tone

Starting your day calmly helps you face whatever comes with greater clarity and ease. Here are some recommended breathing exercises for the morning:

>> **Diaphragmatic breathing (see Chapter 7):** Deepens relaxation and grounds your body.

>> **Alternate-Nostril Breathing (see Chapter 19):** Balances your mind and boosts mental clarity.

>> **Box Breathing (see Chapter 8):** Promotes focus and gentle energy for the day ahead.

Midday: Pausing and resetting your mind

Midday breathing acts as a reset, reducing stress and helping you regain focus. Here are some exercises to try midday:

>> **4-6 Breathing (see Chapter 2):** Reduces stress hormones and lowers blood pressure.

>> **Breathe Light (see Chapter 9):** Refreshes concentration and clarity amid daily tasks.

>> **Extended-Exhale Breath (see Chapter 3):** Quickly shifts your nervous system toward relaxation.

Evening: Unwinding and preparing for restful sleep

Evening breathing helps signal to your body and mind that it's time to relax and release tension. Here are some exercises to try at night:

>> **4-7-8 Breathing (see Chapter 8):** Activates deep relaxation for better sleep.

>> **Ocean Breath (see Chapter 8):** Calms your mind and deeply relaxes your body.

>> **Coherent Breathing (see Chapter 8):** Soothes your nervous system and eases you gently into rest.

Using breathwork to unwind after stress

Stress doesn't always knock loudly. Sometimes it creeps in quietly — during long Zoom calls, after awkward conversations, or while doomscrolling late at night. But your breath can be your ally, especially when you know a few breathing techniques that work for you.

The Pendulum Breath is a calming breath pattern that creates a gentle rhythm between body and mind — especially useful when emotions feel jagged or jarring.

1. **Sit comfortably and close your eyes if you like.**

2. **Inhale softly through the nose for about five seconds.**

3. **Exhale slowly through pursed lips for about five seconds.**

4. **As you breathe, visualize a pendulum gently swinging back and forth with each inhale and exhale.**

5. **Continue for two to five minutes, allowing the rhythm to settle your nervous system.**

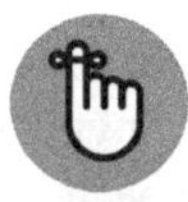

This is similar to the coherent breathing technique, but it involves imaging a pendulum swinging back and forth. It can be very calming for some people.

Breathing in Circles again adds a layer of visual imagination to your breath — great after screen fatigue or when your mind feels scattered.

1. **Begin seated with a long spine, eyes closed or gazing down.**

2. **Inhale slowly through the nose and imagine the breath moving *up* the back of your body (from tailbone to crown).**

3. Exhale gently and imagine the breath flowing *down* the front of your body (from forehead to navel).

4. Feel as though you're tracing a continuous circle of breath energy around your torso.

5. Repeat this circle for one to three minutes, noticing how your awareness shifts from head to body.

If your stress feels frozen in your body and you can't get rid of it, try the Feather Breath. You're not trying to *do* much — just soften and *notice*.

1. Hold your hand in front of your nose, about 2 inches away.

2. Inhale gently through your nose as if you're trying not to disturb anything.

3. Exhale as softly as possible, just enough to *slightly* move an imaginary feather in front of you.

4. Keep your breath light, slow, and quiet — almost like you're barely breathing.

5. Continue for a few minutes, tuning into the stillness it creates within.

By making your breathing light and gentle, you rebalance the levels of carbon dioxide in your bloodstream, calming you down as more oxygen goes into your cells.

Notice if you salivate more or if your hands or feet feel warmer. If so, the breathing exercise is definitely working because your relaxation response is engaging.

Not long ago, I was prepping for a new kind of corporate workshop that had me a little more stressed than usual. I'd overprepared, ironically, and my brain felt cluttered. I noticed my chest was a bit tight. I was tempted to distract myself with emails or yet another cup of tea. (We Brits can't have enough of the stuff!)

Instead, I sat down and did feather breath for about two minutes. At first, it felt like nothing. But gradually, I noticed I wasn't gripping my jaw anymore. My breath slowed on its own. And most importantly, I found enough space between myself and the stress to gently *choose* how to respond, rather than react. I smiled. Then I delivered the session — calm, grounded, and even a little playful.

Enhancing rest through breath

Ahh, rest! That elusive state we all crave but often struggle to achieve in our fast-paced world. Whether it's falling asleep at night or simply finding moments of stillness during the day, rest plays a vital role in your physical and mental well-being. And guess what? Your breath holds the key to unlocking deeper rest.

When I was younger, I had a lot of energy. Too much, really. I'd bounce from one idea to the next, and relaxing felt like a foreign concept. Meditation helped, but it was breathing exercises that really began to soften the restlessness. They taught me how to *feel* calm, not just think about it. And over time, I learned to create rest — not by escaping, but by arriving.

In this section, I show you three simple yet powerful breathing practices that help invite deep rest. They're not flashy, but that's the point. Think of them as slow, gentle bridges from activity into stillness.

Each of these practices invites rest in its own way — whether through soothing the nervous system, guiding the mind with inner sound, or grounding the body through gentle touch. Try one tonight. Or tomorrow after lunch. Let your breath become a quiet companion in your day — not to fix or change anything, but simply to rest with what's already here.

Left-Nostril Breathing

This calming breath is borrowed from yogic traditions. The left nostril is believed to be linked to the parasympathetic nervous system — the part of us that governs rest, digestion, and restoration. Breathing through just the left side can reduce tension and promote a sense of ease, especially useful before sleep or during anxious moments.

1. **Sit or lie down in a relaxed position.**

   Close your eyes if that feels comfortable.

2. **Raise your right hand and gently use your thumb to close off your right nostril.**

3. **Breathe in and out only through your left nostril, slowly and gently.**

4. **Keep your breathing quiet and smooth, aiming for about four to six breaths per minute.**

5. **Continue for two to five minutes, and then release your hand and return to normal breathing.**

You may feel a subtle shift — a cooling sensation, a quieter mind, or a softening of inner effort.

Silent Om Breathing

This is a meditation-style breath that uses internal sound to guide your attention and deepen stillness. Instead of chanting "om" out loud, you imagine the sound as you breathe. It works because the mind has something gentle to focus on — a sound that symbolizes unity, calm, and rest.

1. **Sit or lie down in a comfortable, undisturbed place, and close your eyes.**

2. **As you breathe in through your nose, mentally hear the sound** *ohhh.*

3. **As you breathe out through your nose, mentally hear the sound** *mmm.*

   Let the sound be soft and slow, matching the rhythm of your breath.

4. **Continue for several minutes, allowing the imagined sound to anchor you.**

This practice can be deeply relaxing — almost trancelike — and often leads to a natural stillness without effort.

Weighted Blanket Breathing

Sometimes the body needs more than breath alone — it needs a physical signal that it's safe to rest. This exercise combines breath with gentle pressure on the belly. You can use a folded towel or a light blanket — anything that gives a little weight. It's simple, sensory, and deeply grounding.

1. **Lie down on your back in bed or on a mat, and place a light, folded towel or small blanket over your belly.**

2. **Rest your hands on top of the weight, and feel its presence.**

3. **Breathe in slowly through your nose, directing your breath toward your lower belly.**

4. **Feel the gentle rise of the blanket on each inhale, and its fall on each exhale.**

5. **Continue this slow breathing for five to ten minutes, allowing your whole body to unwind.**

The weight and movement offer a sense of safety and containment — just like being gently held.

Chapter **11**

Breathing for Better Physical Health

Just because you've been breathing your whole life doesn't mean you're doing it in the most beneficial way for your health. The way you breathe can make a huge difference in how you feel, how well your body functions, and even how quickly you recover from illness.

Think of proper breathing as the unsung hero of health practices. It doesn't require fancy equipment, expensive memberships, or special clothes (though you may want to loosen that tight belt before trying some of these exercises). All it takes is a bit of awareness and practice to transform this automatic function into a powerful tool for better physical health.

In this chapter, you discover how to harness the power of your breath to strengthen your respiratory system, boost circulation and immunity, manage pain, and even improve your digestion and posture. Whether you're dealing with a specific health condition or you just want to optimize your overall well-being, these breathing techniques can help you breathe your way to better health. So, take a deep breath (but not yet — you need to learn how first!), and let's dive in.

Breathing for Respiratory Health

When it comes to your lungs, the old saying "Use it or lose it" definitely applies. Just like your biceps need regular workouts to stay strong, your lungs need proper exercise, too. The good news? You don't need to bench-press or do lung push-ups (those aren't a thing, thankfully). Instead, specific breathing exercises can help keep your respiratory system in top shape.

Strengthening the lungs

Your lungs are springy by nature — or at least they should be. Think of them like a screen door with a spring that opens and closes smoothly. Over time, though, especially with conditions like asthma or chronic obstructive pulmonary disease (COPD), your lungs can lose some of that springiness. When that happens, stale air can build up, making it harder for your *diaphragm* (that dome-shaped muscle just below your lungs; see Chapter 2) to do its job properly.

Breathing exercises can help make your lungs more efficient, just like aerobic exercise improves your heart function and strengthens your muscles. They help rid your lungs of accumulated stale air, increase oxygen levels, and get your diaphragm back to full working capacity.

PLAY THIS

This simple exercise, Pursed-Lips Breathing (Track 23), reduces the number of breaths you take and keeps your airways open longer, allowing more air to flow in and out of your lungs:

1. **Sit comfortably with your shoulders relaxed.**

    Avoid hunching for this exercise in particular. Relax your face, shoulders, and jaw if you can.

2. **Breathe in slowly through your nose for a count of two.**

    Remember to breathe into your belly, not your upper chest. No need to lift your shoulders on the inhale. Rest the tip of your tongue on the roof of your mouth just behind your front teeth on each inhale.

3. **Pucker your lips as if you're about to whistle or blow out birthday candles.**

4. **Exhale slowly and gently through your pursed lips for a count of four — twice as long as your inhale.**

    Breathe out gently, as if you're making a candle flame just flicker, but not go out.

5. **Repeat five to ten times.**

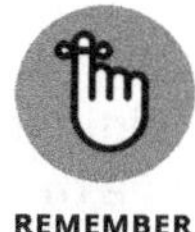

The exhale should be at least twice as long as the inhale. Think "in for three, out for six" as you practice. If three and six don't feel comfortable, adjust to two and four or four and eight, for example.

Other breathing exercises that can help strengthen your lungs are diaphragmatic breathing (Chapter 7), Three-Part Breath (Chapter 3), and breath holds (Chapter 9).

Managing asthma

Asthma is a chronic respiratory condition that affects the airways in the lungs, leading to episodes of wheezing, breathlessness, chest tightness, and coughing. These symptoms occur when the airways become inflamed and narrowed, making it difficult for air to move in and out of the lungs.

The exact cause of asthma remains unclear, but scientists believe it's a combination of genetic and environmental factors. Common triggers that can provoke asthma symptoms include the following:

>> **Airborne allergens:** Pollen, dust mites, mold spores, pet dander, and cockroach waste could bring on symptoms.

>> **Respiratory infections:** Common colds and other viral infections may cause symptoms.

>> **Physical activity:** Exercise can induce symptoms in some individuals.

>> **Cold air:** Exposure to cold weather can exacerbate symptoms.

>> **Air pollutants and irritants:** Smoke, strong odors, and chemical fumes could contribute to symptoms.

>> **Medications:** Certain drugs, including beta blockers and aspirin, may cause symptoms in some people.

>> **Strong emotions and stress:** Intense feelings can lead to hyperventilation, triggering symptoms.

Breathing exercises can be a valuable tool in managing asthma. They aim to improve respiratory muscle strength, enhance airway clearance, and promote relaxation, which can help reduce the frequency and severity of asthma symptoms. Techniques such as diaphragmatic breathing, nasal breathing, and specific methods like the Buteyko Breathing Method or the *Papworth method* (a breathing technique encouraging relaxation and diaphragmatic breathing) focus on developing efficient breathing patterns and reducing hyperventilation.

Breathing through the nose, both during the day and at night, plays a crucial role in managing asthma. The nose acts as a natural filter, warming, humidifying, and cleaning the air before it reaches the lungs. This process helps reduce the risk of airway irritation and *bronchoconstriction* (a narrowing of the airways in your lungs). In contrast, mouth breathing can introduce cold, dry, and unfiltered air directly into the airways, potentially triggering asthma symptoms. Encouraging nasal breathing can, therefore, help in reducing the frequency of asthma exacerbations.

Incorporating breathing exercises into your daily routine can aid in better asthma control. Some recommended techniques include the following:

>> **Diaphragmatic (belly) breathing (Chapter 7):** Focuses on engaging the diaphragm to promote deep and efficient breaths.

>> **Pursed-Lips Breathing (earlier in this chapter):** Involves inhaling through the nose and exhaling slowly through pursed lips, helping to keep the airways open longer.

>> **Buteyko Breathing Method (Chapter 9):** Aims to reduce over-breathing and promote nasal breathing. It's about reducing the volume of air you breathe and practicing light, calm, quiet, regular breathing. This is a powerful and comprehensive method, and my colleagues and friends have helped many people with asthma over the years using this approach.

>> **Papworth method (coming up next):** Combines breathing and relaxation techniques to develop efficient breathing patterns.

>> **Alternate-Nostril Breathing (Chapter 12):** Involves gently breathing through one nostril at a time in a rhythmic pattern to enhance lung function and relaxation.

Developed in the 1960s at Papworth Hospital in England, the Papworth method combines diaphragmatic breathing with relaxation techniques to help individuals with asthma manage their symptoms. This method isn't just for people with asthma — it can help anyone who experiences shallow chest breathing or stress-related breathlessness. With regular practice, you'll find it easier to breathe calmly and efficiently, especially in moments of anxiety or physical tension.

You can practice the Papworth method sitting or lying down — whatever makes you feel most at ease. Here's how to do it:

1. **Find a quiet, comfortable spot.**

   Choose a place where you won't be interrupted.

2. **Relax your body and mind.**

   Gently close your eyes if you like, and take a moment to settle.

3. **Put one hand on your chest and the other on your abdomen.**

   This helps you monitor where your breath is going.

4. **Inhale gently through your nose.**

   Let the air flow into your belly, allowing your lower hand to rise while keeping your chest as still as possible.

5. **Exhale slowly through pursed lips or gently through your mouth.**

   Let your abdomen fall as you breathe out. Make the exhalation longer than the inhalation if you can.

6. **Pause before breathing in again.**

   Allow your breath to settle before the next inhale. This helps prevent over-breathing.

7. **Keep your shoulders and chest relaxed.**

   As you breathe, try to release any tension in the upper body.

8. **Continue for ten minutes.**

   Try to practice daily or anytime you notice yourself becoming breathless or anxious.

There are many benefits of this simple method.

>> **More efficient breathing:** It trains your diaphragm — your main breathing muscle — to do most of the work, reducing strain on accessory muscles in your neck and chest.

>> **Less breathlessness:** Especially helpful for people with asthma or anxiety.

>> **Calm and focus:** Like many breathing practices, it activates your body's relaxation response.

>> **A healthier habit:** Over time, it can help you shift from shallow mouth breathing to deeper nasal breathing.

Breathing exercises aren't meant to replace your rescue medication, but they can complement your asthma management plan. Always follow your doctor's advice about medication.

Improving breath capacity for chronic obstructive pulmonary disease

COPD is an umbrella term for a group of lung conditions — including emphysema and chronic bronchitis — that cause breathing difficulties. These conditions lead to narrowed airways and damaged lung tissue, making it harder for air to flow in and out of the lungs. Common symptoms include shortness of breath, a persistent cough that may produce mucus, and wheezing. Smoking is the primary cause of COPD, but long-term exposure to air pollution, dust, and chemical fumes can also contribute.

The Coordinated Breathing technique helps prevent the anxiety that can make you hold your breath when you're short of air:

1. **Inhale through your nose before beginning an activity that may cause breathlessness.**

2. **Perform the activity while exhaling through pursed lips.**

   For example, when climbing stairs, inhale while standing still, and then exhale through pursed lips while climbing a step or two.

Incorporating specific breathing techniques into your daily routine can help manage COPD symptoms by improving lung function and easing shortness of breath. In the following sections, I cover some commonly recommended exercises.

Try practicing your breathing exercises after using your bronchodilator medication when your airways are more open.

If you experience dizziness, increased shortness of breath, or chest pain while performing any breathing exercises, stop immediately and consult your healthcare provider.

Huff coughing

Huff coughing is a gentler, more controlled way to clear mucus from your lungs. Instead of a strong, forceful cough that can make your airways tighten or collapse, a huff cough uses just enough effort to move mucus without putting too much strain on your body. This makes it especially helpful for people with COPD — it takes less energy and feels more comfortable than regular coughing.

To practice huff coughing, follow these steps:

1. **Sit comfortably with your shoulders relaxed.**

2. **Take a deep breath in (deeper than normal, but not to maximum capacity).**

3. Hold for two to three seconds.

4. Exhale forcefully but not violently, through an open mouth, making a *ha* sound, as if you're trying to fog up a mirror.

5. Repeat two to three times, followed by controlled breathing; repeat the cycle as needed.

Deep breathing

This deep breathing technique for COPD helps you use more of your lung capacity:

1. Sit or stand with good posture to allow maximum lung expansion.

2. Place your hands around the sides of your lower ribs.

3. Breathe in deeply through your nose, feeling your ribs expand outward.

4. Hold for a count of three, if comfortable.

5. Exhale slowly through pursed lips, feeling your ribs return to their resting position.

6. Repeat three to five times, several times per day.

Pursed-Lips Breathing

This technique helps slow your breathing rate, keeps your airways open longer, and promotes better air exchange. It can be particularly useful during physical activity or when you feel short of breath. Read more about how to do Pursed-Lips Breathing earlier in this chapter.

Diaphragmatic breathing

Also known as belly breathing, this exercise strengthens the diaphragm, allowing for more efficient breathing and reducing the effort required to breathe. Read more about how to do diaphragmatic breathing in Chapter 7.

Supporting recovery from pneumonia

After pneumonia, your lungs need some TLC to get back to full function. Recovery times vary (and can take up to six months for complete recovery), but breathing exercises can help clear your lungs and speed up the healing process.

The Active Cycle of Breathing technique helps clear phlegm from your lungs:

1. **Get comfortable in a seated position or lying down.**

2. **Take three to four deep, slow breaths, focusing on full expansion of your lungs.**

3. **Follow with three to four gentle huffs (like the huff cough described earlier in this chapter).**

4. **If needed, end with a controlled cough to clear secretions.**

5. **Repeat the cycle two to three times.**

The Breath Expansion exercise helps restore full lung capacity after pneumonia:

1. **Place your hands on your stomach.**

2. **Take a controlled, deep breath in through your nose.**

   Your hands will rise as your stomach expands.

3. **If possible, hold this breath for a count of two or three.**

4. **Exhale slowly through your mouth.**

5. **Repeat five to ten times, several times a day.**

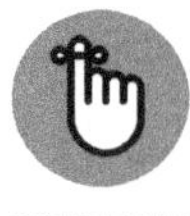

While you're recovering from pneumonia, turn over at least once an hour when you're in bed (and awake) and practice deep breathing followed by huffing or controlled coughing to help clear your lungs.

Improving Circulatory and Immune Health

Who knew breathing could be your cardiovascular system's best friend? The way you breathe affects your heart rate, blood pressure, and even your immune function. Let's explore how you can breathe your way to better circulation and immunity.

Lowering blood pressure naturally

High blood pressure often earns the nickname "the silent killer" because it does its damage without dramatic symptoms. Medication may be necessary for many people, but breathing exercises can be a powerful complementary approach to managing blood pressure.

Incorporating a few minutes of slow, deep breathing into your routine can help lower your blood pressure as effectively as some medications. Research has shown that certain breathing practices can reduce systolic blood pressure — the top number in a reading — by up to 10 points.

For example, practicing slow breathing (typically six to ten breaths per minute) not only calms the nervous system but also increases oxygen delivery and decreases stress hormone levels. Prolonged exhalations, in particular, help the body engage the parasympathetic ("rest-and-digest") response, which can widen blood vessels, slow the heart rate, and ultimately lower blood pressure.

Here are five effective breathing exercises, presented in a simple, practical way, that can help you naturally lower your blood pressure. Begin with the exercise that you find easiest or most enjoyable to do and that you're most likely to do regularly:

>> **Coherent Breathing, six breaths per minute (Chapter 8):** Promotes calmness and balances the body's stress response.

>> **4-7-8 Breathing technique (Chapter 8):** Reduces stress quickly, calming your nervous system and helping to lower blood pressure.

>> **Diaphragmatic breathing (Chapter 7):** Encourages deep relaxation, reducing blood pressure and stress.

>> **Alternate-Nostril Breathing (Chapter 15):** Balances the nervous system, induces calm, and gradually lowers blood pressure.

>> **Extended-Exhale Breathing (Chapter 3):** Activates the parasympathetic nervous system, reducing heart rate and lowering blood pressure.

Regular practice — even just five to ten minutes a day — will gradually make these exercises feel natural, supporting sustained improvements in blood pressure and overall well-being. Obviously, don't change your medication without talking to your doctor — and let them know that you're doing these exercises, too.

Boosting immune function with breath

Your immune system loves oxygen! Proper breathing can help boost your body's natural defenses by improving circulation, reducing stress hormones that suppress immunity, and ensuring that your cells get the oxygen they need to function optimally.

Qi gong breathing combines gentle movement with focused breathing to strengthen what Traditional Chinese Medicine calls *Wei Qi* (defensive energy):

1. Stand with your feet shoulder-width apart in a relaxed posture.

2. Place one hand on your belly and the other on your chest.

3. Begin tapping your chest gently with loose fists, alternating hands.

4. As you tap, breathe deeply into your belly (known as diaphragmatic breathing).

5. Continue for one to two minutes, focusing on the sensation of energy building in your chest.

This technique has been shown to improve heart rate variability (HRV), which is linked to better immune function:

1. Sit comfortably with your spine straight.

2. Inhale through your nose for a count of four.

3. Exhale through your nose for a count of six.

4. Maintain this four-second inhale, six-second exhale pattern for ten minutes.

   Practice twice daily for optimal benefits.

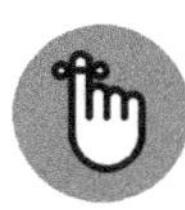

Breathing exercises for immunity work best when combined with other healthy practices like proper nutrition, adequate sleep, and regular physical activity.

Doing breathing exercises after surgery

Surgery puts your body through a lot, and proper breathing afterward is crucial for preventing complications like pneumonia and helping your body heal efficiently.

Diaphragmatic breathing is a great practice for recovery. Another good exercise is breath stacking, which helps increase your lung capacity after surgery. Follow these steps for breath stacking:

1. Inhale normally through your nose, and exhale completely through your nose or pursed lips.

2. On your next inhale, breathe in a little more deeply than before, and exhale normally.

3. Continue this pattern, breathing in a little more deeply each time, until you reach your normal, comfortable capacity.

4. **Hold this breath for three seconds before exhaling completely.**

5. **Repeat ten times, several times a day.**

Check with your doctor if this exercise is a good one for you after surgery. If so, go ahead and gently yet consistently keep practicing.

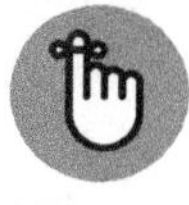

Taking deep breaths doesn't mean over-breathing. It means to breathe low down, in your diaphragm. Your chest doesn't need to expand much — mostly just your belly expands.

Improving circulation and oxygen delivery

Every cell in your body needs oxygen to function, and proper breathing ensures that they get it. Better circulation means better overall health, from your brain to your toes.

The following full-breath sequence helps maximize oxygen intake and distribution throughout your body:

1. **Sit or stand with good posture, shoulders relaxed.**

2. **Place one hand on your belly and one on your chest.**

3. **Inhale slowly through your nose, first filling your lower lungs (your belly will expand) and then your upper chest.**

4. **Hold briefly at the top of the inhalation.**

5. **Exhale slowly through pursed lips, emptying your chest first and then your belly.**

6. **Repeat five to ten times.**

Alternating-Nostril Breathing (Chapter 12) is another good exercise to improve circulation and oxygen delivery.

Breathing to manage long COVID

Long COVID symptoms can persist for months after infection, affecting your energy, breath capacity, and overall well-being. Targeted breathing exercises can help manage these lingering effects.

Research shows that the following resonant breathing technique can help relieve long COVID symptoms:

1. **Find a comfortable seated position.**

2. **Using a ten-second breathing cycle, inhale through your nose for four seconds, and exhale through your nose for six seconds.**

3. **Maintain this 4:6 ratio for ten minutes.**

   Practice twice daily, morning and evening.

If available, using an HRV app on your phone with a chest strap heart rate monitor can help you track your progress with resonant breathing exercises.

The following Gradual Breath Extension exercise helps rebuild lung capacity that may have been diminished by COVID:

1. **Start by taking comfortable breaths, noticing your current breathing pattern.**

2. **Gradually extend your inhale by one count each breath (start with inhaling for two counts, then three, then four).**

3. **When you reach a comfortable maximum inhale length, begin extending your exhale in the same way.**

4. **Work up to a ratio where your exhale is slightly longer than your inhale.**

5. **Practice daily, increasing duration as your capacity improves.**

Managing Pain and Discomfort

Pain has a fascinating relationship with your breath. Notice how you tend to hold your breath when in pain? That actually makes pain worse! Learning to breathe through discomfort can be a powerful tool for pain management.

Reducing physical pain with breathwork

Breathing exercises are among the most effective drug-free pain management techniques available. They work by reducing muscle tension, releasing *endorphins* (natural chemicals your body makes to help reduce pain and boost feelings of pleasure or well-being), and calming your nervous system's pain response.

This simple practice of Focused Breath Awareness for Pain helps shift attention away from pain and toward the soothing rhythm of breath:

1. **Find a comfortable position that minimizes your pain.**

2. **Close your eyes if that helps you focus.**

3. **Breathe normally for a few cycles, simply observing your natural breath.**

4. **Begin to deepen your breath slightly, making it slower and more regular.**

5. **As you inhale, imagine breathing *toward* the painful area.**

6. **As you exhale, imagine breathing *out* from the painful area, releasing tension.**

7. **Continue for five to ten minutes.**

The Breath Counting technique engages your mind, helping to break the pain-focus cycle:

1. **Sit or lie comfortably.**

2. **Breathe naturally and begin counting your breaths.**

3. **Count "one" on your first inhale, "two" on your exhale, "three" on the next inhale, and so on.**

4. **When you reach ten, start over at one.**

5. **If your mind wanders (which is normal), simply return to counting wherever you left off.**

6. **Practice for 5 to 15 minutes when experiencing pain.**

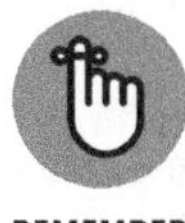

Breathwork for pain management works best when practiced regularly, not just when pain is severe. Daily practice helps train your nervous system to respond more effectively when pain does occur.

Easing headaches

I used to get headaches now and then. Not severe, but enough to disrupt my day. At first, I'd push through, which only made me irritable and less productive. Over time, I noticed my breathing grew shallow and tense during headaches, so I turned to breathing exercises instead of painkillers. A simple pattern — inhale for four, exhale for six, rest for two — calmed my mind and eased tension. I added gentle neck stretches and self-massage, which often brought quick relief. These small practices became my go-to for managing and even preventing headaches.

Try the following headache relief breathing exercise:

1. **Find a quiet, comfortable spot where you won't be disturbed.**

2. **Sit upright in a chair or lie down in a relaxed position; close your eyes, if that feels comfortable, and rest your hands gently on your thighs or stomach.**

3. **Take a moment to notice your natural breathing pattern.**

   Inhale slowly through your nose and exhale gently through your mouth. Don't force the breath — just observe its natural rhythm.

4. **Take a gentle, deep breath in through your nose, counting silently to four.**

   As you breathe in, focus on expanding your belly, rather than your chest. Imagine drawing in soothing, fresh air.

5. **Exhale slowly through pursed lips, as if you're blowing out a candle, for a count of six.**

   Let the breath be longer and more deliberate than the inhale. As you exhale, imagine releasing all tension from your forehead, temples, and neck.

6. **After the exhale, pause for a count of two before starting the next breath.**

   This brief hold helps your nervous system reset and encourages a sense of calm.

7. **Continue with the pattern — inhale for four, exhale for six, pause for two — ten times.**

   With each cycle, allow your shoulders to drop and your facial muscles to soften, feeling the headache tension gradually ease.

8. **After you've completed ten cycles, let go of the counting; simply observe your breath and how it now feels.**

   Stay here for a few minutes, enjoying the calm and relief you've created. If needed, repeat the exercise again.

In one of my workshops, I had a student who suffered from migraines for years. She was taking lots of medication, but she said that after a while, the medication wasn't effective and sometimes made it worse. So, she started doing mindfulness and breathing exercises. Within a few months, her migraines began to ease for the first time in years.

For tension headaches, combine breathing exercises with gentle neck stretches: As you exhale, gently tilt your head to one side, bringing your ear toward your shoulder without raising your shoulder. On the next breath cycle, tilt your head to the other side. Repeat.

Relieving muscle tension

Tense muscles and breathing are in a continual feedback loop — tension leads to shallow breathing, which increases tension. Breaking this cycle with intentional breathing can release chronic muscle tightness.

Just half a minute of focused breathing can begin to release muscle tension:

1. **Identify an area of tension in your body.**

2. **Place one hand on this area if possible.**

3. **Take four gentle, deep, slow breaths, focusing on the tense area.**

4. **With each exhale, mentally direct the muscles to soften and release.**

5. **After the fourth breath, gently move or stretch the area.**

Proper diaphragmatic breathing (see Chapter 7 helps release chronic tension patterns, too.

If muscle tension is accompanied by severe or persistent pain, talk to your health-care provider to rule out serious conditions.

Doing breathing exercises for labor

When labor kicks in, your body is doing one of the most powerful things it can do. That can feel exciting, intense, and sometimes understandably overwhelming. That's where breathing comes in. Although you can't control the contractions, you can control your breath. And that's a game changer.

Breathing exercises during labor help you stay calm, focused, and more in tune with your body. They can ease pain, reduce anxiety, and even help make the pushing phase shorter! Studies show that breathing exercises activate the body's relaxation response, releasing feel-good and pain-relieving hormones like endorphins and reducing stress hormones like cortisol. This helps you ride the waves of contractions with greater confidence and less pain.

There's no need to memorize complicated techniques. In fact, the simpler the better. Think of it as breathing with awareness and intention. Here are a few favorites used by midwives and taught in many prenatal classes:

>> **Deep diaphragmatic breathing:** Breathe in slowly through your nose, keeping your shoulders down and feeling your belly rise. Exhale slowly through your mouth. Do this between contractions to rest and recover. Learn more about how to do this in Chapter 7.

>> **Pursed-Lips Breathing:** Inhale gently through your nose and exhale slowly through pursed lips — like you're blowing gently on a candle flame to make it flicker, but not so much that it goes out. Great for staying calm when contractions build. Get the full instructions in Chapter 11.

>> **Rhythmic breathing for contractions:** As a contraction builds, breathe in for a count of four and out for a count of six or eight. Let your breath be your rhythm. Some people prefer shorter or longer counts — go with what feels natural.

>> **During pushing:** When it's time to push, you can either go with your natural urge to bear down or be coached to take a deep breath, hold it, and push during the contraction. Either way, your breath helps guide the effort.

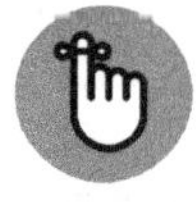

Don't worry if you forget the "right" way to breathe. Labor is not a test. Just come back to your breath, and let it support you, one wave at a time. Many women say that learning to breathe during labor gave them a sense of control and calm, even when things got intense. And that's something you can carry into parenting, too.

Practice these breathing techniques regularly during pregnancy so they become second nature when labor begins. Your birth partner can practice with you and help remind you to use them during labor.

Enhancing Digestive and Postural Health

You may not immediately connect breathing with digestion or posture, but they're surprisingly interrelated. Your breathing pattern affects how your internal organs function and how your body aligns itself.

Supporting digestion through breath awareness

The way you breathe impacts your digestive efficiency by affecting your nervous system, stomach acidity, and the physical movement of your digestive organs.

Taking a few moments to breathe properly before eating helps activate your parasympathetic ("rest-and-digest") nervous system:

1. **Before meals, sit comfortably at the table.**

2. **Close your eyes and place one hand on your belly.**

3. **Take five slow, deep breaths, focusing on the expansion and contraction of your abdomen.**

   Allow each exhale to be slightly longer than each inhale.

4. **Open your eyes and begin your meal in a more relaxed state.**

The following type of breathing provides a gentle massage to your digestive organs:

1. **Sit comfortably or lie on your back after a meal.**

2. **Place both hands on your belly, just below your ribs.**

3. **Breathe deeply into your belly, feeling it expand under your hands.**

   Be gentle if you feel very full. Even a bit of diaphragmatic breathing helps.

4. **Exhale slowly and completely, feeling your belly fall.**

5. **Continue for five to ten minutes to support the digestive process.**

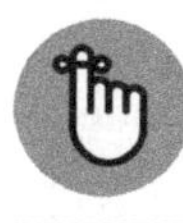

Deep breathing is like giving your digestive system a gentle massage from the inside. When you breathe deeply, your diaphragm moves up and down, creating a massaging action on your stomach and intestines. Additionally, deep breathing flips a switch in your nervous system from "stressed-out" mode to "chill-and-digest" mode. When you're stressed, your body basically says, "Forget about digesting that sandwich — we've got emergencies to handle!" and diverts blood away from your digestive organs. Deep breathing tells your body, "Hey, relax, it's time to properly process that food," which helps with everything from acid reflux to irritable bowel syndrome (IBS) symptoms. So, if your stomach is acting up, try some diaphragmatic breathing — it's free, it has no side effects, and it works better than you'd think!

Improving posture with diaphragmatic breathing

Poor posture can restrict your breathing, and conversely, improper breathing can reinforce poor posture. Breaking this cycle improves both.

The following exercise helps you experience how posture affects your breath capacity:

1. **Sit slumped forward with rounded shoulders and take a deep breath; notice how it feels.**

2. **Now sit up tall with your spine aligned and shoulders relaxed, and take another deep breath.**

3. **Feel the difference in how much air you can inhale in each position.**

4. **Practice breathing deeply while maintaining good posture for two to three minutes.**

The following exercise helps realign your posture while optimizing breath:

1. **Stand with your back against a wall, heels about 6 inches from the wall.**

2. **Press your lower back, your upper back, and the back of your head against the wall.**

3. **Take deep diaphragmatic breaths, focusing on expanding your ribs outward in all directions.**

   Place your hands on the sides of your lower ribs to feel this expansion.

4. **Practice for five minutes daily to reinforce proper breathing and posture.**

Set posture reminders on your phone or computer. When the reminder sounds, check your posture and take three deep, diaphragmatic breaths.

Aligning the body for better comfort

Proper alignment combined with effective breathing can dramatically reduce discomfort from poor posture and restricted breath.

The following exercise helps release tension from misalignment:

1. **Lie on your back on a firm surface, knees bent and feet flat.**

2. **Place a small cushion under your head if needed for comfort.**

3. Allow your spine to lengthen and your shoulders to drop away from your ears.

4. Place one hand on your chest and one on your belly.

5. Take ten slow, deep breaths, focusing on moving only your belly hand.

6. Feel your body settling into the surface with each exhale.

For times when you need to sit for long periods, try this:

1. Sit on a chair with your feet flat on the floor, hip-width apart; position your knees directly above your ankles.

2. Sit tall from your sit bones, imagining a string pulling up from the crown of your head.

3. Drop your shoulders down and back, away from your ears.

4. Take five deep breaths, feeling your ribs expand in all directions.

5. Repeat this posture check and breathing reset every 30 minutes when sitting.

Doing breathing exercises for weight loss

Breathing alone won't melt away pounds, but certain breathing techniques can support weight management by reducing stress hormones, increasing oxygen for metabolism, and improving exercise efficiency.

The Metabolism-Boosting Breath technique enhances oxygen intake, which is crucial for efficient cellular metabolism:

1. Stand or sit with good posture.

2. Inhale deeply through your nose for a count of four, filling your lungs completely.

3. Hold your breath for a count of four.

4. Exhale forcefully through your mouth for a count of four, contracting your abdominal muscles to push all the air out.

5. Without pausing, begin the next inhale.

6. Repeat for ten cycles, one to three times daily.

Stress can trigger weight gain through cortisol release. This calming technique helps manage stress-related eating:

1. Lie on your back in a comfortable position.

2. Place one hand on your chest and the other just below your rib cage.

3. Breathe in slowly through your nose, feeling your stomach rise while keeping your chest still.

4. Exhale slowly through pursed lips, gently contracting your abdominal muscles.

5. Practice for five to ten minutes daily, especially before meals or during food cravings.

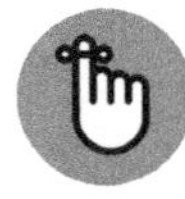

Breathing exercises complement — but don't replace — a healthy diet and regular physical activity for weight management. They work best as part of a comprehensive approach.

This more active breathing practice can help increase energy for physical activity:

1. Stand with feet hip-width apart, arms at your sides.

2. Inhale deeply using your nose while raising your arms out to the sides and up overhead.

3. Hold briefly at the top.

4. Exhale forcefully from your mouth while bringing your arms down and bending forward from the waist (only as far as comfortable).

5. Inhale through the nose while returning to standing, arms rising again.

6. Repeat ten times, moving with your breath.

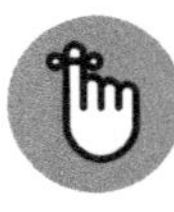

The key to benefiting from these exercises is consistency. Even a few minutes of focused breathing each day can lead to significant improvements in how you feel and function. So, don't hold your breath waiting for better health — breathe your way there instead!

CAN BREATHING HELP WITH DIABETES?

If you've got diabetes, your breath may be more powerful than you think. When you're stressed, your body releases hormones like cortisol and adrenaline, which can raise your blood sugar and make insulin less effective — basically, the opposite of what you want.

That's where breathing exercises come in. Taking slow, deep breaths, especially into your belly, can help switch on your body's "rest-and-digest" system (officially known as the parasympathetic nervous system). This helps calm your mind and reduce stress, and it may even help steady your blood sugar.

Simple techniques like Pursed-Lips Breathing, Alternate-Nostril Breathing, or finding a relaxed, rhythmic pace can all support your body in feeling more at ease. And when your body is more relaxed, it's easier to manage things like blood sugar and even heart health.

Of course, breathing exercises aren't meant to replace your medication, healthy eating, or regular movement. But they can be a helpful extra tool in your diabetes care kit. Just check with your doctor before you start, especially if you've got other health conditions or complications.

Chapter **12**

Energizing Your Day

Ever had one of those mornings when your alarm goes off and you feel like you've been hit by a truck? Or felt that midafternoon slump where your eyelids weigh more than your lunch? We've all been there. In today's world, maintaining energy throughout the day can feel like trying to keep your phone charged without a power bank — nearly impossible.

But what if I told you that your breath — yes, that automatic thing you're doing right now without thinking — could be your personal energy generator? No triple-shot espressos, just your lungs and a few minutes of your time.

In this chapter, you explore how specific breathing techniques can transform your energy levels from "barely functioning" to "ready to conquer the world." Whether you're a morning zombie or an afternoon slumper, these breathing exercises will be your new best friends.

Practicing Energy Breathing Safely

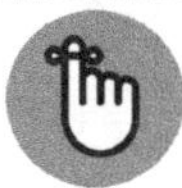

Although breathwork is beneficial, it's crucial to practice safely:

REMEMBER

» **Listen to your body.** If you feel dizzy or uncomfortable, stop and return to normal breathing.

- Before starting, do a quick body scan. Notice your current energy level, tension areas, and overall mood.

- During practice, pay attention to subtle changes in temperature, heart rate, and mental clarity.

- After each session, observe how you feel for five to ten minutes to assess the technique's effectiveness.

- Keep a brief breathwork journal, noting which techniques work best at different times of day or in various emotional states.

- If you feel dizzy or uncomfortable or if you experience any unusual sensations, stop immediately and return to normal breathing.

- Trust your instincts. If something doesn't feel right, it probably isn't right for you at that moment.

>> **Adjust intensity.** Energy breathing isn't one-size-fits-all. Adjust the techniques you use based on your current energy levels and daily requirements:

- On low-energy days, start with gentler techniques like deep belly breathing before progressing to more vigorous practices.

- When you're already feeling energized, focus on balancing techniques, like alternate-nostril breathing (more about that later in the chapter).

- Experiment with the duration and intensity of each technique to find your sweet spot.

>> **Recognize the signs of overexertion.** Energy breathing should invigorate you, but overdoing it can lead to adverse effects. Watch for these signs:

- Persistent lightheadedness or dizziness

- Tingling sensations in your arms, hands, legs, or feet

- Unusual fatigue after practice

- Headaches or nausea

If you experience any of these symptoms, return to normal breathing and reduce the intensity or duration of your practice.

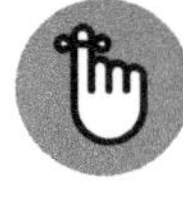

The goal is to energize, not exhaust. Listen to your body and adjust accordingly.

REMEMBER

By incorporating these safe and effective breathing techniques into your daily routine, you can maintain high energy levels, manage stress, and stay focused throughout your day. Your breath is a powerful tool — use it wisely to transform your energy and your life.

Morning Energy Boosters

Everyone wants to start the day feeling positive and energized. One way is to use practices like meditation or even mindful breathing. But what if you're looking for a more direct way to boost your energy? Read on to find out how.

Starting your morning right

Picture this: Your alarm blares at 6 a.m. You groan, hit Snooze three times, and eventually drag yourself out of bed feeling like you've aged 50 years overnight. Sound familiar? Before you stumble to the coffee pot on autopilot, consider this: Your breath may be the most underutilized wake-up tool at your disposal.

The way you breathe in those first few minutes after waking can set the tone for your entire day. Most people wake up breathing shallowly, in just the chest, which keeps them in that groggy, half-asleep state. Your body needs to fire up your systems, and those shallow breaths just aren't cutting it.

TRY THIS

I like to start the day with an equal in and out breath like coherent breathing (see Chapter 8). But you may want something even more energizing. In that case, try this simple morning ritual, the 4-6 Morning Energizer, before your feet even hit the floor:

1. **Upon waking, remain in bed and place one hand on your chest and one on your belly.**

2. **Take five deep, intentional breaths, inhaling through your nose for a count of four.**

3. **Feel your belly rise first, then your chest.**

4. **Exhale slowly through your mouth for a count of six, making a slight "whoosh" sound.**

   With each exhale, imagine releasing the heaviness of sleep.

This simple practice delivers a quick oxygen boost to your brain and tissues, signaling to your body that it's time to wake up and get moving. It's like pressing the "on" switch for your metabolism and alertness.

TRY THIS

But don't stop there. When you're vertical, stand by your bed or near a window and try this energizing stretch-and-breathe combo:

1. **Stand with your feet hip-width apart, arms at your sides.**

2. **Inhale deeply through your nose as you raise your arms overhead in front of you, reaching toward the ceiling.**

3. **Hold for a moment at the top.**

4. **Exhale forcefully through your mouth as you bring your arms down quickly.**

5. **Repeat five times.**

This movement, paired with breath, helps circulate blood and oxygen throughout your body, especially to your brain where you need it most in the morning. It's like turning on all the lights in your house rather than fumbling around in the dark.

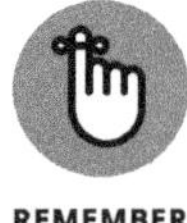

REMEMBER

Morning hydration supports healthy breathing. Your airways need moisture to work well, so before reaching for coffee, drink a glass of room-temperature water to rehydrate after the night's fast. It's like priming the pump before starting the engine.

COFFEE OR BREATHWORK? YOUR BRAIN'S TAKE

Imagine this: It's 3 p.m., your eyelids are staging a protest, and your mouse hand keeps drifting toward the coffee mug like it's magnetic. We've all been there — craving a caffeine hit to power through the afternoon fog. But what if your breath could do the same job, without the jitters?

Turns out, both breathwork and coffee trigger similar chemical changes in the brain. Techniques like Kapalabhati or Breath of Fire (covered in this chapter) stimulate the release of adrenaline and dopamine — those same buzzy neurotransmitters that coffee lovers rely on. But here's the twist: Breathwork gives you the lift without the crash. One study even found that regular controlled breathing boosts focus and alertness better than coffee, and it doesn't mess with your sleep later.

So, next time you're tempted to fire up the espresso machine, try some breathing exercises you enjoy instead. Your nervous system will get a workout, your brain will get a boost, and you'll still be able to fall asleep without counting sheep at 2 a.m. Breath: It's like espresso for the soul.

Energizing techniques

Now that you've mastered some gentle awakening breaths, it's time to shift into high gear with two powerhouse techniques that can rocket your energy levels into the stratosphere. Think of these as your natural energy drinks — no artificial ingredients required, and no afternoon crash, guaranteed.

These techniques aren't ones to approach casually. They're potent tools that require respect, proper technique, and gradual progression. But when practiced safely and consistently, they can become your secret weapons against sluggish mornings and afternoon energy dips.

In the next section, I introduce you to two energizing rapid-breathing techniques: Skull Shining Breath and Breath of Fire. These practices are powerful and stimulating, so it's important that you approach them only if you're in good physical and mental health.

Please avoid rapid-breathing practices such as Skull Shining Breath or Breath of Fire if you:

>> Have heart disease, high or low blood pressure, or cardiovascular issues

>> Have a respiratory condition, such as asthma, bronchitis, or chronic obstructive pulmonary disease (COPD)

>> Have epilepsy, a seizure disorder, or a neurological condition

>> Have had surgery recently, particularly abdominal surgery

>> Have a hernia, gastric ulcer, or spinal disorder

>> Have an eye condition such as glaucoma or a detached retina

>> Have an artificial pacemaker or a blood vessel stent

>> Are at any stage of pregnancy or are trying to conceive

>> Have any other health conditions that could be impacted by stressing your body

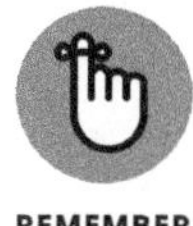

If these warnings leave you in doubt, choose gentler breathing practices. I recommend doing more vigorous exercises only with an experienced, well-qualified practitioner and when you're in good health. I prefer to focus on practicing and sharing slower, gentler breathing exercises with my clients. The benefits of breath can be gained through safer techniques that don't carry these risks.

Shining Skull (Kapalabhati)

If the previous gentle awakening exercises were like turning on your car's engine, Kapalabhati (which means "Shining Skull" in Sanskrit) is like shifting into fifth gear on the highway. This powerful yogic breathing technique is like a natural espresso shot for your system, with a particularly prominent effect on the skull and brain.

Kapalabhati works by rapidly expelling air through quick, forceful exhalations while allowing inhalations to occur passively. This creates a pumping action in your abdominal region that massages your internal organs, increases oxygen circulation, and stimulates your nervous system. The result? A clear mind and energized body in just a few minutes.

Before you do Shining Skull breath, make sure you've read the warning at the beginning of the "Energizing techniques" section to make sure it's safe for you.

You may want to have tissues handy — this exercise is the same as blowing your nose!

Before you try it, keep this in mind to practice safely:

>> Start with short sessions (for example, just five breaths to begin with).

>> Focus on the forceful exhalation, letting the inhalation happen naturally.

>> Keep your shoulders and face relaxed.

>> Stop immediately if you feel lightheaded or dizzy.

>> Especially avoid this exercise if you have high blood pressure, have a medical condition, or are pregnant.

>> Practice on an empty stomach

Here's how to practice Kapalabhati for beginners:

1. **Sit comfortably with a straight spine, either cross-legged on the floor or in a chair with feet flat on the ground.**

2. **Place your hands on your knees or in your lap.**

3. **Take a deep breath in through your nose.**

4. **Begin with a forceful exhalation through your nostrils by contracting your diaphragm and pulling your lower abdomen inward.**

   Think of tucking your tummy in to generate the power to force the air out in one big spurt.

5. **Allow your inhalation to happen automatically through your nose too, relaxed as your belly naturally returns to its normal position.**

   Don't put any effort into breathing in.

6. **Repeat this pattern for five cycles.**

   One exhalation plus one passive inhalation equals one cycle.

7. **At the end of your round, take a deep inhalation through your nostrils, hold your breath for as long as comfortable, and then exhale and observe your natural breathing.**

8. **After relaxing for a bit, perform another round of five cycles, followed by the breath holding and relaxation.**

9. **Complete up to three total rounds, allowing plenty of time to relax between each one.**

Very gradually work up to three rounds of 30 breath cycles over some weeks or months, if it feels comfortable and safe to do so. With experience, you can do three rounds of 30 breaths each morning, for example.

When you first try Kapalabhati, you may feel a bit dizzy or light-headed. That's normal — it's just your body adjusting to the increased oxygen and reduced carbon dioxide. If this happens, stop and return to normal breathing until you feel steady again.

TIP

Here's a great tip most practitioners don't realize: Kapalabhati can be done at different levels: mild, medium, or strong. It can be done as mildly as a normal breathing pace. Be flexible and adjust the exercise to your body and needs today. Every day and every moment is different.

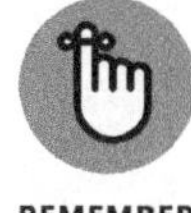

REMEMBER

The power in Kapalabhati comes from the exhale, not the inhale. Focus on making your exhalations sharp and strong, like you're blowing out a candle from a foot away.

The benefits of making Kapalabhati part of your morning routine are numerous:

>> It clears mucus from the lungs and sinuses. (Goodbye, morning congestion!)

>> It stimulates the liver, spleen, pancreas, and digestive organs.

>> It increases metabolism. (Hello, calorie burning!)

>> It improves focus and mental clarity.

>> It energizes the nervous system.

>> It strengthens the abdominal muscles. (You get a mini workout while sitting still!)

Many practitioners report that regular Kapalabhati practice reduces their dependence on caffeine. I'm not suggesting you throw away your beloved coffee maker just yet, but you may find yourself naturally reaching for that second cup less often.

For maximum benefit, practice Kapalabhati before eating breakfast. On a full stomach, this exercise can be uncomfortable and less effective. Think of it as preparing your digestive system for the day ahead — like preheating an oven before baking.

Breath of Fire (Agni Pran)

If Kapalabhati is like driving on the highway, Breath of Fire is like taking your sports car onto the racetrack. This technique, borrowed from Kundalini yoga traditions, is one of the most powerful energizing breaths in our respiratory toolkit.

Make sure you've read the warning at the beginning of the "Energizing techniques" section before trying this one.

Breath of Fire (also called Agni Pran) involves continuous, rapid breathing through the nose with equal emphasis on the inhale and exhale. While it might look similar to Kapalabhati at first glance, there's a key difference: in Breath of Fire, both the inhale and exhale are active and equally forceful, creating a continuous, rhythmic pumping of the belly.

Before you start, keep this in mind to practice safely:

>> Begin with 30-second intervals.

>> Ensure equal force in both inhalation and exhalation.

>> Maintain a steady rhythm without strain.

>> Especially avoid if you have high blood pressure, have a medical condition, or are pregnant.

Here's how to ignite your inner fire:

1. **Sit with a straight spine, either cross-legged or in a chair.**

2. **Rest your hands on your knees or in your lap.**

3. **Begin by taking a few normal breaths to center yourself.**

4. **Start breathing rapidly through your nose, making both inhales and exhales equal in duration.**

   Your belly should move in with each exhale and out with each inhale. Usually, a pace of about two or three breaths per second is recommended (yes, that's fast!). But as a beginner, it's much better to do whatever feels right for you — perhaps breathe in for one second and breathe out for one second. Keep your upper body, shoulders, and face relaxed despite the rapid pace.

   Begin with 10 seconds and gradually increase your duration.

5. **After about 30 seconds, take a deep breath in and hold it for as long as you can**

6. **Now breathe out consciously through your nose and continue to breathe naturally to give yourself time to recover.**

7. **After about a minute, repeat this cycle two more times.**

   Finish the exercise with some slow, deep breathing for a few breaths to center yourself.

When practiced correctly, Breath of Fire creates heat in the body (hence, the name) and produces a sensation of alertness and readiness. It's particularly effective on cold mornings when you need both physical warmth and mental clarity.

Over time and with experience, you can increase to doing one minute of this vigorous exercise, and then taking a break to observe your breathing. This whole cycle can be repeated three to five times.

Breath of Fire is powerful medicine! Start slowly and build up gradually. If you feel dizzy, develop a headache, or experience tingling in your extremities, stop immediately and return to normal breathing. The same warnings for Kapalabhati, count for Breath of Fire. Only practice this exercise if you're in good health.

The benefits of adding Breath of Fire to your morning routine include the following:

» It rapidly increases core body temperature.

» It expands lung capacity.

» It strengthens the nervous system.

» It filters the blood. (The rapid breathing increases circulation.)

» It balances the *glandular system* (the parts of your body that make and release hormones).

» It provides a natural "high" through increased oxygen and endorphin release.

>> It can clear your nasal passages, allowing you to breathe more freely after the exercise.

>> It can help build your core strength as it works your abdominal muscles and diaphragm.

TRY THIS

For an extra energy boost, try combining Breath of Fire with simple arm movements:

1. **Begin Breath of Fire as described earlier.**

2. **While maintaining the breath, extend your arms straight out in front of you at shoulder height.**

3. **Make fists with your hands.**

4. **Continue the breath while holding this position for 30 seconds.**

5. **Relax and breathe normally.**

This combination creates what practitioners call a "full system reset" — engaging your respiratory system, cardiovascular system, and muscular system simultaneously. It's like pressing Ctrl+Alt+Delete on your body's computer!

TRY THIS

To maximize the benefits of these morning breathing practices, try creating a sequence:

1. **Start with the gentle awakening breaths while still in bed.**

2. **Move to the stretch-and-breathe combo when you're up.**

3. **Practice a round of Kapalabhati.**

4. **Practice 30 to 60 seconds of Breath of Fire.**

5. **Finish with a couple of minutes of light, slow, deep breathing to channel your energy.**

The entire sequence takes less than ten minutes but can transform your morning experience from groggy and reluctant to energized and ready. And unlike that triple-shot latte, these techniques won't leave you crashing two hours later.

Staying Energized Midday

Starting your morning energized is all well and good, but you need to manage the afternoon, too. In this section, I explain how your breath can help.

Boosting midday energy with breathwork

It's 2:30 p.m. You've had lunch, you're staring at your computer screen, and your eyelids feel like they're being pulled down by invisible weights. The afternoon energy crisis has hit, and you're seriously considering crawling under your desk for a nap. Before you set up that makeshift pillow fort, consider how breathwork can rescue you from the notorious midday slump.

The post-lunch energy dip is actually a natural part of your *circadian rhythm* (your body's internal clock). Your core temperature drops slightly, and your brain produces a bit more *melatonin* (the sleep hormone). You can't eliminate this natural cycle completely, but strategic breathing can help you navigate through it without face-planting onto your keyboard.

I work from home quite often, so I like to do some calming breathing exercises while lying down in the afternoon. If I fall asleep, I end up having a rejuvenating power nap. I set a timer for 30 minutes so I don't fall asleep for too long and to prevent myself from waking up groggy. Usually, I feel much more energized after the breathing/nap, and I'm ready for what the afternoon has in store for me.

One way to energize yourself is a powerful breathing technique from yoga called Bhastrika, or bellows breathing. It's named after the bellows used to fan flames in a fire. Just as bellows draw in air and push it across hot coals to stoke heat, this breathwork pumps air in and out using the abdominal muscles and diaphragm, stimulating circulation and building inner heat. The result? More energy, improved digestion, and a stronger nervous system.

Before you jump in, keep in mind that this is a vigorous breathing practice. It's best done on an empty stomach. Don't force anything. Start small, build gradually, and listen to your body.

Follow these steps:

1. **Sit upright in a comfortable position with your spine straight. Rest your hands on your knees or lap. Gently close your eyes if that feels comfortable.**

2. **Begin by breathing slowly and deeply, allowing your abdomen to expand as you inhale.**

3. **When you're ready, exhale sharply through your nose by quickly pulling your abdominal muscles in; then allow a quick, automatic inhalation as your belly relaxes and your diaphragm draws air back in.**

4. **Repeat this rhythm — one strong exhale followed by a natural inhale.**

Try one breath per second, completing three rounds of seven to ten breaths, with a short rest of relaxed breathing between rounds.

Over time, you can increase the speed to two breaths per second, and work toward up to 120 breaths per round — but only if your breath stays smooth, even, and powerful.

The challenge is to synchronize your diaphragm and abdominal muscles. After the exhale, the diaphragm contracts to draw air in; then as the diaphragm relaxes, the abdominal muscles contract again for the next exhale. Both the inhale and exhale should feel equal in force and speed — and you'll hear both.

WARNING

Skip this practice if you're pregnant; you're menstruating; or you have high blood pressure, a heart condition, an ulcer, a hiatal hernia, or chronic constipation or panic disorder. And as always, if you're unsure, check in with your health-care provider.

This technique mimics the way you naturally breathe when you're excited or alert. By consciously adopting this breathing pattern, you're essentially telling your brain, "Hey! This is no time for sleep! Something exciting is happening!" Your brain responds by releasing stimulating neurotransmitters that increase alertness.

TRY THIS

For a quick energy reset that won't have your coworkers raising their eyebrows, try the Silent Energizing Breath:

1. **Sit or stand tall.**

2. **Inhale through your nose for a count of four, imagining you're drawing energy up from the ground through your feet.**

3. **Hold for just a moment at the top.**

4. **Exhale forcefully but silently through your nose for a count of four, imagining you're expelling fatigue and staleness.**

5. **Repeat ten times.**

This technique is subtle enough to use in a meeting or shared workspace but effective enough to give you a noticeable energy boost. The visualization component engages your mind, which helps break the cycle of afternoon drowsiness.

Reenergizing at your desk with breathing breaks

Let's face it: Many of us spend our workdays tethered to a desk, which is basically energy kryptonite. Sitting for prolonged periods reduces circulation, compresses your diaphragm, and encourages shallow chest breathing — all recipes for fatigue. But with strategic breathing breaks, you can transform your desk from an energy drain to an energy station.

The key is to schedule regular breathing breaks throughout your day. Set a timer on your phone or computer to remind you to take a two-minute breathing break every hour. These micro-interventions can prevent energy depletion before it happens, instead of trying to recover after you're already dragging.

Here's a simple desk-friendly breathing sequence:

1. **Set a timer for 2 minutes.**

2. **Push your chair back slightly from your desk.**

3. **Place both feet flat on the floor.**

4. **Rest your hands on your thighs.**

5. **Close your eyes (or lower your gaze if closing your eyes feels uncomfortable).**

6. **Take five deep "rectangle breaths": Inhale for a count of four, hold for a count of two, exhale for a count of four, hold for a count of two.**

7. **Follow with ten "energy sniffs": Inhale sharply through your nose in three quick sniffs to fill your lungs; then exhale in one long breath through your mouth.**

8. **Finish with five more rectangle breaths.**

This sequence takes just two minutes but provides multiple benefits: The rectangle breaths calm your nervous system, the energy sniffs increase oxygen intake, and the bookending effect creates a complete mini-reset for your system.

For an even more effective desk break, combine breathing with subtle movement:

1. **While seated, inhale deeply as you roll your shoulders up toward your ears.**

2. **Hold your breath briefly at the top.**

3. **Exhale completely as you roll your shoulders back and down.**

4. **On the next inhale, gently arch your back and look slightly upward.**

5. **On the exhale, round your spine slightly and look down.**

6. **Continue this breathing-movement coordination for one to two minutes.**

This technique counteracts the forward-hunched position most of us adopt at computers, which compresses the lungs and restricts breathing. By opening your chest and shoulders while breathing deeply, you're literally creating more space for oxygen — like upgrading from a studio apartment to a penthouse suite for your lungs.

Don't underestimate the power of a simple change in breathing location. If possible, take one of your breathing breaks near an open window or outdoors:

1. **Find a spot with fresh air.**

2. **Stand tall with feet hip-width apart.**

3. **Inhale deeply through your nose for five counts, raising your arms overhead in whatever way you want.**

4. **Hold for two counts at the top.**

5. **Exhale forcefully through your mouth for five counts, bringing your arms down.**

6. **Repeat ten times.**

The combination of fresh air, full-body movement, and intentional breathing creates a triple-threat energy boost. Plus, the brief exposure to natural light helps reset your circadian rhythm and reduce that afternoon melatonin surge that makes your eyelids heavy.

Resetting during afternoon slumps

Even with regular breathing breaks, sometimes the afternoon slump hits hard. Maybe you had a particularly heavy lunch or stressful morning, or maybe you're just not getting enough sleep at night. When you feel yourself sliding into that 3 p.m. energy crater, it's time to pull out the big guns — breathing techniques specifically designed for deep energy resets.

The Breath Walking technique is perfect for those moments when you feel like you may actually fall asleep at your desk:

1. **Get up and find a place where you can walk (even if it's just up and down a hallway).**

2. **Coordinate your breathing with your steps: Inhale for four steps, and exhale for four steps.**

3. **After a minute, shift to inhaling for four steps and exhaling for six steps.**

4. **Continue for three to five minutes.**

This technique combines the energizing benefits of movement with the focusing power of rhythmic breathing. The slight increase in carbon dioxide created by the longer exhalations increases the amount of oxygen getting into your cells, triggering your body's natural alertness response. Plus, the change in scenery and posture breaks the monotony that contributes to afternoon fatigue.

When you can't leave your desk but need a serious energy intervention, try the Coffee Breath (and no, it doesn't involve breathing coffee fumes):

1. **Sit up straight with your feet flat on the floor.**

2. **Place your hands in your lap or on your knees.**

3. **Inhale deeply through your nose.**

4. **Purse your lips as if you're drinking through a straw.**

5. **Exhale forcefully through this small opening, creating a focused stream of air.**

   Make the exhale audible — it should sound a bit like a whistle or the steam from an espresso machine.

6. **Repeat for 20 breaths.**

This technique creates back pressure in your respiratory system, which increases oxygen absorption in your lungs. The forceful exhalation also engages your core muscles, improving circulation and waking up your body. The auditory component — hearing your own breath — helps maintain focus and prevents your mind from drifting into sleepiness.

For those desperate moments when you're fighting to keep your eyes open during an important meeting or presentation, try this discreet technique called the Invisible Energizer:

1. **While seated normally, press your tongue firmly against the roof of your mouth.**

2. **Keeping your mouth closed, breathe rapidly in and out through your nose.**

3. **Simultaneously, tense the muscles in your feet and legs on the inhale; then release on the exhale.**

4. **Continue for 30 seconds.**

This combination of breathing, tongue pressure (which stimulates acupressure points), and muscle tension sends multiple awakening signals to your brain. The beauty of this technique is that it's nearly undetectable to others — your secret weapon against public drowsiness.

Another great, gentle technique to boost your energy is Light Slow Deep Breathing (see Chapter 9). Combine it with visualizing yourself breathing energy into all the cells in your body.

Managing Stress While Staying Energized

We've all been there — your boss drops a last-minute project on your desk, your presentation is in 20 minutes, and the projector just died, or you're stuck in gridlock traffic when you're already late. Your heart races, your breathing becomes shallow, and your energy scatters in a thousand directions. In these moments, you need techniques that both calm your stress response and maintain focused energy.

Staying calm during stressful situations

The challenge is finding that sweet spot: Too much calming breathwork may make you sleepy, while purely energizing techniques may amplify your stress. The solution? Balanced breathing techniques that simultaneously soothe your nervous system while maintaining alertness.

The Reset Button Breath is your first line of defense when stress hits:

1. **Wherever you are, pause and straighten your spine.**

2. **Place one hand on your chest and one on your belly.**

3. **Close your eyes if appropriate, or soften your gaze.**

4. **Inhale slowly through your nose for four counts, directing the breath first to your belly and then to your chest.**

5. **Hold for one count.**

6. **Exhale through slightly pursed lips for six counts, emptying your chest first and then your belly.**

7. **At the end of the exhale, contract your abdominal muscles to squeeze out the last bit of air.**

8. **Repeat three times.**

This technique works because the extended exhale activates your parasympathetic nervous system (the "rest-and-digest" response), while the complete emptying at the end of each breath cycle ensures full oxygen exchange and prevents shallow breathing patterns that often accompany stress. The gentle abdominal contraction also engages your core muscles, creating a physical anchor that helps ground you in the present moment.

Discovering Alternate-Nostril Breathing (Nadi Shodhana) for balance energy and focus

I still remember the first time I tried Alternate-Nostril Breathing. I was struggling to sit cross-legged on a yoga mat, unsure whether I was about to experience inner peace or accidentally poke myself in the eye. But as I settled into the rhythm, something subtle shifted. My thoughts slowed down, my mind felt clearer, and no injuries occurred — a bonus!

Alternate-Nostril Breathing (called Nadi Shodhana in yoga traditions) is a classic and popular exercise. It's easy to see why — the technique is simple yet profound. You gently close one nostril with your finger, inhale through the open side, switch fingers, then exhale through the other side. It sounds confusing — a bit like playing a nose flute — but you'll get used to it quickly.

This practice is believed to balance the left and right hemispheres of the brain, support the nervous system, and improve mental clarity. Whether or not you believe in the ancient energy channels it's based on, science is catching up: Studies show that Alternate-Nostril Breathing can lower stress, reduce heart rate, and improve attention.

Use Alternate-Nostril Breathing whenever you need a combination of calm and focus — for example, when you're feeling mentally scattered, you want to calm down before a meeting or performance, you need a natural energy boost without another cup of coffee, or you're transitioning between tasks and want to reset your focus.

PLAY THIS

Follow these steps to do the ancient and powerful exercise of Alternate-Nostril Breathing the easy way (or listen to Track 24):

1. **Get comfortable. Sit upright but relaxed, and rest one hand on your lap.**

2. **With your other hand, your thumb to close one nostril and your ring finger to close the other.**

    If that doesn't feel good, use your thumb and any of your other fingers.

3. **Start the cycle:**

    - Close your right nostril and inhale through the left.

    - Switch nostrils: Close the left nostril and exhale through the right.

    - Inhale through the right, and then switch and exhale through the left.

    That's one full round.

4. **Repeat for three to five minutes, or longer if you're enjoying it.**

TIP

Breathe light, slow, and deep for the most powerful effect. No need to force or strain yourself. The idea is to ease into balance, not blast your brain with air.

It may feel awkward at first, but that's completely normal. With a little practice, the movement becomes smooth and even soothing. Some people use a *mudra* (hand gesture) for elegance; others just do it in pajamas while watching TV. Both are valid.

As you practice, you may feel calmer, with more "centered" energy, as well as a weird sense of accomplishment from just breathing differently! If nothing happens right away, that's fine, too. Sometimes the magic is subtle. Think of it like adjusting a radio dial — getting the static out so you can hear yourself more clearly.

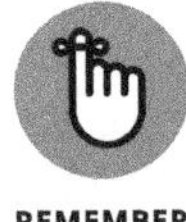

REMEMBER

If you're busy, doing just one or two cycles is fine, too. Notice how your body feels — you may be able to feel the difference even with one round of Alternate-Nostril Breathing.

Using the Infinity Breath to stay calm, centered, and balanced

In our fast-paced world, finding a balance between energy and focus can be a real challenge. Breathwork offers a simple yet powerful way to bring your body and mind into harmony, boosting your alertness while keeping you grounded.

One of the most accessible techniques for this is the Infinity Breath, also known as Figure-Eight Breath. It's a calming, rhythmic practice that gently recharges your system while sharpening mental clarity:

1. **Start by sitting or lying down comfortably.**

   If it feels okay, let your eyes rest or close.

2. **Begin to notice your breath coming in and going out.**

   There's no need to control anything at first. Just observe.

3. **Begin to gently adjust the rhythm so that your inhale and your exhale are roughly the same length.**

   Don't worry about counting — let it be intuitive. Like a gentle sway or a seesaw, allow your breath to find a steady rhythm that feels good to you.

4. **When the breath feels even and natural, imagine it forming a smooth circle.**

   As you breathe out, picture tracing one half of the circle. As you breathe in, complete the other half. There's no break between the two — just a soft, seamless flow. Let the image of the circle guide your breath and give your mind something to rest on. The simplicity of the shape helps settle your thoughts and draws you gently into the present.

5. **Now let the circle open out into a sideways figure eight — like the symbol for infinity.**

   As you breathe out, follow one loop of the eight. As you breathe in, trace the other. Let your breath move like a slow, graceful wave, flowing through the curves of the shape. There's no right or wrong way to imagine it. Your infinity may be small or wide, moving left to right or up and down. Go with whatever feels natural. Let it become a quiet rhythm that carries your attention with it.

This technique works by linking the breath with gentle visualization, which calms the nervous system and invites flow into both your body and your mind. The continuous, looping pattern helps smooth out erratic thoughts and brings a gentle rhythm that's both energizing and grounding. It's ideal when you want to feel present, focused, and lightly uplifted, without pushing or effort.

Avoiding burnout with restorative breathing

When you're burned out, even slowing down can feel exhausting. Forest Breath offers a gentle, imaginative way to restore calm, clarity, and rootedness, even if you're far from a forest.

The beauty of Forest Breath is that it combines mindful breathing with visualization, tapping into the healing power of nature through the imagination. It's especially helpful for people who feel overwhelmed or depleted but still want something soothing, light, and accessible.

Follow these steps:

1. **Sit or lie down somewhere quiet, where your body feels supported.**

    Let your shoulders drop and your hands rest gently in your lap or by your sides.

2. **Close your eyes or soften your gaze, and picture yourself standing in a peaceful forest.**

    It could be pine, oak, or whatever comes to mind. Visualize tall trees stretching above you, soft earth beneath your feet, and the scent of moss, bark, or cool air. Imagine light filtering through the canopy, dappled and golden.

3. **Inhale slowly through your nose for a count of four.**

    As you breathe in, imagine drawing in the scent of the forest — fresh, earthy, and calming.

4. **Hold the breath gently for a count of four, letting it settle in your body like mist clinging to the trees.**

5. **Exhale slowly through your nose for a count of six.**

    As you breathe out, imagine a breeze passing through the leaves or the quiet hush of forest stillness.

6. **Continue this breath cycle — inhaling for four, holding for four, exhaling for six — for several minutes.**

    Let the rhythm soothe your body and your mind. If thoughts arise, gently return to the imagery of the forest and the rhythm of your breath.

I shared this practice with a corporate coaching client who had worked in health care for more than two decades. She came to me completely burned out — physically, emotionally, and mentally drained from years of high-stress work. When I introduced her to Forest Breath, she was hesitant. "I'm not usually the visualization type," she said. But she agreed to try. A week later, she told me she'd begun doing it every evening before bed and sometimes midday to reset. She described it as a "mini-retreat," saying the forest imagery with the slow breath brought a peace she hadn't felt in years. Over time, Forest Breath became a key part of her healing, helping her reclaim stillness even on her busiest days. She later said, "That breath helped me come back to myself."

LAUGHTER: A SURPRISING BOOST FOR ENERGY . . . AND LUNG HEALTH

It turns out that laughter really *is* good medicine, not just for the soul, but for the lungs, too. When you laugh, your diaphragm and chest muscles tighten, giving your lungs a mini workout. This helps you exhale more fully, clearing out stale air and making room for fresh oxygen to flow deeper into the lungs. Laughter is thought to expand the tiny air sacs in your lungs (called the *alveoli*), improving oxygen exchange and boosting respiratory efficiency.

But there's more! Laughing lowers stress, improves mood, and triggers the release of *endorphins,* your body's natural feel-good chemicals. For people with chronic lung conditions like asthma or COPD, laughter may improve emotional well-being and, in some cases, even reduce *air trapping* (a major issue in COPD that leads to shortness of breath).

In fact, one leading lung doctor compared a hearty belly laugh to using a medical breathing device after surgery. It helps clear mucus and expands the lower lungs. So, if you needed an excuse to watch your favorite comedy, giggle with friends, or even attend a local laughter yoga class (yes, that is a thing), this is it. Your lungs will thank you.

Chapter **13**

Sleeping Soundly with Breathwork

Have you ever found yourself staring at the ceiling at 3 a.m., mentally calculating how many hours of sleep you would get if you dozed off "right now"? Or perhaps you fall asleep easily but wake up feeling as though you've spent the night running a marathon rather than resting? If so, you're not alone — I've had those experiences, too — and your breath may be the key to transforming your nights.

In this chapter, I explore how something as simple as changing the way you breathe can lead to profound improvements in your sleep quality. From falling asleep faster to staying asleep longer, the right breathing can make the difference between waking up like a zombie and waking up refreshed. I offer practical, effective, and sometimes surprising ways you can use your breath as your personal sleep medicine.

Understanding the Connection Between Breath and Sleep

When it comes to sleep, your breathing pattern is essentially a control switch for your nervous system, capable of signaling your body whether it's time for action or relaxation.

How breathing patterns influence sleep quality

The way you breathe directly impacts your sleep experience — the various stages and cycles your sleep goes through each night. When I first began researching sleep issues, I was astounded to discover how many people sabotage their sleep without realizing it, simply through dysfunctional breathing patterns.

Until I became aware of the power of healthy breathing, I kept waking up with a dry mouth and a slight headache. I thought it was normal. After tracking my sleep for a week, I noticed I was breathing through my mouth all night — hence, the dry mouth and headache. When I started using nasal strips at night, which helped open up my nostrils, and practicing some of the techniques I share later in this chapter, I started nose breathing all night. So all those morning headaches virtually disappeared. And no more dry mouth. I wake up feeling more fresh and rejuvenated. This small change in my breathing pattern transformed my sleep quality and subsequent energy levels throughout the day.

Here's what happens when your breathing pattern supports healthy sleep:

>> Your heart rate slows down as you exhale fully.

>> Your blood pressure stabilizes at lower levels.

>> Stress hormones like cortisol decrease.

>> *Melatonin* (the sleep hormone) can work more efficiently.

>> Your brain waves shift toward patterns associated with deep relaxation.

Conversely, rapid, shallow breathing keeps your body in a state of alertness — exactly what you don't want at bedtime. This type of breathing pattern is often associated with the fight-or-flight response, which evolved to keep our ancestors safe from predators but now keeps us awake worrying about tomorrow's presentation or an unanswered email.

The role of the nervous system in relaxation and sleep

Your autonomic nervous system has two main branches: sympathetic ("fight-or-flight") and parasympathetic ("rest-and-digest"). Think of these two branches, respectively, as the accelerator and brakes for your body. The sympathetic nervous system speeds things up — increasing heart rate, boosting alertness, and preparing you for action. The parasympathetic nervous system does the opposite — slowing things down, promoting digestion, and setting the stage for sleep and recovery.

Here's where breath comes in as a powerful tool: By changing how you breathe, you can switch from sympathetic being more dominant to parasympathetic being more dominant. Slow, deep breathing activates the vagus nerve, which is like the main control wire of your parasympathetic system. When stimulated through proper breathing, the vagus nerve broadcasts relaxation signals throughout your body.

One night, during a particularly stressful period when I had to give a presentation to thousands of people the next day, I found myself wide awake at 1 a.m., mind racing with thoughts of everything that could go wrong. Instead of reaching for my phone (the worst thing I could do!), I remembered my own teachings and began a slow breathing pattern, extending my exhales longer than my inhales. Within about ten minutes, I felt my thoughts slowing, my muscles relaxing, and sleep gently approaching. I've used this emergency sleep reset countless times since.

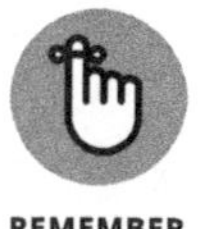

If you find all these breathing exercises confusing and want to relax, just breathe gently and try to breathe out for longer than you breathe in.

Common breathing mistakes that disrupt rest

Before I dive into what works, let me explain what doesn't. The following common breathing habits can sabotage your sleep before your head even hits the pillow:

>> **Chest breathing:** Many people breathe primarily using their chest muscles rather than their diaphragm. This shallow breathing pattern keeps the body in a mild stress state and reduces oxygen exchange efficiency. When you're in a stressed state, you can't sleep well.

>> **Mouth breathing:** Breathing through the mouth during sleep can lead to snoring, *sleep apnea* (a sleep disorder characterized by pauses in breathing or shallow breathing during sleep, which can lead to fragmented sleep and

daytime fatigue), dry mouth, tooth decay, and increased risk of respiratory infections. Humans evolved to breathe through the nose, which filters, warms, and humidifies the air before it reaches the lungs.

>> **Irregular breathing patterns:** Erratic breathing with random pauses, gasps, or changes in rhythm disrupts the steady flow of oxygen your brain needs during sleep.

>> **Breath holding:** Some people unconsciously hold their breath when stressed or focused — a habit that can continue during sleep, creating micro-awakenings you may not even remember.

>> **Over-breathing (also known as hyperventilation):** Breathing too deeply or too rapidly can actually reduce carbon dioxide levels below their optimal range, leading to symptoms like dizziness, numbness, and even insomnia.

A student in one of my workshops shared that she would wake up every morning feeling exhausted despite sleeping for eight hours. After using a phone app to record herself sleeping, she discovered she was mouth-breathing all night. Taping her mouth closed with special sleep tape transformed her sleep quality within days. Sometimes the simplest interventions yield the most dramatic results!

USING MOUTH TAPE SAFELY (YES, REALLY!)

You may have come across the idea of *mouth taping* on social media or wellness podcasts. It sounds a bit strange at first — like something your little brother or sister may have done to you as a prank — but there's a good reason it's become a hot topic in the world of breathing.

Whether mouth taping at night is a good idea is still being researched. Some experts say it is. Others say there isn't enough evidence yet, so let's wait and see. Anecdotal evidence suggests that, for some adults, it seems to totally transforms their sleep for the better.

Mouth taping at night is simply a tool to gently encourage breathing through your nose during sleep. Why? Because nasal breathing supports better oxygen uptake, helps humidify and filter the air, and may even reduce snoring. Some people find that taping their mouth shut at night leads to deeper, more restful sleep and fewer dry-mouth mornings.

But — and it's a big but — safety comes first.

If you have sleep apnea or suspect you might (especially if you snore loudly, wake up gasping, or feel exhausted in the morning), completely sealing your mouth shut with tape can be dangerous. And around 80 percent of people with sleep apnea don't even know they have it.

So, instead of using a full strip of tape across your mouth, many experts recommend a gentler option like a tiny piece of medical tape or something called MyoTape. This kind of tape surrounds the mouth instead of sealing it shut. It encourages nasal breathing but still allows your mouth to open if needed — which is ideal for those who may have undiagnosed sleep-disordered breathing. Another option is to use a tiny square piece of medical tape and use it in the middle of your lips, so you can breathe through the sides of your mouth if you need to.

Here's how to use mouth tape safely:

- **Choose the right tape.** Look for mouth tape designed specifically for sleep, like medical tape, MyoTape, or something similar. No strong adhesive tapes from the hardware store!

- **Apply the tape to clean, dry skin.** Make sure your lips and surrounding skin are clean and dry so the tape sticks properly. You may want to reduce the strength of the stickiness of the tape by sticking it on your hand and removing it a few times. If it's too sticky, it'll hurt when you remove it from your lips.

- **Start slow.** Try using mouth tape for 10 to 15 minutes during the day while reading or watching TV to get used to it.

- **Use it only if you can breathe well through your nose.** If you're congested or feel panicky with the tape on, stop. It's not for everyone.

- **Don't use it if you've been diagnosed with sleep apnea without speaking to a medical professional.** Safety first, always.

Warning: Never tape a child's mouth shut unless a medical professional says it's safe. Children with even mild nasal congestion, allergies, or undiagnosed sleep issues could be put at risk. Instead, focus on encouraging nasal breathing during the day — using gentle reminders, fun games, and breathing exercises to help build the habit naturally. Mouth tape can be a tool, but it's never a substitute for proper medical advice.

The goal isn't to *force* your body but to gently *nudge* it toward healthier breathing habits. As always, experiment mindfully and listen to your body.

Breathing exercises for sleep apnea

Sleep apnea is a big issue: It's estimated to affect a billion people worldwide. Serious cases require medical intervention, but the following breathing exercises can help strengthen the muscles involved in keeping airways open during sleep:

>> **Didgeridoo Breathing:** Research published in the *British Medical Journal* found that didgeridoo playing reduced sleep apnea symptoms. You don't need one of these Australian musical instruments, though — simply purse your lips and make a continuous humming sound while breathing out, creating resistance similar to playing the didgeridoo. Added bonus: This vibration will stimulate the vagus nerve, promoting relaxation.

>> **Tongue Slide:** Press your tongue flat against the roof of your mouth, and slide it backward while keeping contact with the roof of the mouth. Do this five to ten times before bed to tone the muscles that help keep airways open.

>> **Soft-Palate Stretch:** Open your mouth wide, saying "Ahhhh" for about 20 seconds. This stretches and strengthens the soft palate, helping to prevent collapse during sleep.

>> **Balloon Breathing:** Inflate a balloon with five long breaths (through your mouth), taking a brief rest between each breath. The resistance of the balloon strengthens your airway muscles. Start with one set and build up to five sets daily.

>> **Tiger Breath:** Extend your tongue out as far as is comfortable. Then breathe through your mouth with a slight constriction in your throat for ten breaths. This unusual technique tones multiple airway muscles simultaneously.

Switching to nasal breathing can help reduce the risk of sleep apnea, where the airway collapses during sleep. Mouth breathing can make this worse by allowing the tongue to fall back and block the airway. Some people use gentle mouth tape alongside their continuous positive airway pressure (CPAP) machine — a device that keeps your airway open by blowing a steady stream of air through a mask. In fact, studies suggest that mouth taping may help people stick with CPAP therapy more consistently. Just be sure to use tape that still allows for *mouth puffing* (in which small bursts of air escape through the lips during sleep), especially if you have sleep apnea or suspect you may have it.

These exercises aren't instant fixes, but regular practice can improve mild to moderate sleep apnea symptoms over time.

Research shows that specific breathing exercises can help reduce symptoms of obstructive sleep apnea, especially in mild to moderate cases. Exercises like inspiratory and expiratory muscle training (using special resistance devices) and *oropharyngeal* (mouth and throat) exercises strengthen the muscles involved in breathing and keeping the airway open, leading to improvements in sleep quality and reductions in snoring and apnea severity. Techniques such as diaphragmatic breathing and slow, controlled breathing may also support better sleep by calming the nervous system and promoting more stable breathing patterns. Currently, the strongest evidence supports muscle-strengthening approaches.

For severe cases, always follow your doctor's primary treatment recommendations while using these techniques as complementary approaches.

YOGA NIDRA: THE ANCIENT ART OF YOGIC SLEEP

Centuries ago, in the serene ashrams of India, yogis sought a state of consciousness that transcended ordinary sleep. They discovered *yoga nidra*, or "yogic sleep," a profound practice that induces deep relaxation while maintaining a thread of awareness.

In yoga nidra, practitioners lie in *Shavasana* (corpse pose) and are guided through a series of steps: setting a personal intention, rotating consciousness through the body, observing the breath, experiencing opposite sensations, and visualizing vivid imagery. This journey leads to a state between wakefulness and sleep, known as the *hypnagogic state,* in which the body rests deeply and the mind remains lucid.

Regular practice of yoga nidra has been shown to reduce stress, improve sleep quality, and enhance overall well-being. It's a testament to the timeless wisdom of ancient yogic practices, offering a sanctuary of rest in our modern, fast-paced world.

Here's how to do it in short form. To practice it properly, reach out to a yoga teacher or yoga nidra teacher, or find a guided audio on YouTube or in the Insight Timer app to take you through it.

1. **Lie down comfortably on your back, arms at your sides, palms facing upward.**

   Close your eyes and take a few deep breaths, allowing your body to relax completely.

2. **Mentally state a positive affirmation or heartfelt desire.**

   This intention plants a seed in the subconscious, guiding personal growth and transformation.

(continued)

(continued)

3. **Systematically bring awareness to different parts of your body, starting from the right hand thumb and moving through the body in a specific sequence.**

   This process promotes physical relaxation and mental stillness.

4. **Focus on the natural rhythm of your breath, observing the inhalation and exhalation without altering it.**

   This anchors your awareness and deepens relaxation.

5. **Engage in guided imagery, such as envisioning tranquil landscapes or experiencing contrasting sensations like warmth and coolness.**

   These techniques help release emotional tension and foster inner peace.

Looking at the Long-Term Benefits of Sleep-Focused Breathwork

Incorporating breathwork into your sleep routine isn't just about tonight's rest — it's an investment in your long-term health and well-being. Let's explore the lasting benefits of making breathing exercises a regular part of your bedtime ritual.

Improving energy and focus during the day

Quality sleep translates directly to better daytime performance. When I began teaching breathing exercises to corporate executives, many were skeptical about the connection between breath and productivity. However, after just two weeks of practicing presleep breathing techniques, most reported significant improvements in their energy levels, decision-making abilities, and creative thinking.

One notable case was a high-level banker who'd been relying on six cups of coffee daily to function. After implementing a ten-minute bedtime breathing routine for a month, he found himself naturally waking before his alarm and needing only one or two cups of coffee. His quarterly performance metrics showed an improvement of about 20 percent, which he attributed directly to better sleep quality.

The science supports these anecdotal results:

>> Proper sleep helps your brain clear waste through something called the *glymphatic system,* which is ten times more active during deep sleep.

>> Memory consolidation happens primarily during deep sleep phases, which are enhanced by proper breathing.

>> Emotional regulation centers in the brain restore themselves during quality sleep.

>> Hormones that control hunger and metabolism are balanced during proper sleep cycles.

Without quality sleep, these processes remain incomplete, leaving you operating at a fraction of your potential. The breathing exercises I cover don't just help you fall asleep — they enhance the quality of each sleep stage, maximizing these restorative benefits.

TECHNICAL STUFF

The *glymphatic system* (your brain's natural cleaning crew) is most active during deep sleep. That's why getting enough of all stages of sleep, especially the deeper one, is so important. Lighter, disrupted sleep, often caused by dysfunctional breathing, can interfere with this process, leaving your brain less able to clear out waste. When the glymphatic system can't do its job properly, toxins like amyloid-beta and tau proteins start to build up. These are the same proteins linked to Alzheimer's disease and other neurodegenerative diseases.

Reducing chronic sleep issues with regular practice

Consistency is key when it comes to using breathwork for sleep improvement. Think of it like exercise — one trip to the gym won't transform your fitness, but regular workouts over time create lasting change.

Many sleep issues develop gradually as poor breathing habits become ingrained. The good news is that positive breathing patterns can become automatic through regular practice. And improved daytime breathing habits impact nighttime breathing habits. Here's what you could expect to happen when you commit to sleep-focused breathwork over time:

>> **One to two weeks:** Initial improvements in falling asleep; occasional better nights.

>> **One month:** More consistent good nights; reduced time to fall asleep.

>> **Two to three months:** New breathing patterns becoming automatic; fewer nighttime awakenings.

>> **Six months:** Significant reduction in chronic sleep issues; breathing regulation occurring automatically during sleep.

>> **One year+:** Transformed sleep quality and potential resolution of long-standing sleep problems.

I witnessed this progression firsthand with a client recovering from her own sleep issues. After years of poor sleep following a particularly stressful period in her life, she committed to practicing specific breathing techniques every night before bed. The first week, she saw minimal improvements, but by the third month, her sleep was better than she'd experienced in decades.

The key is *neuroplasticity* — the brain's ability to rewire itself based on repeated experiences. Each time you practice optimal breathing before sleep, you strengthen the neural pathways that support healthy sleep patterns. Eventually, your breathing regulation during sleep improves automatically, without conscious effort.

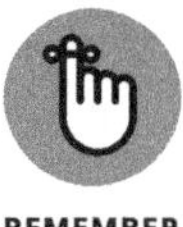

There's no hard-and-fast rule here. Some people notice a big improvement within just a few days — especially when using nasal strips or a little mouth tape. Even those with obstructive sleep apnea sometimes report almost immediate benefits. For many others, though, gentle, consistent breathwork over time is what really makes the difference.

Preparing Your Body for Restful Sleep

Creating the right conditions for sleep begins long before you climb into bed. Your presleep routine sets the stage for how quickly you'll drift off and how deeply you'll sleep through the night. Let's explore how to prepare your body and breathing for optimal rest.

Establishing a presleep breathing routine

The transition from daytime activity to nighttime rest isn't like flipping a switch — it's more like slowly dimming the lights. Your body needs clear signals that it's time to shift gears, and a dedicated breathing routine provides exactly that.

A few years ago, I was working with around a hundred team members at a corporate organization who struggled with sleep due to busy schedules. We developed what we called the 5-5-5 routine: five minutes of gentle movement, five minutes of journaling, and five minutes of structured breathing exercises. Within three weeks, 83 percent of attendees reported falling asleep faster and waking less during the night, despite their challenging schedules.

Here's a presleep breathing routine you can adapt to your own needs:

>> **Thirty-five to 40 minutes before bed**

- Begin limiting exposure to bright lights and screens (or use blue light filters).

- Do two to three minutes of gentle stretching, focusing on shoulders, neck, and back.

- Practice the Humming Breath (Bhramari Pranayama; see Chapter 6) for two minutes.

>> **Twenty to 25 minutes before bed:**

- Sit comfortably and practice Ocean Breath (Ujjayi; see Chapter 8) for three to five minutes, creating a soft restriction in the back of your throat to produce a gentle ocean sound.

- Follow with Alternate-Nostril Breathing (see Chapter 12 for three minutes to balance your nervous system.

>> **Ten minutes before bed:**

- Lie in bed and practice Wave Breathing — visualizing your breath as a wave that rises on the inhale and falls on the exhale, gradually making the exhales longer than the inhales.

- Transition to one of the sleep-inducing techniques I cover later in this chapter.

The beauty of this routine is its flexibility — you can shorten it to just five to ten minutes when time is limited, or expand it when you have more time to unwind. The key is consistency in signaling to your body that sleep is approaching.

Creating a calm environment with breath awareness

Your physical environment and your breathing pattern influence each other. A chaotic space can disrupt breathing, and irregular breathing can make even a calm environment feel stressful. Creating harmony between your space and your breath multiplies the benefits of both.

Consider these environment-breath pairings for optimal sleep preparation:

>> **Temperature regulation:** Keep your bedroom slightly cool (65°F to 68°F/18°C–20°C). Practice Cooling Breath by curling your tongue (or pursing your lips if tongue curling isn't possible), inhaling slowly through your mouth, and then exhaling through your nose. This ancient technique, called Sitali in yoga traditions, literally cools your body from the inside.

>> **Sound management:** If noise disrupts your sleep, try Droning Breath by cupping your hands lightly over your ears and breathing slowly and deeply, focusing on the natural sound of your breath. This creates a gentle sound barrier that masks external noises while promoting relaxation.

>> **Light control:** As you dim the lights, practice Darkness Cultivation Breath by closing your eyes and breathing normally while imagining each exhale carrying tension away and each inhale bringing in peaceful darkness, preparing your brain for sleep.

>> **Scent optimization:** If you're using sleep-promoting essential oils like lavender or chamomile, you can enhance their effect with Aroma Breath. Inhale slowly and quietly through your nose for a count of four, hold briefly at the top, and exhale through your nose for a count of six, imagining the calming scent traveling throughout your body.

One participant in my online breathing exercise workshop had a breakthrough when she realized her "calming" bedtime routine — checking email one last time, setting multiple alarms, and making to-do lists for the next day — was actually activating her stress response right before bed. By replacing these habits with environmental adjustments paired with specific breathing techniques, she transformed her presleep experience from anxiety-producing to genuinely relaxing.

Pairing stretching and relaxation techniques with breathwork

The mind-body connection is powerful — physical tension often leads to disrupted breathing, and vice versa. Combining gentle stretches with specific breathing patterns creates a synergistic effect, releasing physical tension while calming the mind.

To practice Seated Forward Bend with Extended Exhale, follow these steps:

1. **Sit on the edge of your bed with your legs extended.**

2. **Inhale for a count of four, lengthening your spine.**

3. **Exhale for a count of six, gently folding forward.**

4. **Continue for five to seven breaths, focusing on releasing back tension.**

To practice Child's Pose with Wave Breathing, follow these steps:

1. **Kneel with big toes touching, knees apart.**

2. **Fold forward, extending your arms or resting them alongside your body.**

3. **Breathe into your back, creating a gentle "wave" motion.**

4. **Make each exhale slightly longer than the inhale.**

5. **Continue for one to two minutes.**

To practice Legs-Up-the-Wall with Belly-Heart Breath, follow these steps:

1. **Lie on your back with your legs extended up a wall.**

2. **Place one hand on your belly and the other on your heart.**

3. **Breathe into your belly for three counts, and then continue the inhale into your chest for three more counts.**

4. **Exhale from your chest to your belly for a total of eight counts.**

5. **Continue for three to five minutes.**

To practice Supine Spinal Twist with Alternate-Side Breathing, follow these steps:

1. **Lie on your back, knees bent.**

2. **Let your knees fall to the right while turning your head to the left.**

3. **Breathe deeply into the left side of your rib cage for three to five breaths.**

4. **Return to the center briefly, and then repeat on the right side.**

5. **Continue alternating sides for two to three minutes.**

I discovered the power of these combined techniques during a particularly stressful speaking tour. After long days of travel, presentations, and meeting new people (all fun as well as stimulating activities), I found it nearly impossible to wind down in hotel rooms. Developing this sequence of four stretches with specific breathing patterns became my portable sleep solution, effectively resetting my nervous system regardless of the environment.

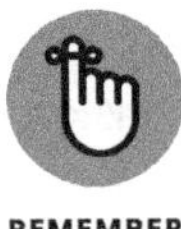

For best results, move slowly through these stretches, synchronizing movement with a comfortable breathing rate for you. Listen carefully to your body and what feels good. The goal isn't to achieve the perfect pose — it's to create a mind-body connection that signals safety and relaxation to your nervous system, preparing it for deep, restorative sleep.

Finding Techniques to Fall Asleep Faster

Now let's get to the heart of what many people struggle with: how to actually fall asleep when your head hits the pillow. These specialized breathing techniques are designed to override the racing thoughts and physical tension that often delay sleep onset.

Practicing 4-7-8 Breathing for relaxation

The 4-7-8 Breathing technique, often shared by Dr. Andrew Weil, has gained popularity for good reason: It works remarkably well for many people. This method acts like a natural tranquilizer for the nervous system by forcing it to shift from sympathetic to parasympathetic dominance — in other words, from stressed to chilled.

Here's how to practice it properly:

1. Sit with your back straight or lie in a comfortable position.

2. Place the tip of your tongue against the ridge behind your upper front teeth, keeping it there throughout the exercise.

3. Exhale completely through your mouth, making a whooshing sound.

4. Close your mouth and inhale quietly through your nose for a mental count of four.

5. Hold your breath for a count of seven.

6. Exhale completely through your mouth with a whoosh for a count of eight.

   This completes one cycle.

7. Repeat for a total of four cycles.

What makes this technique so effective is the extended exhalation — the eight-count exhale is twice as long as the four-count inhale. This extended exhale activates the parasympathetic nervous system, reducing heart rate and blood pressure while increasing feelings of relaxation.

During a retreat I led in the UK, an insomniac participant was skeptical about this technique, having tried "everything" previously. I suggested she modify the counts to fit her lung capacity (starting with 2-3-4 instead of 4-7-8) and gradually work up to the full count. By the third night, she reported falling asleep within minutes of using the technique — a first in her two decades of sleep struggles.

Although 4-7-8 Breathing is powerful, it may cause lightheadedness when you first start practicing it. Always start in a seated or lying position, and if you feel dizzy, return to normal breathing. Over time, your body will adjust to the pattern.

Using extended exhalation to calm the mind

The 4-7-8 Breathing technique is structured and precise, but sometimes a more flexible approach works better, especially if counting itself keeps your mind too active. Extended exhalation breathing gives you the benefits of parasympathetic activation without rigid counting.

In the 1:2 Ratio Breath, instead of focusing on specific counts, you simply make your exhale twice as long as your inhale. For example, if you naturally breathe in for three to four seconds, your exhale would be six to eight seconds. The beauty of this approach is that it works with your natural breathing rhythm.

1. **Lie down in bed, ready for sleep.**

   Make yourself cozy. You don't need to sit up or do anything special.

2. **Let your eyes gently close.**

   Or soften your gaze — whatever feels most restful.

3. **Notice your natural breathing.**

   No need to change anything at first. Just notice: Breathing is happening.

4. **Begin to gently extend your exhale.**

   As you breathe in (for maybe three to four seconds), let your out-breath be roughly twice as long — maybe six to eight seconds.

   No counting needed. Just feel it out. Think of your exhale like a long, slow sigh of relief.

5. **Continue for a few minutes.**

   Let each exhale melt you deeper into the bed. If you lose track, no worries —
   you're probably relaxing already.

6. **Let go of trying to fall asleep.**

   Simply rest in the rhythm of your breath. Often, sleep sneaks in through the
   long exhale.

If you'd like something more engaging for your mind as well as your breath, try
the Descending Count Method. Just follow these steps:

1. **Start by breathing normally for a few cycles.**

2. **Begin counting your natural inhale length.**

   For example, let's say it's three seconds.

3. **Exhale double the length of your natural inhale.**

   For example, if your natural inhale was three seconds, make your exhale
   six seconds.

4. **On the next breath, keep the inhale the same but add one second to
   your exhale.**

   In this example, your exhale would now be seven seconds.

5. **Continue adding one second to each exhale until you reach a comfortable
   maximum.**

6. **Gradually return to your starting ratio.**

   This progressive extension allows your nervous system to downshift gradually,
   like slowly applying brakes rather than slamming them. Many people find they
   fall asleep before completing the sequence.

The Wave Exhale focuses on the quality of the exhale rather than its precise length.
Ideal for beach lovers! To practice it, follow these steps:

1. **Breathe in naturally through your nose.**

2. **As you exhale through your nose, imagine your breath as a wave receding from shore.**

   Make the exhale slow, steady, and complete — like a wave that gradually
   loses momentum.

3. **At the end of the exhale, pause briefly before inhaling again.**

4. **With each breath cycle, try to make the exhale slightly smoother and
   more complete.**

You can combine this technique with the Ocean Breath (Ujjaji; see Chapter 8). The natural sound you make sounds like the ocean, so it's particularly relaxing. Ocean Breath is one of my favorites to do anytime I want to rest, sleep, or simply recharge.

I discovered the power of this approach while guiding a group of mindfulness students who struggled with overthinking at bedtime. Many of them found traditional counting techniques too rigid or mentally activating, but the gentle, image-based wave exhale helped them shift from doing to being — allowing their minds and bodies to soften into rest without effort.

Practicing simple breathing exercises to ease racing thoughts

Sometimes the biggest barrier to sleep isn't physical tension but mental activation — the infamous "monkey mind" that jumps from thought to thought. The specialized breathing techniques in this section are designed specifically to interrupt thought patterns and create mental space.

Practice the 5-5-7 Breathing Reset by following these steps:

1. **Inhale for five seconds, focusing solely on the sensation of air entering your nostrils.**

2. **Hold your breath for five seconds, creating a deliberate pause in mental activity.**

3. **Exhale for seven seconds, imagining your thoughts flowing out with your breath.**

4. **Repeat eight to ten times.**

The mid-breath pause in this technique interrupts thought patterns more effectively than continuous breathing exercises, creating brief but powerful moments of mental stillness.

Practice the Color Breathing technique by following these steps:

1. **Choose a color you associate with calmness.**

   People often choose blue, green, or purple, but there is no "right" color.

2. **As you inhale, visualize this color filling your body.**

3. **As you exhale, visualize a color representing tension leaving your body.**

   People often choose red or green to represent tension, but again, there's no "right" color.

4. **Focus entirely on this color transformation, giving your thinking mind a simple, absorbing task.**

5. **Continue for five minutes or until you notice your thoughts slowing down.**

To practice Alphabetical Breathing, follow these steps:

1. **As you inhale, think of a calming word beginning with *A* (like *abundance* or *angel*).**

2. **Exhale completely.**

3. **On your next inhale, move to *B* (for example, *balance* or *beach*).**

4. **Continue through the alphabet.**

   If you notice your mind wandering, gently return to the last letter you remember.

This technique is particularly effective for analytical thinkers, because it gives the mind a structured task that gradually becomes more challenging (finding words for uncommon letters like *Q*, *X*, or *Z*), which paradoxically often leads to drifting off to sleep before completing the alphabet.

I once struggled with severe jet lag while teaching in the Far East, finding myself wide awake at 3 a.m. with an important retreat the next day. Using the Alphabetical Breathing technique, I only made it to *H* before falling asleep, and I awakened refreshed despite the time zone disruption.

One-Minute Breath is an advanced technique, but it's good fun if you find the other breathing exercises easy to do. Follow these steps:

1. **Gradually extend your inhale, hold, and exhale until each complete breath takes about one minute.**

   A good starting pattern is 20 seconds inhale, 20 seconds hold, 20 seconds exhale.

   Focus completely on the breath, making it smooth and controlled.

2. **Practice for three to five minutes.**

This advanced technique requires practice but can be extraordinarily effective for breaking thought patterns. The extended breath cycle requires such concentration that it crowds out other mental activity, creating space for sleep to arise.

Using Breathwork to Stay Asleep through the Night

Falling asleep is only half the battle for many people — staying asleep is equally important. Let's explore breathing techniques specifically designed to prevent nighttime awakenings and help you get back to sleep quickly if you do wake up.

Maintaining a slow and steady breathing rhythm during sleep

Your breathing pattern during sleep significantly impacts sleep quality and continuity. You can't consciously control your breath while sleeping, but you *can* train respiratory patterns that continue during sleep through presleep programming and consistent practice.

TRY THIS

To fall asleep more easily, sleep more deeply, and wake up refreshed, train your body and nervous system to downshift into rest mode each night through gentle breathing:

1. **Each night, spend five to ten minutes lying down or seated comfortably in bed, breathing at a calming pace of six breaths per minute (for example, inhale for four seconds and exhale for six seconds).**

   Focus on:

   - Breathing through the nose only

   - Using the diaphragm so your belly gently rises and falls

   - Keeping the breath silent, light, slow, and regular

2. **Make the exhalation slightly longer than the inhale (for example, four counts in and six counts out, or five counts in and seven counts out).**

   This activates your parasympathetic nervous system, helping your body wind down and prepare for sleep.

3. **As you drift off, let go of any effort or control.**

   Allow the slow breathing rhythm to continue naturally and effortlessly, like a lullaby for your nervous system

4. **If you want, add a body scan.**

   As you breathe, gently bring awareness to each part of the body — from your feet up to your head — releasing tension with each outbreath.

If you like the idea of a body scan, you may enjoy the high-quality guided meditation audio track that comes with my book *Mindfulness For Dummies* (published by John Wiley & Sons). Many people have found it especially helpful for winding down and drifting off to sleep. Or, if you'd like to try one for free first, just enter **Body Scan Shamash Alidina** into YouTube and you'll find a few options there.

Over time, this practice helps establish a healthy breathing rhythm that your autonomic nervous system maintains during sleep. Research has shown that respiratory patterns practiced consistently before sleep can influence breathing patterns during sleep itself.

Think of it this way: Imagine your breath as a gentle tide washing onto the shore. When you slow the waves before bed — calm, steady, rhythmic — they continue flowing quietly through the night. But when the tide is choppy at dusk, it tends to stay restless until morning. Over time, the body begins to remember these softer waves, settling into deeper, more restorative waters.

For maximum benefit, practice Coherent Breathing (five to six breaths per minute) not just before bed, but at intervals throughout the day:

>> Five minutes upon waking

>> Five minutes before lunch

>> Five minutes midafternoon

>> Five minutes before dinner

>> Five to ten minutes before bed

This consistent practice helps recalibrate your default breathing pattern, making it more likely that you'll maintain healthy breathing during sleep.

Drawing on breathing techniques if you wake up in the middle of the night

Middle-of-the-night awakenings can be frustrating, but having a specific breathing protocol ready can help you return to sleep quickly instead of spiraling into wakefulness.

Try the 4-4-6-2 Return to Sleep Sequence:

1. **Inhale for four seconds.**

2. **Hold for four seconds.**

3. **Exhale for six seconds.**

4. **Hold the exhale (empty lungs) for two seconds.**

5. **Repeat until you drift back to sleep.**

The brief pause after exhaling creates a subtle air hunger that can help redirect attention away from thoughts and back to the body, facilitating a faster return to sleep.

If you wake feeling anxious, restless, or too alert to fall back asleep, try the gentle Breathing Body Scan for Sleep. You can imagine your breath like a soft golden light that fills each area of your body, bringing warmth and ease as it moves through you.

1. **Lie comfortably on your back, with your hands resting where they feel most natural.**

2. **Begin by bringing your awareness to your feet: Inhale as if you're drawing breath into the soles of your feet, and exhale and let them soften completely.**

3. **Move your attention to your lower legs: Imagine breathing in and out of your calves and shins, letting the golden light melt away any tension.**

4. **Shift your focus to your upper legs and thighs, breathing in gently, exhaling slowly.**

   Feel the muscles relax and release.

5. **Bring your awareness to your hips and pelvis, breathing into this foundation of your body, inviting stillness and support.**

6. **Breathe into your lower back and belly, feeling the breath expand gently with each inhale and settle with each exhale.**

7. **Continue to your rib cage and midback, letting the breath radiate through the space around your heart.**

8. **Move to your upper chest and shoulders, allowing them to soften and drop with every exhale.**

9. **If you're still awake, bring the golden breath to your arms, hands, neck, and finally your face and head, relaxing the jaw, eyes, and forehead.**

I sometimes use this practice myself — and honestly, I rarely make it to my head! I'm usually fast asleep by the time I get to my chest or shoulders. Hopefully, it works just as well for you, too.

This calming breath-based scan helps quiet the nervous system and ease your body back into rest.

Left-Nostril Breathing is a specialized technique from yoga traditions. According to yogic tradition, Left-Nostril Breathing activates the parasympathetic nervous system more strongly. Modern research suggests this may be related to the fact that the left and right sides of the nasal cavity have different blood flow patterns that alternate throughout the day (known as the *nasal cycle*), potentially influencing brain activity patterns. Follow these steps:

1. **Lie on your right side.**

2. **Use your right thumb to gently close your right nostril.**

3. **Breathe slowly and exclusively through your left nostril for 8 to 12 breaths.**

I discovered the effectiveness of this technique quite by accident when I had a blocked nose and one nostril was congested. Breathing just through my left nostril, I noticed I fell back asleep much more quickly. I've since recommended this method to many insomnia sufferers with some very positive feedback.

If mental chatter is keeping you awake, try Silent Mantra Breathing:

1. **Choose a simple, calming word or phrase (for example, peace, letting go, or rest now).**

   The key is choosing a word that feels neutral or positive — avoid mantras that remind you of daytime responsibilities or goals.

2. **Silently repeat your mantra on each exhale.**

   Keep your breathing slow and even. When thoughts arise, gently return to your mantra.

If you're looking for something relaxing to listen to, I have more than 150 free guided meditations and breathwork sessions available for free on YouTube. Most are 30 minutes long, so you can practice them as you lie down in bed. Just head to www.youtube.com/@shamashmindful. If you'd like to listen to them ad-free, get in touch with me or join our Daily Mindfulness Club.

Balancing carbon dioxide and oxygen for deeper rest

Few people realize that the balance between oxygen and carbon dioxide in the blood significantly impacts sleep quality. Contrary to popular belief, slightly elevated carbon dioxide levels (within a healthy range) promote deeper sleep by:

>> Enhancing blood flow to the brain during sleep

>> Facilitating the transition between sleep cycles

>> Preventing micro-awakenings due to breathing disruptions

>> Supporting proper oxygen delivery to tissues

>> Avoiding over-breathing

Many breathing techniques focus heavily on deep inhalation, but excessive breathing can actually lower carbon dioxide levels too much, causing sleep disruptions. The following balanced approaches help maintain optimal gas exchange.

TRY THIS

Try Cupped Hands for Calm Breathing (Paper Bag Simulation):

1. **Cup your hands loosely over your nose and mouth (not airtight).**

2. **Breathe normally into this small space for 10 to 12 breaths.**

3. **Remove your hands and breathe normally for five breaths.**

4. **Repeat once or twice.**

This exercise gently rebalances oxygen and carbon dioxide levels without the dramatic effects of actually breathing into a paper bag (which should only be done under medical supervision because you could easily overdo it, which would be dangerous).

TRY THIS

The gentle Buteyko Breathing Method for Sleep technique is based on the Buteyko Breathing Method and is designed to calm the nervous system and reduce over-breathing — a common contributor to restless sleep. Follow these steps:

1. **Close your mouth and breathe only through your nose.**

2. **Allow your breath to become quiet, light, and soft — so gentle that it feels like you're hardly breathing at all.**

3. **Gradually take slightly smaller breaths than normal.**

   Don't hold your breath — just reduce the size of each inhale and exhale.

   You're aiming to create a very mild feeling of *air hunger* (a subtle desire for more air). This is a sign that carbon dioxide levels are gently rising, which helps relax your body and promote sleep.

4. **Continue with this pattern for two to three minutes, and then return to a natural breath.**

This practice helps shift your body into a parasympathetic state — the rest-and-digest mode — making it easier to fall asleep and stay asleep.

A sign you're doing this right is sensing more saliva in your mouth, or warming of the hands or feet, or just a feeling of relaxation.

I offered some exercises from the Buteyko Breathing Method to an entrepreneur I was coaching who said he had quite severe sleep apnea. While continuing his prescribed medical treatment, he added Buteyko breathing practices. Within three weeks, his sleep-tracking data showed a measurable reduction in breathing disturbances during sleep. His sleep doctor was impressed enough to ask for more information about the breathing techniques.

Supporting overall health and recovery through better sleep

Your breath has a quiet but powerful influence on the quality of your sleep — and by extension, your physical and mental well-being. When you breathe lightly, slowly, and gently through your nose at night, you're setting the stage for deep rest and recovery.

The good news? You don't need a complicated routine. What matters most is consistency and simplicity. The core principles are:

>> **Nasal breathing:** Breathe in and out through your nose as much as possible.

>> **Slow breathing:** Aim to slow your breath down, especially your exhalation.

>> **Light breathing:** Let your breath be quiet and soft — almost like you're not breathing at all.

>> **Rhythm and relaxation:** Find a pace that feels calming and natural, not forced.

If you'd like to, you can explore techniques like gentle humming, lengthened exhales, or light breath holds to deepen your experience — but they're optional tools, not requirements.

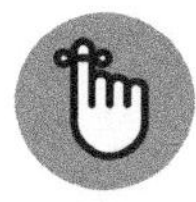

You don't need to "get it right." There's no perfect way to breathe for sleep. What matters most is creating a calm and kind environment within yourself. If you drift into sleep, wonderful. If not, remember: The breathing itself is doing you good. You're training your body and nervous system to settle, heal, and recover.

Personally, I've found that when I focus too much on "trying to sleep," it often backfires. But when I shift my attention to gently enjoying the breath — welcoming sleep as a bonus if it comes — I almost always rest more deeply. Even when sleep takes its time, I wake up more refreshed than I'd expect.

Be patient with yourself. Let go of the idea of success or failure. You may even want to explore mindful approaches to sleep in my book *Mindfulness For Dummies* or *Acceptance & Commitment Therapy For Dummies* (both published by John Wiley & Sons), which offer more guidance on how to befriend wakefulness and find peace, even in the middle of the night.

Sleep well — or just breathe well. Either way, you're giving your body and mind exactly what they need.

Chapter **14**

Breathing Exercises for Kids

I remember a particular day when I was a schoolteacher, and a young student was having a meltdown in my classroom. Red-faced and hyperventilating, he was beyond reason. With 29 other children watching wide-eyed, I tried everything in my teacher toolkit — calm talking, distraction, even the classic "count to ten" approach — but nothing worked.

Looking back, I wish I'd known what I know now about the power of breathing exercises. A simple, engaging breathing exercise may have helped my young student regulate his emotions and return to a calm state. Instead, it took nearly 30 minutes of traditional behavioral management techniques to help him settle.

Breathing exercises aren't just for yoga studios or meditation retreats — they're powerful tools that can help children navigate their emotional worlds, improve focus, ease anxiety, improve friendships, and even boost physical health. The best part? Kids actually enjoy them when they're presented in the right way!

In this chapter, I guide you through the world of children's breathing exercises — from introducing basic concepts to implementing age-appropriate techniques for everyone from infants to teenagers. You discover how to make breathing fun (yes, really!), integrate it into daily routines, and use it as a powerful tool for managing those big emotions that can overwhelm little bodies.

Introducing Breathing Exercises to Children

One of my favorite client stories comes from a frustrated mom who attended one of my workshops. Her 6-year-old son had been labeled "difficult" at school. After learning some simple breathing techniques, my client began a five-minute daily practice with him. Two weeks later, she received a note from his teacher asking what had changed. The "difficult" child was now raising his hand instead of shouting out answers and using his "breathing breaks" when he felt frustrated. Small changes, remarkable results.

This section introduces key principles for sharing breathing exercises with children and teens.

Teaching breathing techniques early

Children are natural breathers. Babies especially demonstrate perfect breathing patterns before they're influenced by stress, poor posture, and other habits that affect breathing. By introducing breathwork early, you are

- **Building lifelong skills:** The breathing patterns established in childhood often persist into adulthood. Teaching proper breathing early helps develop healthy habits that last a lifetime.

- **Taking advantage of brain plasticity:** Young brains are incredibly adaptable. The neural pathways formed during childhood breathing exercises create foundations for self-regulation that become more automatic with practice.

- **Preventing breathing problems:** Many children develop mouth breathing habits or irregular breathing patterns that can lead to sleep issues, reduced concentration, and even facial development problems. Early intervention helps prevent these issues.

- **Creating a foundation for emotional regulation:** Children who learn to connect with their breath develop an internal resource they can access anywhere, anytime, without special equipment or adult assistance.

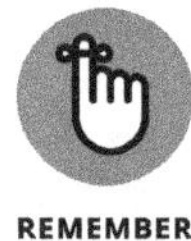

Research shows that children as young as 4 years old can learn simple breathing techniques that help them manage emotions and improve focus.

Finding simple ways to explain breathing to kids

When I first tried explaining breathing exercises to my nephew, I launched into a technical explanation about oxygen, carbon dioxide, and the nervous system. His eyes glazed over faster than a doughnut at Krispy Kreme. Lesson learned!

Here are better approaches I've discovered along the way:

>> **Use their language.** For example, you may say, "Breathing is how your body gets its superpower. When you breathe in a special way, you're giving your body and brain extra strength!"

>> **Make it visual.** For example, "Imagine your tummy is a balloon that fills up when you breathe in and gets smaller when you breathe out."

>> **Connect it to feelings.** For example, "When you feel wobbly inside [anxious] or hot and angry, your breathing can help your body feel calm and cool again."

>> **Keep it simple.** Focus on the sensation rather than the science. For example, "Can you feel the cool air coming in through your nose? Now feel the warm air going out."

>> **Use analogies they understand.** For example, "Your breath is like a remote control for your body. It can turn the volume down when feelings get too loud."

Always demonstrate the breathing technique yourself first. Children learn by watching even more than by listening to instructions.

Making breathing fun and engaging

The key to successful breathing exercises with kids isn't perfection — it's engagement. If it's not fun, they won't do it. Here are some approaches that have worked wonders with children in my practice:

>> **Turn it into a game.** For example, "Let's see who can make their stuffed animal rise the highest on their belly when they breathe."

>> **Use props.** Pinwheels, bubbles, feathers, or light scarves all respond to breath in visible ways that fascinate children.

>> **Create characters.** For example, "Let's breathe like different animals!" Snake hisses, lion roars, and rabbit sniffs all involve different breathing patterns.

>> **Incorporate movement.** Adding simple hand movements to breathing exercises helps *kinesthetic learners* (those who learn best through movement and hands-on activities) stay engaged.

>> **Tell stories.** Create breathing adventures where each breath is part of a journey. For example, "We're climbing a mountain with each breath in, and sliding down with each breath out."

>> **Make it competitive (in a healthy way).** For example, "Let's see if we can make our breathing slower and quieter than last time."

One of my community members transformed her son's resistance to bedtime by creating "The Breathing Challenge." Each night they tried a different breathing exercise, and he got to rate it from 1 to 10 and add it to their "Breathing Champions" chart. Not only did he start falling asleep faster, but he also began *requesting* his breathing time!

Avoid making breathing exercises feel like a chore or punishment. Never say, "You need to do your breathing because you're being too wild!" Instead, offer it as a tool: "Would some dragon breathing help you feel stronger right now?"

Setting everyday breathing habits for kids

Before we dive into specific exercises, let's explore the breathing habits that form the foundation of respiratory health for children. Creating awareness of these basics can make a huge difference in a child's well-being.

Making sure they're breathing through their nose

When a client, a mother, told me about her daughter's tiredness and focus issues, I gently suggested checking her breathing. We discovered she was mouth breathing. With just a few weeks of simple nasal breathing practice, her energy and focus noticeably improved — even her teacher commented on the change.

Nasal breathing (covered in detail in Chapter 6) isn't just a preference — it's how the respiratory system functions best. Nasal breathing filters out allergens and germs, warms and moistens the air to protect the lungs, and even produces nitric oxide, which helps the body absorb oxygen more efficiently. It also supports better sleep by reducing snoring and nighttime disruptions.

Surprisingly, consistent mouth breathing can even affect the way a child's face develops over time, so encouraging nose breathing early on can make a big difference in their overall health and well-being.

To encourage nasal breathing:

>> **Check for obstructions.** If your child struggles with nasal breathing, consider having them checked for allergies, excessively enlarged *adenoids* (tissue located behind the nose and above the roof of the mouth), or other obstructions.

>> **Give gentle reminders.** Create a secret signal with your child to remind them to close their mouth and breathe through their nose.

>> **Practice.** Have "nose breathing minutes" where everyone focuses on breathing through their nose.

>> **Build in nighttime awareness.** For children who mouth-breathe at night, consult with a healthcare provider about gentle solutions.

Some practitioners experiment with gentle mouth-tape strips. These strips have a gap for breathing through the mouth, if necessary, but they encourage the mouth to close in order to reinforce nasal breathing during sleep. Evidence in children is preliminary, and we don't yet know the long-term safety of this technique. But if you're curious, consult a pediatric sleep-medicine specialist and avoid taping without a professional's consent. They're usually not recommended for children under 5.

The Smell the Flower, Blow the Candle exercise (described in the "Young Children" section, later in this chapter) is excellent for developing awareness of nasal breathing for kids, because the cue to "smell the flower" naturally invites a nasal inhale.

Encouraging proper posture for healthy breathing

If you've ever seen a slumped-over teenager trying to take a deep breath, you'll understand how posture affects breathing. When I taught in schools before becoming a mindfulness and breathing coach, I noticed how differently my students breathed when they sat up straight versus when they hunched over their desks.

Good posture creates space for the lungs to expand fully. For children, whose bodies are still developing, establishing good posture habits early is crucial. Here are some tips for helping kids have good posture:

>> **Make it playful.** Turn posture into a game, like imagining a string pulling you tall.

>> **Be a role model.** Kids copy what they see — sit tall yourself.

>> **Set up their space.** Create a comfy, posture-friendly study area.

A simple exercise I teach is Royal Breathing:

1. **Ask your child to imagine they're a prince or princess sitting on a throne.**

2. **Have them sit with their "royal posture" — straight back, shoulders relaxed, head balanced.**

   Encourage them not to strain themselves so they're not tensed up. Just aim for an elegant, regal, yet relaxed posture.

3. **In this position, have them take five slow breaths through their nose.**

4. **Ask them to notice how much easier it is to breathe deeply in this position.**

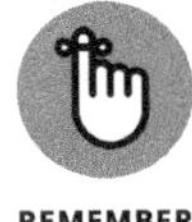

A child who slumps is using their accessory breathing muscles (shoulders and neck) instead of their diaphragm. Over time, this can lead to shallow breathing patterns, increased stress and anxiety, and perhaps even attention deficit hyper-activity disorder (ADHD).

Recognizing and addressing common breathing issues

After an online breathing workshop last year, a participant approached me about his 5-year-old daughter who frequently complained of being tired despite sleeping ten hours a night. After discussing her breathing patterns, he realized she may be experiencing sleep-disordered breathing. A visit to their pediatrician confirmed mild sleep apnea, which they addressed with breathing exercises and minor interventions.

Being aware of common breathing issues can help you spot potential problems early, including the following:

>> **Mouth breathing:** Mouth breathing can indicate nasal obstructions or simply be a habit.

>> **Rapid, shallow breathing:** This practice may become habitual for some children, particularly those who experience anxiety.

>> **Breath holding:** Some children unconsciously hold their breath during concentration or stress.

>> **Irregular breathing patterns:** Noticeable pauses or irregular rhythms may indicate sleep apnea or other concerns.

>> **Chest breathing:** Ideally, children should primarily breathe using their diaphragm (belly breathing), not just their chest.

>> **Frequent sighing:** This can indicate insufficient regular breathing.

Signs that may warrant a conversation with your healthcare provider include the following:

>> Snoring

>> Pauses in breathing during sleep

>> Restless sleep (lots of tossing and turning)

>> Bedwetting

>> Waking up frequently to pee

>> Morning headaches

>> Excessive tiredness during the day

>> Difficulty paying attention

>> Behavioral issues, including hyperactivity or irritability

>> Regular mouth breathing (especially during sleep)

>> Frequent colds or respiratory infections

Consider keeping a simple breathing journal for a week or so if you're concerned about your child's breathing patterns. Note when issues occur and under what circumstances.

Finding Breathing Techniques for Different Age Groups

Children's breathing needs evolve as they grow. What works for a toddler probably won't engage a teenager. In this section, I explore age-appropriate techniques that meet children where they are developmentally.

Babies and toddlers

In my coaching and community, I often get questions about meditations or breathing exercises for parents or teens. Parents are sometimes surprised when I suggest breathing exercises they can do with their babies and toddlers, too. These early experiences lay important foundations.

Gentle exercises to calm and soothe

The most natural breathing exercise for infants is one where you synchronize your breath with theirs. Synchronicity Breath is a very simple and enjoyable exercise for parent and baby to do together. It's often soothing for both.

1. **Hold your baby in a comfortable position where you can feel their chest or belly move.**

2. **Begin to notice their breathing rhythm.**

3. **Gradually match your breathing to theirs.**

4. **As you establish synchrony, slowly extend your exhales, making them slightly longer.**

   Your baby will often naturally begin to match your more relaxed pattern.

Try Tummy Breathing by following these steps:

1. **Place a small, lightweight toy on your baby's belly.**

2. **As they breathe, point out how the toy moves up and down.**

   Even though they won't understand the words, this brings attention to the breath.

3. **For slightly older babies, make a gentle "whoosh" sound as they exhale.**

You can incorporate breathing patterns into lullabies, too. Try Lullaby Breathing:

1. **Rock your baby gently to the rhythm of a calm breath.**

2. **Sing on the exhale, pause on the inhale.**

   The combination of breathing rhythm, gentle movement, and your voice is incredibly soothing.

Games and rhythms to encourage natural breathing patterns

For mobile toddlers, try the Feather Flying technique:

1. **Hold a feather or a small piece of tissue paper at an appropriate distance.**

2. **Demonstrate blowing it gently.**

3. **Let your child try blowing it themselves using their nose or mouth.**

   This encourages controlled exhalation and is endlessly fascinating for toddlers.

Try Balloon Face with your toddler:

1. **Make your cheeks big like a balloon, and then slowly let the air out.**

2. **Make a gentle hissing sound as you release the air.**

   Your toddler will naturally want to copy this playful breathing game.

Play Teddy Bear Rides with your toddler to playfully introduce the concept of belly breathing:

1. **Have your toddler lie on their back and place a small stuffed animal on their tummy.**

2. **Encourage them to make the teddy go up and down with their breath.**

   Use phrases like "Teddy up" (inhale) and "Teddy down" (exhale).

To create an unconscious pattern of deeper breathing, try Bubble Watch with your toddler. Blow bubbles between you and your toddler, and encourage your toddler to watch the bubbles float. Their natural instinct will be to take a deeper breath as they watch in anticipation.

If they can take a deep breath in through their nose with you, and blow the bubbles themselves, that's even more fun and powerful for them.

When to use breathing to ease discomfort

If your baby is crying and isn't stopping, you could try the following technique:

1. **Hold your baby in the "tiger in the tree" position (tummy down, supported along your forearm).**

   Every baby is different, so experiment to figure out if a particular posture works best for yours. It may also differ from day to day.

2. **Gently pat their back while making a rhythmic *shhhh* sound that mimics a long exhale.**

   The combination of position, movement, and sound soothes the nervous system.

If your baby is struggling to sleep, it can be very stressful. Try this to help them fall asleep:

1. **Dim the lights, lower the noise, and snuggle your baby in the same cozy spot each night.**

   A calm, familiar environment helps their nervous system begin to wind down.

2. **Match your breathing with your baby's natural rhythm for a minute or two, and then gently slow your exhale.**

   Babies often mirror your calmer pace.

3. **Gently sway side to side like ocean waves, whispering a soft *shhhh whoosh* on each exhale.**

   You can also place your palm on their belly and tap lightly every few breaths to anchor attention and ease tension.

4. **Gradually reduce movement, soften your sounds, and let your hand simply rest.**

   This gentle fade-out signals it's time to sleep, helping your baby drift off peacefully.

If you're going to be apart from your baby for a while, breathing exercises can help soothe them. Before separation, hold your toddler close and take three slow breaths together. This creates a sense of connection that lingers after you've left.

Some parents leave a recorded "breathing message" that caregivers can play if the child becomes distressed. This message can be anything you already say to your child when doing some breathing with them.

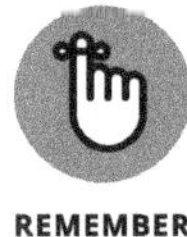

Babies and toddlers won't "do" breathing exercises in a structured way. Instead, you create environments and interactions that naturally encourage healthy breathing patterns.

Young children

A 5-year-old girl's teacher was concerned about the little girl's emotional outbursts. The girl's mother learned the Animal Breathing techniques in this section and made them part of their daily routine. Within three weeks, the little girl was using them independently at school and asking for her "turtle breathing" when she felt overwhelmed.

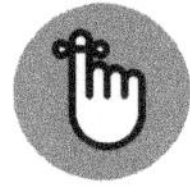

Young children thrive with concrete, imaginative exercises that engage their natural playfulness.

Using simple techniques

This classic technique, Smell the Flower, Blow the Candle, works brilliantly with young children:

1. **Have the child hold an imaginary flower in one hand and an imaginary candle in the other.**

2. **Instruct them to smell the flower deeply (inhale through the nose).**

3. **Then blow out the candle gently (exhale through the mouth).**

4. **Repeat three to five times.**

For added engagement:

>> Use a real flower for smelling (not lit candles, for safety reasons).

>> Draw pictures of flowers and candles they can use as visual cues, or give them coloring in sheets of flowers and candles.

>> Create paper flowers that have a pleasant scent.

Promoting relaxation with humming breaths

Humming creates gentle vibrations that are naturally calming for children. Bumble Bee Breath is a helpful exercise to try:

1. **Have the child sit comfortably with their shoulders relaxed.**

2. **Ask them to inhale through the nose.**

3. **On the exhale, make a humming sound like a bee with lips closed.**

   Challenge them to make their bee sound last as long as possible.

Making sounds of trains is fun for kids. Try Train Breath to help kids learn breath control while having fun:

1. **Have the child inhale through the nose.**

2. **Have the child exhale, making a *choo-choo* sound, moving from louder to softer.**

For another playful way to help your child practice humming, try Motorcycle Mouth Breathing. This one is ideal if you live in a city and often hear that sound:

1. **Have the child breathe in slowly through the nose.**

2. **Have them close their lips lightly and exhale while making motorcycle sounds.**

   The vibration in the lips is soothing and helps release facial tension.

Children often find this one hilarious — that's fine! Laughter and breathing exercises go well together.

Playing fun games to teach breathing awareness

Children absolutely love games. So if you can link and associate breathing exercises with games, you're both winning!

Here are some fun animal-themed breathing exercises you can share with young children:

>> **Bunny Breath:** Take three quick sniffs through the nose and one long exhale through the mouth.

>> **Snake Breath:** Take one long inhale through the nose and one long exhale with a hissing sound.

>> **Lion Breath:** Inhale through the nose, open the mouth wide, stick out the tongue, and exhale with a *haaa* sound.

>> **Elephant Breath:** Let the arms hang down like an elephant trunk, inhale through the nose while raising the "trunk" up, and exhale through the mouth while swinging the "trunk" down between the legs.

Over time, get your child breathing in and out using their nose. Breathing out with the nose helps to gently clear it, making the next in breath easier. But for these breathing games, it's okay for them to breathe out through their mouths, especially if they're combining it with sounds.

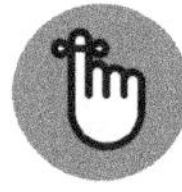

If your child has a stuffy nose or allergies and *they're finding* it hard to breathe through their nose, you can teach them the nose unblocking exercise (you'll find the full version in Chapter 6). In short, it involves a gentle breath in and out through the nose, followed by holding the breath for as long as feels comfortable, and then repeating that several times until their nose is clear. To make it more *kid*-friendly, invite them to imagine they're diving underwater — "Let's see how long you can stay under before coming up for air!" This playful approach not only engages their imagination but also helps clear nasal passages naturally.

Animal breathing doesn't have to be the only source of your inspiration. The weather works well, too:

>> **Rainbow Breath:** Extend the arms in a rainbow shape while inhaling; then return the arms to your sides while exhaling.

>> **Thunder Breath:** Inhale deeply, then exhale with a loud *boom!* while gently drumming on the floor.

TRY THIS

>> **Gentle Rain Breath:** Inhale through the nose; then exhale while fluttering the fingers downward like raindrops.

>> **Wind Breath:** Inhale through the nose; then exhale through the mouth with varying intensity to mimic different wind strengths.

Children love blowing bubbles, so Bubble Wand Breathing will be fun for them:

1. **Use a bubble wand but without bubble solution to start with (to avoid inhaling chemicals).**

2. **Have children practice slow, controlled exhales through the wand.**

   Challenge them to make their exhale last longer each time.

3. **When they've mastered control and are doing it calmly, use real bubbles as a reward.**

TRY THIS

Children can easily become overwhelmed by big emotions — and they often need support to manage them. Breathing exercises are an ideal way to help. Because kids are naturally visual and imaginative, try this technique I call Breathing Colors for Calming Emotions whenever they need a gentle way to release a difficult feeling:

1. **Invite your child to sit comfortably with one hand on their belly and one on their heart.**

2. **Say, "Let's take a little breath journey using colors."**

3. **Ask, "What's your favorite color today?"**

   This is their *calm color*.

4. **Gently guide them to notice the feeling that's most present right now by asking, "What feeling is strongest in your body right now? Is it sadness? Anger? Worry? Something else?"**

5. **Ask, "If your big feeling had a color, what would it be?"**

   That's their *release color*.

6. **Guide them like this: "Breathe in [calm color] calm. Fill up with it. Now breathe out your [release color] [the feeling]. Let it float away like a balloon."**

   For example, "Breathe in blue calm. Fill up with it. Now breathe out your red anger. Let it float away like a balloon."

7. **Repeat three to five times with slow, gentle breaths.**

   They can move their arms with the breath if they like.

8. **Finish by asking, "How do you feel now?" or "What color do you feel inside?"**

For young children, keep breathing sessions short (two to three minutes) and end while they're still engaged. This builds positive associations with the practice.

Teens

Teenagers face unique pressures, and their breathing exercises need to respect both their developmental stage and their desire for autonomy. When I was offering mindful coaching to a mother of a 15-year-old who struggled with test anxiety, the breakthrough came when I encouraged her to stop "teaching" him breathing exercises and instead helped him design his own practice that felt relevant to his life.

Present these exercises to teens as "performance hacks" or "stress management techniques" rather than "breathing exercises" to increase buy-in.

Improving focus during study and exams

Exams are a top source of stress for teens — and stress hijacks the brain. But with simple breathwork, they can shift from panic to presence in under a minute. Light, slow, deep nasal breathing doesn't just calm the mind — it optimizes oxygen delivery to the brain, improving focus, memory, and emotional control. It's not just about feeling better — it's about learning better.

Before studying, spend one minute prepping your brain with this pattern:

1. **Inhale gently through the nose for four counts.**

2. **Pause briefly.**

3. **Exhale slowly through the nose for six counts.**

4. **Repeat for five to ten breaths.**

This activates the parasympathetic nervous system, improving mental clarity and focus. Quiet, nasal breathing is key.

When your attention drifts or your screen starts calling, reset with this 5-5-5-5 Focus Reset:

1. **Close your eyes or soften your gaze.**

2. **Take five light, slow breaths — five seconds in, five seconds out.**

3. **Return to work with a clearer head.**

It's faster than scrolling Instagram — and it actually resets your nervous system.

Syncing breath with study can boost memory encoding. The trick? Keep it nasal and calm.

1. **Inhale for a count of four, hold for a count of two (while recalling info), exhale for a count of six.**

2. **Repeat for three to five cycles at the start or end of a study block.**

This style of breathing optimizes brain oxygenation and locks in learning.

Feeling jittery before an exam? Over-breathing or shallow mouth breathing can spike stress. Reverse it in under a minute.

1. **Place one hand on your belly (or just imagine it if you're in public).**

2. **Take three to five slow nasal breaths, extending the exhale gently.**

   Focus on light, silent breathing.

This balances carbon dioxide and oxygen — key to calming the nervous system.

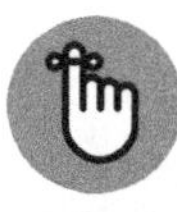

Light breathing is calm breathing.

WHAT TEENS SECRETLY THINK

"Breathing exercises? That's so lame."

That's often their first thought. But here's the twist: Many of the world's most successful performers — from elite athletes to global music icons and even pro gamers — rely on breathwork as a powerful tool to stay focused, manage anxiety, and perform at their best.

Take Billie Eilish, for example. Known for her raw honesty about mental health, she's spoken openly about using breath awareness and meditation to calm her nerves before shows and interviews.

(continued)

(continued)

Or look at Cristiano Ronaldo. Beyond his intense physical training, he uses slow, deliberate breathing to stay composed during penalty shootouts and high-pressure moments on the pitch.

Even in the gaming world, the Ninja (Tyler Blevins), one of the most popular streamers on the planet, uses deep breathing to stay calm and focused during competitive matches — where one slip in attention can cost everything.

And in the world of tennis, Novak Djokovic credits mindful breathing as a key part of his mental training. His ability to recover between points and maintain laserlike focus during marathon matches is no accident.

Breathing is no longer just a wellness thing. It's a mental performance strategy used by people at the top of their game.

So, if your teen ever rolls their eyes at a breathing exercise, invite them to try it not as a relaxation technique, but as a mental hack.

Managing emotional ups and downs

Teenagers experience intense emotions due to hormonal changes and developing brain structures. The techniques in this section help.

For processing anger or frustration, try Volcano Breath:

1. **Inhale deeply through the nose, gathering tension.**

2. **Hold briefly at the top.**

3. **Exhale forcefully through the mouth with a *ha* sound, releasing the tension.**

   Gradually make each exhale longer and quieter until reaching a calm state.

You can combine the *ha* sound with punching in the air, cycling between left and right hands. As you start to calm down a little, open up your hands and reduce the speed of punching.

This is a lovely, calming one. For calming intense emotions without drawing attention, try the Whisper Breath:

1. **Inhale normally through the nose.**

2. **Exhale through slightly parted lips with a tiny whisper sound, like you're silently blowing on a candle, very calmly.**

3. **Make each exhale longer than the last.**

   This exercise can be done discreetly anywhere, even in class.

Square Breathing with Finger Tracing is a clever, discreet technique for public settings. It involves not only doing the breathing exercise but making tiny movements with your finger or leg.

1. **Trace a square on your leg or desk with one finger.**

2. **Breathe in while tracing up one side.**

3. **Hold while tracing across.**

4. **Exhale while tracing down.**

5. **Hold while tracing across to complete the square.**

   You can breathe for a count of three, four, or five for each side of the square (for example, in for three, hold for three, out for three, hold for three).

Another great exercise for teens for emotional regulation is Alternate-Nostril Breathing, described in Chapter 12.

Finding breathing practices for sports and physical activities

Many professional athletes use breathing techniques to enhance performance. This angle often engages teen interest.

This is an ideal Pre-Game Breathing exercise to optimize oxygen levels and focus:

1. **Inhale through the nose for six counts, expanding the belly.**

2. **Hold for two counts.**

3. **Exhale through the nose for six counts.**

4. **Repeat ten times.**

TRY THIS

The following exercise is great to use between plays or during breaks. This pattern helps you clear lactic acid and return to baseline faster.

1. **Inhale through the nose for two counts.**

2. **Exhale through the nose for four counts.**

3. **Gradually slow down the in and out breaths and make them quieter as you start to recover.**

TRY THIS

Coordinating breath with movement is a great technique for running and improving your time. Find a breathing pattern that matches footfalls (for example, inhale for three steps, exhale for two steps). This creates a meditative state and optimizes oxygen uptake.

TIP

When running, breathe in and out using your nose. If you can't do it, slow down your running. Over time, you'll be able to run faster and for longer, all while breathing with your nose! You just need to be patient with yourself as you readjust.

TRY THIS

After intense physical activity, try the Cooldown Cascade:

1. **Start with shorter breaths, matching the current elevated breathing rate.**

2. **Gradually extend each exhale.**

3. **Aim to reach a normal breathing pattern within three to five minutes.**

This systematic approach helps the nervous system regulate more efficiently.

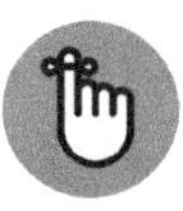

REMEMBER

For teens, the "why" matters as much as the "how." Briefly explain the physiological benefits of each technique to increase motivation.

Managing Stress and Anxiety with Breathwork

One of my corporate clients was worried about his seven-year-old son, who was so anxious about school that he refused to go. Skeptical but desperate, my client agreed to try daily Balloon Breathing with his son. Within three weeks, the boy had not only returned to school but created his own "Worry Wizard Breathing Kit" — and even started sharing the techniques with his classmates. This is the power of breath!

Identifying signs of stress in children and teens

Children often can't articulate feeling "stressed" or "anxious" — they simply know they feel "bad," "scared," or "weird." As adults, we need to recognize the signals:

The physical signs of stress include the following:

- Headaches or stomachaches with no medical cause
- Changes in appetite
- Sleep disturbances
- Bedwetting or other regressions
- Restlessness, fidgeting, or an inability to sit still
- Frequent illness due to lowered immunity

Emotional signs include the following:

- Increased irritability or moodiness
- Excessive worrying
- New fears or phobias
- Clinginess or separation anxiety
- Withdrawal from activities they previously enjoyed
- Aggressive behavior

Behavioral signs include the following:

- Decreased academic performance
- Reluctance to attend school
- Difficulty concentrating
- Negative self-talk
- Nervous habits (nail biting, hair twisting, and so on)
- Avoidance of certain situations

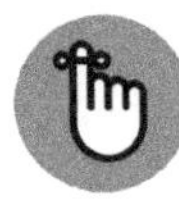

Stress isn't the only potential cause of these symptoms, but stress could be a factor. So, keep an open mind and keep observing if you notice these symptoms or if your child shares them with you. Stress is a normal part of growing up, but kids need to learn the skills to manage stress so it doesn't get out of hand.

Create a "feelings check-in" routine where everyone in the family shares how they're feeling or rates their stress level on a scale of 1 to 10. This normalizes discussing emotions and creates awareness of when breathing techniques may be helpful.

Sharing exercises to help them relax

Many of the deep, slow breathing exercises are good to help kids relax. In this section, I offer some more exercises to help children and teens calm down that stress response.

Balloon Breathing

This popular visual technique helps children understand diaphragmatic breathing. You could also call it teddy bear breathing.

1. Have the child lie on their back with a small stuffed animal on their belly.

2. Ask them to pretend their belly is a balloon.

3. When they breathe in, the balloon inflates (belly rises).

4. When they breathe out, the balloon deflates (belly falls).

5. Challenge them to make the stuffed animal rise and fall with their breath.

For older children and teens, this can be done sitting up, with their hands on their abdomen to feel the movement.

4-4-4 Triangular Breathing

Triangular Breathing is like drawing a gentle triangle with your breath. It's easier than box breathing and helps kids feel calm and focused.

1. Imagine drawing a triangle in the air with your finger.

   You can also draw the triangle on paper or in the air with your whole arm for fun!

2. Breathe in for four counts as you trace up one side of the triangle.

3. Hold your breath for four counts as you trace the second side across the top.

4. **Breathe out for four counts as you trace down the final side back to where you started.**

5. **Repeat three to five times, keeping the triangle shape and rhythm.**

For younger children, start with a 3–3–3 pattern. For teens or those ready for more, try 4–4–6 (longer exhale). You can also "color" each side of the triangle with words like *calm*, *still*, and *release*.

Five-Finger Breathing

Five-Finger Breathing is a calming and grounding breath practice using your hand. Challenge your child or teen to breathe as quietly as possible.

1. **Hold up one hand in front of you, fingers spread wide.**

   This is your breathing hand — the one you'll trace.

2. **Use the index finger of your other hand to slowly trace your thumb: As you breathe in, trace up the side of your thumb, and as you breathe out, trace down the other side.**

3. **Continue this pattern for each finger: Breathe in as you trace up a finger, and breathe out as you trace down that finger.**

4. **Move slowly across all five fingers.**

   By the end, you'll have taken five full, mindful breaths.

5. **If you feel calmer and more focused, you can stop. If not, do another round!**

Combine this technique with a humming out breath, or making the sound of the ocean by pursing their lips as they breathe out, to deepen the calming experience.

Using breathwork to navigate big emotions

In my daily mindfulness club, I once shared what I call the CALM Breath Technique, a sequence designed specifically for emotional overwhelm. One mother whose 12-year-old daughter struggled with intense emotional reactions reported that implementing this approach transformed their home environment.

Here's how to do the CALM Breath technique:

1. **Connect: Before helping your child, take a moment to connect with your own breath and body.**

   A calm adult presence is the strongest co-regulator.

Take one steady breath and soften your shoulders. Just this small pause can shift the energy.

2. **Aware and Anchor: Guide your child to notice what's happening inside and around them.**

   For example, "Can you name three things you see and three things you hear?" "Where do you feel that big feeling in your body?" This anchors attention in the present moment and starts calming the nervous system.

3. **Long Outbreaths: Breathe together slowly.**

   Emphasize longer exhales to trigger the relaxation response. For example, "Inhale for three, exhale for five." Or simply say, "Let's blow the worry out like a balloon."

4. **Meet with kindness: When they're calmer, offer gentle presence and connection.**

   Ask with warmth: "What are you feeling right now?" or "What would help you feel better?" Hold space without rushing to fix. A kind word or a hand on the heart goes a long way.

For specific emotional states, try these targeted breathing techniques:

>> **For anger:** Dragon Fire Breath. Follow these steps:

   1. **Inhale deeply through the nose.**

   2. **Exhale forcefully through the mouth with an audible *haa* sound.**

   3. **Optional: Add arm movements pushing outward on the exhale.**

   4. **Repeat until the intensity subsides.**

>> **For worry or fear:** Starfish Breath, which is similar to Five-Finger Breathing. Follow these steps:

   1. **Hold up one hand and imagine it's a starfish.**

      They can gently move their hand as if it's in the ocean.

   2. **With the index finger of the other hand, trace up one finger while inhaling.**

   3. **Trace down the other side while exhaling.**

   4. **Continue tracing each finger up and down.**

      The tactile element provides grounding while regulating breath.

>> **For sadness:** Heart Blossom Breath. Follow these steps:

1. **Place both hands over the heart, one on top of the other.**

2. **Breathe into the heart space, imagining it warming up.**

3. **On the exhale, bloom the hands outward like a flower opening.**

   This creates a physical expansion that counteracts the contraction of sadness.

>> **For overwhelm:** 5-4-3-2-1 Grounding Breath. Follow these steps:

1. **Take a deep breath while noticing five things you can see.**

2. **Take another deep breath while noticing four things you can touch.**

3. **Continue with three things you can hear, two things you can smell, and one thing you can taste.**

   Each sensory awareness is paired with a conscious breath.

Practice these techniques during calm times so they become accessible during emotional moments. The body remembers what you repeatedly do.

Integrating Breathwork into Daily Routines

The most successful breathing practice isn't the one with the fanciest techniques — it's the one that actually happens regularly. When I first started teaching breathing to families, I created elaborate 20-minute sessions that looked impressive but rarely got done. Now I focus on simple, integrated approaches that become part of the family culture.

Breathing at bedtime for better sleep

Sleep challenges are among the most common concerns parents bring to my coaching or community. A mother of twins shared how implementing a breathing-based bedtime routine transformed their evening struggles into a peaceful transition that everyone actually enjoyed.

Create a breathing bedtime ritual:

1. **Choose a consistent time to begin the wind-down process.**

2. **Dim the lights to signal to the body that it's time for melatonin production, which helps you sleep.**

3. **Start with active breathing to release residual energy:**

- **For younger children:** Three to five Dinosaur Stomps (big inhale, raising arms, loud exhale, stomping feet).

- **For older children:** Five to ten Wave Breaths (inhale, raising arms like a wave, exhale, folding forward).

4. **Move to calming breathing (choose one):**

- **Sleep Countdown:** Starting from ten and count down with each exhale.

- **Stuffed Animal Rise:** Place a small stuffed animal on their belly and watch it rise and fall with each breath.

- **Starlight Breath:** Inhale, imagining drawing golden light in, exhale, spreading it throughout the body.

5. **Finish with listening breath: Simply pay attention to the natural breath for 10 to 30 seconds.**

TIP

For sleep-specific breathing:

>> Make exhales longer than inhales to activate the parasympathetic nervous system.

>> Keep the jaw relaxed.

>> Encourage breathing at a slower rate.

>> Use a sound machine synchronized to breathing rates (ocean waves work well).

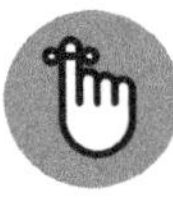

REMEMBER

Consistency matters more than perfection. Even a two-minute breathing routine, done reliably, creates powerful sleep associations.

Starting the day calmly with morning breaths

The first minutes after waking set the tone for the entire day. I learned this lesson personally when I noticed how my own morning rush was affecting my nervous system regulation. Now, the parents I work with report that morning breathing is often their most impactful practice.

TRY THIS

This simple Morning Minute routine takes just 60 seconds but can transform the day:

1. **Before getting out of bed, take three deep breaths.**

2. **Sit up and do five Sunrise Breaths: Inhale arms up like the rising sun, exhale arms down.**

3. **Set an intention for the day with one final deep breath.**

For children who resist structure in the morning, try these playful alternatives:

» **Stretch and Breathe Animal Wakeups:**

- "Let's wake up like a lion!" (Lion Breath)

- "How does a snake stretch in the morning?" (Snake Breath)

Rotate through different animals each day of the week.

» **Breathing Games:**

- "Can you blow this feather to the door?" (Controlled exhale practice)

- "Let's see whose belly balloon can get biggest!" (Deep diaphragmatic inhale)

» **Breath-Centered Morning Song:** A simple melody with movements timed to breath creates a joyful routine.

For school-age children, create a "morning breath card" they can keep by their bed as a reminder. Let them decorate it to increase ownership of the practice.

TIP

Using breathwork in challenging situations

Some of the most powerful moments that are shared in my community come when parents realize they can transform habitual stress points in the day using targeted breathing interventions.

Here are some common challenging situations and breathing solutions:

» **For morning rush/transitions:**

- **Transition Breath:** Before leaving the house or car, everyone takes three synchronized breaths together.

- **Ready, Set, Breathe:** Before entering a new environment (school, store, activity), take one giant breath in and "power exhale."

» **For tantrums/meltdowns:**

- **Co-regulation Breath:** Parents breathe audibly and obviously, modeling calm for the dysregulated child.

- **Dragon Fire Breath:** Channel overwhelming emotions through powerful exhales.

- **Bubble Emergency Kit:** Keep a small bubble container for "breathing emergencies." The act of blowing bubbles naturally regulates breathing.

» **For school stress:**

- **Test-Taking Power Breath:** Before exams, five cycles of four-count inhales, six-count exhales.

- **Homework Helper:** Set a timer for 20-minute work sessions with 2-minute breathing breaks between.

- **Locker Breath:** One calm breath while opening the locker creates a micro-moment of centering.

» **For social anxiety:**

- **Friendship Breathing:** Before entering social situations, imagine breathing in courage, exhaling doubt.

- **Worry Shrink Breath:** Inhale normally, and then exhale with a whispered *whoosh,* imagining worries shrinking.

» **For sibling conflicts:**

- **Peace Pause:** When arguments escalate, call a "peace pause" for one minute of breathing.

- **Back-to-Back Breath:** Siblings sit back-to-back, feeling each other's breathing rhythm.

After successfully using breathing to navigate a challenging situation, create a quick positive reinforcement by naming what happened: "You used your Dragon Breath and calmed your body down. That's using your breathing power!"

Encouraging consistency with fun tools

Even the most beneficial practice won't help if it isn't done consistently. Here are creative ways to make breathing exercises a regular part of family life:

» **Visual reminders and charts:**

- **Breathing Buddy System:** Designate special stuffed animals as "breathing buddies."

- **Breathing Wheel:** Create a paper wheel that children can turn to select different breathing exercises.

- **Breathing Jars:** Fill jars with different colored items representing different breathing techniques.

- **Growth Charts:** Track consistent breathing practice with stickers or stamps.

>> **Stories and personification:**

- **Breathing characters:** Create characters who embody different breathing techniques (for example, Eddie the Elephant for elephant breath).

- **Breathing adventure books:** Read stories that incorporate breathing, like *Breathe Like a Bear* by Kira Willey (Rodale Kids).

- **Creating your own book:** Have children illustrate their favorite breathing techniques.

>> **Making it social:**

- **Family breathing moments:** Designate specific times when everyone pauses for a breathing break.

- **Breathing challenges:** "Can everyone remember to do morning breaths for seven days straight?"

- **Breathing show-and-tell:** Each family member demonstrates their favorite technique at dinner.

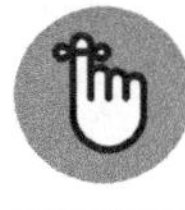

REMEMBER

The best breathing practice is the one that actually happens. Focus on enjoyment and integration rather than perfection.

As one of my clients wisely said, "We stopped trying to 'do breathing exercises' and started simply 'being a breathing family.' That's when everything changed."

When breathing becomes part of your family culture rather than another task to complete, the benefits multiply exponentially. Children develop a lifelong skill that will serve them through every challenge and celebration.

These aren't miracle cures — they're the natural results of giving children tools to connect with their own innate capacity for regulation and well-being.

So, start simple. Start today. Breathe together. And watch what unfolds.

4

Advanced Breathing Practices

Here you explore advanced breathing techniques to strengthen your lungs, enhance performance, and unlock deeper levels of physical and mental resilience, as well as how to go beyond any one technique. You start by finding out how to expand your lung capacity, practice extended breath holds, and use recovery techniques to improve breathing efficiency in everyday life and high-intensity situations.

Next, you discover how breathwork can boost physical and mental performance. You find out how to balance energy and relaxation for peak performance, use pre-event breathing routines to stay calm and focused, and integrate breathing techniques into endurance training and high-intensity activities.

I introduce you to a wide range of breathwork styles designed for deeper physical, emotional, or spiritual exploration, from calming practices like Sudarshan Kriya to intense techniques like Holotropic Breathwork and the Wim Hof Method. You see how different methods evoke different experiences — from emotional release to altered states of consciousness — and how to choose a practice that suits your needs, temperament, and safety.

Finally, you discover how to shift from controlling your breath to simply allowing it — seeing that breathing can be a natural, effortless path to presence, peace, and a deep sense of connection. By letting go of the need to "do it perfectly," you realize that breath can become your best friend — a steady reminder that you are already enough, already home.

Chapter **15**

Strengthening Your Lungs

Welcome to the lung gym! In this chapter, you discover how to assess your current lung capacity (without any expensive medical equipment), warm up your breathing muscles safely, build impressive respiratory endurance, and recover like a pro. These techniques go beyond your basic "breathe in, breathe out" instructions — they're specially designed to strengthen your respiratory system from the inside out.

Preparing Your Lungs for Advanced Exercises

Before you start bench-pressing air with your diaphragm, you need to know where you're starting from and how to prepare your lungs safely. You wouldn't try to run a marathon without checking your fitness level or warming up first, and you shouldn't jump into advanced breathing exercises without proper preparation.

Assessing your current breathing capacity

How do you know if your lungs are working at their full potential? Medical tests like *spirometry* (a test that measures how much air you can breathe in and out and how quickly you can do it) can give you precise measurements, several do-it-yourself methods can give you a good idea of your current breathing capacity.

The Body Oxygen Level Test (BOLT), a term coined and developed by Patrick McKeown, is a simple yet effective way to assess your breathing efficiency. It's the same as the Control Pause used in the Buteyko Breathing Method (see Chapter 9), but it can be used by everyone, even if not doing the Buteyko Breathing Method. Think of it as a fitness test for your lungs that you can do anywhere, anytime. Here's how to do it:

1. **Sit comfortably with your back straight.**

   Wait for a few minutes if you've been talking or moving around to ensure you're fully at rest before taking the test.

2. **Take a normal breath in and out through your nose.**

3. **After the exhale, pinch your nose closed and start a stopwatch.**

4. **Hold your breath until you feel the first clear desire to breathe — not until you're gasping for air.**

   It can be a bit tricky to know when to stop holding your breath. If you have to take a much bigger breath than usual after your breath hold, you held your breath too long. Take a break and try again. You should be able to breathe in the same way as prior to the measurement. The number of seconds you can comfortably hold your breath is your BOLT score. A BOLT score of 25 seconds or more indicates good breathing function. Below 25 seconds suggests room for improvement.

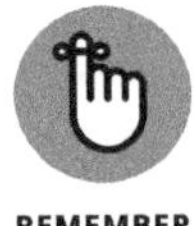

Don't worry if your score is on the lower side — that's why you're reading this chapter! By doing the exercises I recommend daily, your BOLT score is highly likely to improve.

Learning warm-up techniques for lung expansion

Now that you know where you stand (or breathe), it's time to warm up those lungs before diving into the heavyweight breathing exercises.

The Accordion warm-up helps increase the mobility of your rib cage, allowing for greater lung expansion:

1. **Stand or sit with good posture.**

2. **Place your hands on the sides of your lower ribs.**

3. **Breathe in slowly through your nose, feeling your ribs expand outward against your hands.**

4. **Exhale completely through your mouth, feeling your ribs contract.**

5. **Repeat five to seven times, focusing on expanding your ribs in all directions — front, sides, and back.**

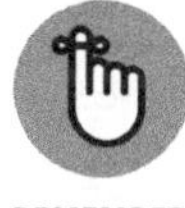

Think of your rib cage as an accordion that needs to be stretched and contracted regularly to maintain flexibility. The more mobile your ribs are, the more space your lungs have to expand.

The Progressive Lung Inflation warm-up gradually increases your breathing depth:

1. **Take five breaths at 25 percent of your maximum capacity.**

2. **Take five breaths at 50 percent of your maximum capacity.**

3. **Take five breaths at 75 percent of your maximum capacity.**

4. **Take five breaths at 100 percent of your maximum capacity.**

5. **Reverse the process, gradually decreasing back to shallow breathing.**

You may wonder how to gauge 25 percent, 50 percent, or 75 percent of your breath. Think of 100 percent as a full inhale, 75 percent as three-quarters, 50 percent as half, and 25 percent as a gentle sip. No need for precision, just explore the depths gradually.

This progressive approach helps prevent strain while preparing your lungs for more challenging exercises.

The Whispered Ha is a subtle technique that's perfect for warming up your breathing muscles:

1. **Inhale slowly through your nose.**

2. **Exhale through your mouth while making a whispered *ha* sound.**

   Focus on extending the exhale to twice the length of the inhale.

3. **Repeat ten times, gradually increasing the length of both inhale and exhale.**

The resistance created by the whispered sound helps activate your diaphragm and *intercostal muscles* (the muscles between your ribs, assisting your rib-cage movement when you breathe), preparing them for more intensive work.

Ripple Breath, sometimes also called the Three-Part Breath, is an ideal warm-up exercise. I prefer the name Ripple Breath because it gives you a nice visual image of ripples expanding in a lake as you do it:

1. **Start by breathing into your lower abdomen, seeing it rise.**

2. **Continue the same breath, feeling it move into your lower ribs, expanding them outward.**

3. **Finally, allow the breath to fill your upper chest.**

4. **Exhale in reverse: The upper chest deflates first, then the lower ribs, and finally the abdomen.**

5. **Repeat five to seven times, visualizing a wave of breath moving through your torso.**

This warm-up helps engage all parts of your respiratory system and increases awareness of the different regions of breathing.

Recognizing signs of overexertion

When it comes to breathing exercises, the "No pain, no gain" mentality can be dangerous. Your lungs aren't biceps, and pushing them too hard can lead to problems.

Here are some of the warning signs that you need to ease up:

>> Dizziness or lightheadedness (beyond mild)

>> Tingling in your fingers or toes or around your mouth

>> Unusual headaches during or after practice

>> Heart palpitations or irregular heartbeat

>> Excessive fatigue following breathing exercises

>> Chest pain or tightness

>> Feeling anxious or panicky during exercises

>> Fainting

>> Nausea/cold sweat

>> Blurred vision

>> Muscle cramps

>> Persistent cough/wheeze and/or blue lips

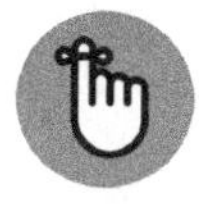

You may experience another symptom not listed here. Listen to your body and take a rest if you feel uncomfortable. Breathing exercises should make you feel better, not worse!

One of my clients got so eager about breathwork that he practiced breath holds for nearly an hour, ending up with tingling hands, dizziness, and confusion. "More is better, right?" he joked. I explained that with breathing, consistency beats intensity; 10 to 15 minutes of steady daily practice works far better than marathon sessions that strain the lungs.

Before each breathing practice session, ask yourself:

>> Am I in a safe environment where I can focus? (For example, you should *not* do these exercises in water or while driving.)

>> Have I waited at least two hours after a heavy meal?

>> Do I have any medical conditions that may be affected by breathing exercises?

>> Am I well rested enough to practice effectively?

If you answer "No" to any of these questions, consider modifying your practice or choosing a better time.

If you have uncontrolled asthma, a flare of chronic obstructive pulmonary disease (COPD), recent chest surgery, cardiovascular disease, pregnancy complications, or a history of panic attacks, check with your doctor before doing these exercises.

If you experience any of the following symptoms, here's what to do:

Symptom	What to Do
Lightheadedness	Stop and return to normal breathing immediately.
Chest pain	Stop and consult a healthcare provider.
Gasping	Pause and rest.
Irregular breathing	Pause and rest.
Increasing tension in the shoulders, jaw, or face	Pause and rest.

When it comes to lung strengthening, progress is gradual. Your respiratory system adapts over weeks and months, not days. Patience is your friend here!

REMEMBER

Building Strength and Capacity

Now that you've assessed your starting point and learned how to warm up properly, it's time to build those lung muscles and expand your breathing capacity. These exercises may feel challenging at first, but with consistent practice, they'll become easier as your respiratory system strengthens.

Exploring extended breath holds for endurance

Breath holding isn't just for underwater swimmers and breathwork masters. When done correctly, it can significantly increase your lung capacity and respiratory muscle strength. Think of it as resistance training for your breathing system.

The Incremental Hold is the most well-proven of the exercises in this chapter. This progressive technique helps you safely extend your breath-holding capacity:

1. Sit comfortably with good posture.

2. Take three normal breaths through your nose.

3. After a normal exhale (not forced), hold your breath for a comfortable count (start with half your BOLT score; see "Assessing your current breathing capacity," earlier in this chapter).

4. Resume normal breathing for 30 seconds.

5. Repeat, adding 2 seconds to each hold.

6. Continue until you reach a challenging but manageable duration.

7. Perform five rounds three times per week.

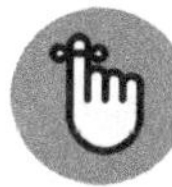

The key here is gradual progression. Don't try to double your time in one session!

The Recovery Hold Method simulates the oxygen demands of physical exertion:

1. March in place or do jumping jacks for 30 seconds to slightly elevate your heart rate.

2. Immediately sit down and take one deep breath.

3. Exhale normally and hold your breath.

4. Hold until you feel the first urge to breathe (not to your maximum).

5. Resume normal breathing for one minute.

6. Repeat five times.

This method trains your body to manage oxygen more efficiently during and after physical activity.

The Expansive Hold is a unique technique that combines breath holding with rib-cage expansion:

1. Inhale fully into your lower abdomen, lower ribs, and upper chest.

2. Hold this breath while actively expanding your rib cage in all directions.

3. Hold for a comfortable duration (start with five to ten seconds).

4. Exhale slowly through pursed lips.

5. Rest for two normal breaths.

6. Repeat five times.

This exercise not only improves your breath-holding capacity but also increases the flexibility of your rib cage, allowing greater lung expansion over time.

Practicing Pursed-Lips Breathing for lung efficiency

Pursed-Lips Breathing isn't just for people with respiratory conditions — it's a powerful technique for anyone looking to improve lung efficiency. This technique creates back pressure in the airways, helping to keep them open longer and allowing for more complete air exchange.

The 2:1 Pursed-Lips Ratio is a fundamental technique that improves lung efficiency:

1. Sit upright with relaxed shoulders.

2. Inhale through your nose for a count of two.

3. Purse your lips as if drinking through a straw or whistling.

4. Exhale through pursed lips for a count of four.

5. Gradually increase both counts while maintaining the 1:2 ratio (3:6, 4:8, and so on).

6. Practice for five minutes daily.

Even doing just three to five breath cycles of this has been found to have measurable benefits. So, feel free to do it anytime you have a moment.

The back pressure created by the pursed lips helps the *bronchioles* (branches inside your lungs) stay open longer, allowing more air to exit and reducing the work of breathing.

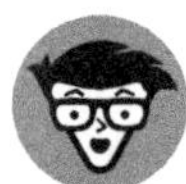

The Walking Pursed-Lips Method is a practical application that helps build stamina:

1. While walking, inhale through your nose for two steps.

2. Exhale through pursed lips for four steps.

3. Continue this pattern throughout your walk.

4. As you build strength, try exhaling for six or eight steps.

This technique is particularly valuable for hills or stairs, helping you maintain efficient breathing during exertion.

The Resistant Pursed-Lips technique adds an element of resistance for greater strength building:

1. **Place a drinking straw between your pursed lips.**

2. **Inhale normally through your nose.**

3. **Exhale completely through the straw, creating resistance.**

4. **Focus on maintaining a steady, controlled exhale.**

5. **Repeat for ten breaths.**

6. **As you progress, use narrower straws for greater resistance.**

This technique strengthens your *expiratory muscles* (the group of muscles that help you breathe out) and trains you to exhale more completely, reducing stale air in the lungs.

Trying the Lung-Strengthening Nostril Cycle for balance

Alternate-Nostril Breathing (called Nadi Shodhana in yoga) is often practiced for its mental benefits, but it also offers significant advantages for lung strength and respiratory balance when modified with specific parameters. Turn to Chapter 12 for how to do the basic Alternate-Nostril Breathing.

The Lung-Strengthening Nostril Cycle is a modification that focuses specifically on lung development. The key difference is that you breathe in and out fully and completely through each nostril:

1. **Sit comfortably with an upright spine.**

2. **Close your right nostril with your right thumb.**

3. **Inhale slowly and completely through your left nostril.**

4. **Close your left nostril with your right ring finger, release your thumb.**

5. **Exhale slowly and completely through your right nostril.**

6. **Inhale through your right nostril.**

7. **Close your right nostril, release your left.**

8. **Exhale through your left nostril.**

   This completes one cycle.

9. **Start with five cycles and build to ten.**

Breathe as quietly and gently as you comfortably can to enhance the experience and quality. One nostril may be more blocked than the other. Don't worry about that — that's normal.

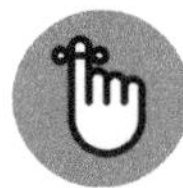

The key difference for lung strengthening is to focus on complete inhalations and exhalations, using your full lung capacity with each breath.

The following Resistance Variation technique adds mild resistance to strengthen breathing muscles:

1. **Follow the same alternate-nostril pattern as the Lung-Strengthening Nostril Cycle (earlier in this section), but slightly constrict the open nostril by gently pressing the side of your nose.**

   Create just enough resistance to feel the breath, but not enough to strain.

2. **Practice for five minutes, gradually increasing the resistance as your strength improves.**

This added resistance works like weight training for your breathing muscles.

The following Extended Ratio Method is a variation that uses timing to increase lung efficiency:

1. **Begin the same alternate-nostril pattern as the Lung-Strengthening Nostril Cycle (earlier in this section).**

2. **Inhale for a count of four.**

3. **Hold the breath gently for a count of two.**

4. **Exhale for a count of six.**

5. **Progress to a 4:4:8 pattern as your capacity increases.**

The extended exhale is particularly effective for strengthening the lungs and training them to expel more air.

In a corporate workshop I was running, a senior executive struggled with public speaking anxiety tied to her breathing. I taught her Alternate-Nostril Breathing with calming visualization to use before presentations. Two months later, she wrote to say her breathing had improved, her confidence had soared, and she'd even been promoted. "I thought I needed speech therapy," she said. "Turns out I needed breathing therapy!"

Enhancing Lung Health with Recovery Techniques

You've learned how to assess, warm up, and strengthen your lungs. Now let's focus on recovery — an often-overlooked aspect of respiratory health that's crucial for long-term improvement and maintaining healthy lung function.

Breathing after exercise or high-intensity activity

How you breathe immediately after exertion significantly impacts your recovery and lung health. These techniques help optimize the recovery process and train your lungs to return to baseline more efficiently.

Do you find yourself breathing heavily for too long after exercise? If so, try the Pursed-Lips Recovery Ladder, a progressive technique to help your breathing system recover methodically:

1. Immediately after exercise, stand or sit tall.

2. Begin with slightly pursed lips, exhaling fully.

3. Inhale through your nose for a count of two.

4. Exhale through pursed lips for a count of four.

5. Repeat five times.

6. Transition to equal-length breaths (3:3) for five more breaths.

7. Allow your breathing to normalize naturally.

This cascade approach helps prevent the common post-exercise "breathing debt," in which you continue to breathe heavily long after you've stopped moving.

The Lateral Recovery Breath technique engages the often-neglected *lateral aspects* (sideways expansion and contraction) of breathing:

1. After exercise, stand with your feet shoulder-width apart.

2. Place your hands on the sides of your lower ribs.

3. Inhale through your nose, focusing on expanding your ribs sideways against your hands.

4. **Exhale slowly through your nose.**

5. **Repeat for ten breaths.**

This lateral expansion helps engage different parts of your lungs during recovery, improving overall gas exchange efficiency.

Recovery Breath Counting is a mindful technique that combines recovery with awareness:

1. **Find a comfortable position after exercise.**

2. **Begin counting your breaths backward from 20 to 1.**

   Focus on making each breath slightly slower and deeper than the last.

3. **By the time you reach 1, your breathing should be close to your resting rate.**

This technique not only facilitates physical recovery but also helps transition your mind from the aroused exercise state to a more relaxed condition.

Using slow breathing to reduce breathlessness

Feeling breathless can be frightening, whether it's from exertion, anxiety, or environmental factors. These specialized slow breathing techniques help you regain control and comfort.

The 4-2-6 Rescue Breath quickly addresses breathlessness. You don't have to stick to these exact numbers of 4-2-6. Ideally, you want to aim for around ten seconds for the in and out breath combined.

1. **Inhale through your nose for a count of four.**

2. **Hold briefly for a count of two.**

3. **Exhale through pursed lips for a count of six.**

4. **Repeat until breathing normalizes.**

The extended exhale helps prevent air trapping and reduces the feeling of breathlessness.

The Cyclic Sighing for Recovery technique uses the natural mechanism of sighing to reset breathing patterns:

1. Inhale slowly through your nose into your lower lungs.

2. Without exhaling, take a second, shorter breath to fill your upper lungs.

3. Exhale slowly and completely through your mouth with a slight sighing sound.

4. Repeat five to ten times.

Research at Stanford University has shown this technique to be very effective in reducing anxiety and improving mood, in addition to addressing breathlessness.

The Hand Breathing technique is a tactile method that helps manage breathlessness through sensory feedback:

1. Place one hand on your abdomen and one on your upper chest.

2. Focus on moving only the lower hand during inhalation.

3. Keep the upper hand relatively still.

4. Exhale slowly through pursed lips.

5. Repeat until breathing stabilizes.

The tactile feedback helps redirect your breathing pattern from chest-dominant (which often occurs during breathlessness) to diaphragm-dominant.

Seated Lean-Forward Breathing is a position-based technique that's particularly helpful during episodes of breathlessness:

1. Sit on the edge of a chair with feet flat on the floor.

2. Lean forward slightly, keeping your back straight.

3. Rest your elbows on your knees or on a table in front of you; keep your shoulders relaxed.

4. Breathe in through your nose.

5. Exhale through pursed lips for twice as long as the inhale.

This position naturally engages your diaphragm and reduces the work of breathing. This technique is shared in clinics for acute breathlessness.

Supporting respiratory health in everyday life

Strengthening your lungs isn't just about dedicated exercise sessions — it's about incorporating healthy breathing habits into your daily life. These practical techniques help maintain and continue building your respiratory health throughout your day.

Transform waiting at traffic lights from frustration to a respiratory opportunity with the Traffic Light Breath:

1. **When stopped at a red light, take a deep breath in.**

2. **Hold briefly as the light remains red.**

3. **Begin exhaling after five or six seconds or when the light turns green.**

4. **Continue a controlled exhale as you begin accelerating.**

Not only does this improve your breathing, but it also reduces traffic stress!

Create environmental cues for better breathing with the Desktop Breathing Station:

1. **Place a small object on your desk or in your work area as a breathing reminder.**

2. **Every time you notice the object, take three conscious breaths.**

   For the first breath, focus on inhaling fully. For the second breath, focus on exhaling completely. For the third breath, focus on the pause between inhale and exhale.

This micro-practice accumulated throughout the day significantly improves breathing habits.

Use doorways as triggers for breathing awareness with the Doorway Breath Reset:

1. **Choose specific doorways in your home or workplace.**

2. **Every time you pass through these doorways, take one full, conscious breath.**

   Vary the breathing pattern for different doorways (some for deep breathing, others for exhale emphasis).

This technique integrates breathing practice into your environmental transitions.

TRY THIS

End your day with the Before-Sleep Breathing Ritual:

1. **Lie in bed and place one hand on your abdomen.**

2. **Take ten slow, deep breaths, through your nose, feeling your hand rise and fall.**

   With each exhale through your nose, allow your body to sink deeper into the mattress. Imagine your lungs cleaning and rejuvenating as you breathe.

This practice not only supports respiratory health but also improves sleep quality.

I recently received a message from a client who joined my private community after recovering from pneumonia. His doctor had told him his lung function might be permanently reduced. He faithfully practiced the meditation and breathing techniques I share daily, particularly the everyday life integrations. Six months later, his lung function tests showed remarkable improvement. "My doctor was very pleased," he told me. "He asked what I'd been doing, and when I told him about these simple daily practices, he was reminded of the power of breathing exercises."

REMEMBER

Strengthening your lungs takes time. Gentle, consistent practice brings better results than occasional intensity. Notice small improvements in stamina, stress, and well-being. Your lungs adapt beautifully with steady training.

Chapter **16**

Enhancing Performance

In this chapter, you supercharge your abilities through the power of breath! If you've ever watched elite athletes or top performers in action, you've probably noticed how they seem to have an almost magical ability to stay calm under pressure, access explosive energy when needed, and maintain laserlike focus. Here's their secret: They've mastered the art of breathing for performance. After reading this chapter, you'll have a toolkit of breathing techniques that can help you perform better — whether you're running a marathon, giving a presentation, or just trying to stay mentally sharp during a day full of meetings.

I've seen firsthand how transformative these techniques can be. One of my clients, a surgeon, went from struggling with hand tremors during lengthy procedures to performing with rock-steady precision after implementing the breathing strategies in this chapter. Another client took up and excelled in running marathons after learning how to implement breathing exercises. These people aren't anomalies — they're examples of what happens when you harness the remarkable power of your breath.

Appreciating the Role of Breath in Physical and Mental Performance

You may think that breathing harder or deeper during exercise or stressful situations is always better — after all, more oxygen must be good, right? Well, hold that thought (along with your breath, but I get to that later).

Understanding how oxygen impacts stamina and focus

Here's something that may surprise you: Breathing too much can reduce your performance. I know, it sounds backward, but stick with me. This phenomenon, known as the *oxygen paradox*, is a game-changer for understanding performance breathing.

When you breathe excessively (what experts call *over-breathing*), you blow off too much carbon dioxide. Many people think of carbon dioxide as just a waste gas, but it actually plays a crucial role in helping oxygen detach from the blood cells and enter the tissues where it's needed most — the muscles, brain, and organs.

When carbon dioxide levels drop from breathing too much (known as the *Bohr effect*), oxygen binds more tightly to hemoglobin in the blood, making it harder for that oxygen to reach the muscles and brain. The result? Decreased stamina, brain fog, and poor focus — exactly what you *don't* want during performance!

I once coached a client who came to my online workshop complaining about brain fog during important meetings as an executive. "Shamash," he told me, "I take these huge, deep breaths before speaking to get more oxygen, but I still feel lightheaded and my thoughts scatter." After explaining the oxygen paradox, I taught him to breathe more lightly through his nose. Within weeks, he reported dramatic improvements in his mental clarity during presentations. His colleagues even commented on how much more articulate and focused he seemed.

More breathing doesn't equal more oxygen delivery to your tissues. Balanced breathing that maintains appropriate carbon dioxide levels optimizes oxygen release where it's needed.

REMEMBER

Balancing energy and relaxation for peak performance

Have you ever noticed how some people seem perpetually wired and anxious, while others appear so relaxed they may fall asleep mid-conversation? Neither extreme makes for peak performance. The sweet spot lies in between — what psychologists call the *optimal arousal zone* or what athletes know as being "in the flow."

Your breath is your body's most direct path to finding this balance because it connects directly to your autonomic nervous system. Think of your breath as having two essential gears:

>> **Sympathetic (fight-or-flight):** Faster, upper-chest breathing activates your body for action.

>> **Parasympathetic (rest-and-digest):** Slower, deeper breathing promotes recovery and calm focus.

The trick is knowing which gear to engage and when. For a sprinter at the starting blocks, a few powerful breaths may help channel productive tension. For a golfer lining up a crucial putt, slow, measured breathing helps steady the hands.

In my Daily Mindfulness Club, I often guide participants through three different breathing exercises. Over time, they discover which breathing exercises energize them, which exercises calm them, and which exercises create a balance of just the right combination of energy and calm.

Try this three-step process when deciding what breathing exercise to do at any time:

1. **Notice your current breathing pattern.**

2. **Decide what state would serve you better for the task at hand.**

3. **Shift your breathing accordingly (quicker for energy, slower for calm).**

Surprisingly simple, yet remarkably effective.

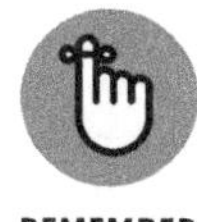

If you're tired and you have a few minutes or more, you may want to practice some soothing and calming breathing exercises. This will both relax and restore your energy, so when you're done, you feel rested and energized.

Measuring your breathwork progress

"How do I know if I'm getting better at breathing?" This is a common question I get. Unlike strengthening your biceps, where you can see and measure progress, breathing improvements can seem nebulous — but they don't have to be.

One of the best ways to measure your breathing efficiency, apart from using professional equipment, is to do the Body Oxygen Level Test (BOLT). Developed by breathing expert Patrick McKeown and adapted from the Buteyko Breathing Method, this simple test provides clear feedback on your carbon dioxide tolerance and overall breathing efficiency. (You can learn how to do it in Chapter 15.)

When I first took the BOLT test myself, I scored just 15 seconds. This was probably part of the reason why I was struggling to sleep deeply at night and waking up tired. After a few weeks of practicing the techniques in this chapter, my score rose to around 25 seconds. The improvement wasn't just a number. I noticed better endurance during my hikes, clearer thinking during teaching, better sleep, and less afternoon fatigue.

THE LEGENDARY RUNNER WHO WON THREE GOLD MEDALS . . . WITH HIS NOSE

Long before wearable tech, Emil Zátopek — known as the "Czech Locomotive" — became one of the greatest long-distance runners in history. He won three gold medals at the 1952 Helsinki Olympics in the 5,000 meters, 10,000 meters, and marathon — all in the same Games. No other athlete achieved this for the next 70 years.

But here's the lesser-known part of his story: Zátopek trained using nasal breathing, decades before it became trendy. He would often run with his mouth closed, focusing on controlling his breath, even during high-intensity intervals. His goal wasn't just endurance — it was calm under pressure.

Zátopek realized early on that he needed to train not just his body, but his breath. Modern breath experts like Patrick McKeown now teach similar methods — and research confirms that nasal breathing during running helps maintain better carbon dioxide tolerance, improves oxygen uptake, and reduces fatigue.

So, whether you're training for a 10K or chasing your kids round the park, take a page from Zátopek's book: Close your mouth, calm your breath, and run like a legend.

Measure your BOLT score weekly to track progress. Morning measurements provide the most consistent results. Record your scores to stay motivated as you improve.

Practicing Pre-Event Breath Routines

The minutes before a performance — whether physical or mental — often determine success or failure. Your breath is your best tool for creating an optimal pre-performance state.

Breathing to calm pre-performance nerves

We've all felt those pre-performance jitters: the racing heart, sweaty palms, scattered thoughts. Instead of trying to fight these sensations (which often makes them worse), you can use specific breathing techniques to transform nervous energy into focused readiness.

One great technique to deal with this is 4-2-6 Breathing. This is a gentle, controlled breathing pattern designed to turn anxious "nerves" into focused "drive." With a longer exhale, it works wonders to calm your body, center your mind, and get you feeling ready for action rather than overwhelmed. Here's how to do it:

1. **Sit or stand tall — shoulders soft, feet firm.**

    Imagine you're at the starting line of calmness.

2. **Inhale smoothly through your nose for a slow count of four.**

    Try to fill up your lower abdomen and lower chest. Keep your shoulders down.

3. **Gently hold your breath for a count of two.**

    Use this pause to imagine gathering your energy and focus.

4. **Exhale slowly and steadily through your mouth or nose for a count of six.**

    Let your shoulders drop if they raised. Imagine tension pouring out with your breath. If you want, you can picture little cartoon worries floating away.

5. **Repeat for three to five rounds.**

    Each exhale sends a signal to your nervous system: "Relax, you've got this."

If the counts feel too long, shorten them (for example, 3-1-5). Comfort, not heroics!

The extended exhale (six counts) taps your relaxation system, leaving you calm but not sluggish. The short hold builds a little inner momentum. Perfect for transforming nerves into laser-sharp focus.

I taught this technique to a concert pianist who struggled with performance anxiety. Before discovering this technique, she'd often have memory lapses during recitals despite flawless practice sessions. "The difference is remarkable," she told me after using 4-2-6 Breathing before her next performance. "My hands were steady, my mind clear. I actually enjoyed performing instead of dreading it."

For situations requiring a deeper focus, together with the calm, try this Mindful Body Scan Coherent Breathing:

1. **Sit comfortably.**

2. **As you inhale for five to six seconds and exhale for five to six seconds, mentally scan and relax your forehead and face.**

3. **As you inhale for five to six seconds and exhale for five to six seconds, soften your throat and tongue.**

4. **As you inhale for five to six seconds and exhale for five to six seconds, relax your hands.**

5. **As you inhale for five to six seconds and exhale for five to six seconds, soften your belly.**

6. **As you inhale for five to six seconds and exhale for five to six seconds, soften your hips and pelvis area.**

7. **As you inhale for five to six seconds and exhale for five to six seconds, relax your feet.**

8. **Repeat, gently moving your attention through these common areas of tension and letting go with every breath.**

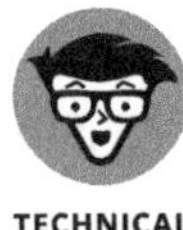

Coherent Breathing, as shared by Stephen Elliott, isn't just about slow, steady breath. You can go deeper if it's paired with consciously relaxing six key regions in the body, which he dubbed the "Six Bridges." These bridges are: the face, the tongue and throat, the hands, the diaphragm, the pelvic floor, and the feet. Elliott discovered that each of these areas is under both voluntary and automatic (dual) control, making them special levers for calming the whole system. By systematically relaxing these six bridges as you breathe, you connect your mindful intention with your body's built-in relaxation wiring, helping the breath and nervous system reach a state of true coherence and deep calm.

If you struggle to relax any area, that's absolutely fine and nothing to worry about. Just simply become aware of the sensations and tension in that part of your body. The mindful awareness will have a beneficial effect, even if that body part isn't relaxed. This is one of the amazing things mindfulness research has discovered.

Energizing techniques for physical events

Sometimes you don't need calm — you need energy! For those situations, you need breathing techniques that prime your body for explosive action without the jittery side effects of caffeine or pre-workout supplements.

One highly effective pre-event energizing technique is what I call the Triple-Pump Primer.

You need to be in good health to practice this technique. If you're prone to hyperventilation, panic attacks, or certain heart conditions, avoid this one — or start *very slowly.*

Here's how to do the Triple-Pump Primer:

1. **Stand tall with your feet shoulder-width apart.**

2. **Take three quick, powerful inhalations through your nose without exhaling, progressively filling your lungs.**

3. **Exhale forcefully through your mouth.**

4. **Repeat five to eight times, resting with normal breathing for 15 seconds between each set.**

This technique mimics the breathing pattern observed in many explosive animal movements in nature. It temporarily increases oxygen intake while activating your sympathetic nervous system in a controlled manner.

I used this technique before going for a run. The Triple-Pump Primer helped channel my energy and got me into the right state of mind.

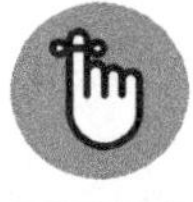

This exercise is a stressor and raises your heart rate and blood pressure.

For high-intensity physical events like sprinting or weightlifting, try the following Power-Up Breath:

1. **Take a full, deep breath through your nose.**

2. **Hold for two seconds.**

3. **Exhale forcefully through pursed lips, engaging your core.**

4. **Repeat three to five times.**

5. **On the final breath, inhale deeply and hold briefly as you begin your activity.**

Breathing in through your nose helps oxygenate your body. The brief breath hold helps build up carbon dioxide, which helps get the oxygen into your muscles. And the pursed-lips exhale helps activate your deepest abdominal muscles and creates a pressure between your diaphragm and pelvic floor. This protects your lower back, stabilizes your spine, boosts explosive power, and helps with posture and balance. Win-win-win!

Using visualization with breath for mental focus

Elite performers often pair breathing with visualization to create a state of focused readiness. When combined, these techniques become more powerful than either practice alone.

Here's a pre-event focus routine I call Performance Breath Imaging:

TRY THIS

1. **Find a quiet spot and sit or stand comfortably.**

2. **Close your eyes and establish a smooth, rhythmic breathing pattern.**

3. **As you inhale, imagine drawing in your optimal performance state — confidence, focus, strength.**

4. **As you exhale, imagine releasing tension, doubt, and distraction.**

5. **Begin visualizing yourself performing successfully, syncing your breath with the rhythm of your imagined performance.**

6. **For three to five minutes, immerse yourself in this visualization, always anchoring to your breath.**

When visualizing, go through all your senses. What would you see, hear, smell, taste, or feel?

TIP

I used this technique with an executive who struggled with focus during her meetings and presentations. She really enjoyed visualization. "The corporate world can be chaotic," she explained, "and I found my attention pulled in a dozen directions." After practicing Performance Breath Imaging before going into a challenging meeting, she reported a remarkable shift: "It's like creating a bubble of calm and focus around me. The chaos is still there, but it doesn't penetrate my concentration anymore."

Record a guided version of this visualization on your phone, using your own situation.

Training for Strength and Stamina

Pre-performance breathing helps optimize your immediate state, but systematic breath training develops capacities that stay with you all the time. Think of it as the difference between putting on armor before battle (helpful) versus strengthening your body year-round (transformative).

Breathing exercises for running and endurance activities

Most runners focus entirely on leg strength, heart capacity, and training plans, but they often neglect the very thing that limits performance: breathing efficiency. Incorporating specific breathing exercises into your training routine can dramatically improve endurance without adding more miles.

One powerful technique that transformed my own running (okay, slow jogging in my case!) is Nasal-Only Running:

1. **During an easy run, breathe exclusively through your nose.**

   If you feel you need to mouth-breathe, slow down until nasal breathing feels comfortable again.

2. **Gradually increase either distance or pace each week, always maintaining nasal breathing.**

3. After four to six weeks, you'll likely be able to run at your previous pace while breathing only through your nose.

If your nose is too blocked to be able to do nasal breathing when running, try wearing a nasal dilator. You can find skin-color or transparent ones.

Nasal-Only Running forces your body to become more efficient at oxygen utilization and carbon dioxide tolerance. When you return to "normal" breathing during a race, you'll find your endurance has improved substantially.

For rhythmic endurance activities like cycling or swimming, try Cadence-Matched Breathing:

1. **Establish a comfortable breathing-to-movement ratio (for example, one breath cycle every four pedal strokes).**

   Focus on maintaining this rhythm regardless of intensity. If maintaining the rhythm becomes difficult, reduce intensity slightly

2. **Gradually extend the duration you can maintain this synchronized pattern.**

This technique trains your nervous system to coordinate breathing with movement, reducing the energy cost of both.

I guided a client through these methods as he prepared for his first marathon. "I was skeptical at first," he admitted. "It seemed too simple to make a real difference." Six weeks later, his tune had changed dramatically: "I'm not gasping during hard efforts anymore, and my recovery is much faster. I wish I'd learned this years ago!"

Controlled hyperventilation for short, high-intensity moments

Chronic hyperventilation is problematic, but brief, intentional periods of increased ventilation can benefit specific high-intensity situations when used strategically.

Never practice hyperventilation techniques near water, while driving, or if you have cardiovascular concerns, have epilepsy, or are pregnant. These techniques are for healthy individuals during specific training contexts only.

The Power Breathing Surge technique can be valuable immediately before or during intense efforts. This technique is mostly suitable for efforts under one to two minutes, like sprints, power lifts, and high-intensity interval training (HIIT) sessions.

1. **In 30 to 40 seconds, take 20 to 30 slightly faster and deeper breaths through your nose.**

   Make each breath deliberate but not maximal.

2. **Follow immediately with your high-intensity effort.**

This technique temporarily increases oxygen availability while preparing your body for the oxygen debt that comes with all-out effort. The key difference between this and dysfunctional hyperventilation is that it's brief, controlled, and purposeful.

For sports with intermittent sprints (like soccer or basketball), the Recovery Accelerator helps you bounce back more quickly:

1. **Immediately after a sprint, take five quick, strong nasal inhalations.**

2. **Follow with one long exhale through pursed lips.**

3. **Return to normal nasal breathing.**

This accelerates carbon dioxide clearance while quickly restoring normal breathing patterns.

Wondering how this works? Taking five quick breaths in through your nose acts like a reset button for your breathing after you've pushed yourself hard. Then breathing out slowly through pursed lips helps your body switch into recovery mode, calming your heart rate. Going back to slow, gentle nose breathing trains your body to handle more carbon dioxide and keeps you from breathing too fast or feeling lightheaded.

Breath holds for increased oxygen efficiency

Perhaps counterintuitively, one of the most effective ways to improve breathing efficiency is to practice *not* breathing. Controlled breath-holding exercises, when done safely and progressively, can dramatically improve your body's oxygen utilization.

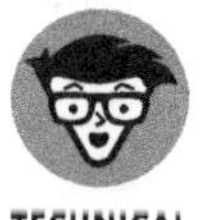

The science is fascinating: Brief, intermittent *hypoxia* (oxygen reduction) stimulates adaptations similar to altitude training, while increased carbon dioxide levels help recalibrate your breathing center's sensitivity. The result? Better performance with less breathlessness.

Here's a progressive training protocol I've used with numerous clients, called Carbon Dioxide Tolerance Builders:

1. **Sit comfortably and relax with normal breathing for two minutes.**

2. **Take a normal breath in and out through your nose (not deep, not shallow).**

3. **Hold your breath after the exhale for a comfortable duration (start with 50 percent to 60 percent of your BOLT score — see Chapter 15).**

4. When you resume breathing, breathe normally for 30 to 45 seconds.

5. Repeat for five to ten rounds, gradually increasing hold time as comfort allows.

For a more functional application, try Walking Breath Holds:

1. While walking at a comfortable pace, exhale normally and hold your breath.

2. Continue walking until you feel a moderate air hunger; then resume nasal breathing.

3. Recover with normal breathing for one to two minutes.

4. Repeat five to eight times.

As you progress, try increasing your walking pace during the holds.

I practiced this technique extensively before a hiking trip to a high altitude. When I reached the summit, where many others struggled with the thin air, I was able to maintain steady breathing and energy levels throughout the climb. The adaptation to intermittent hypoxia through breath holds had prepared my body for the challenging conditions.

One of my memorable client success stories involved a purpose-driven entrepreneur who was juggling multiple projects and constantly feeling breathless — not just physically, but mentally. Despite his success, he hit a wall: His energy dipped midday, his focus wavered, and stress was creeping in more than he liked to admit.

We started incorporating breath-hold training into his morning routine and daily walks. Within a few weeks, he reported a surprising shift: "It's like I've unlocked this hidden gear," he said. "I feel calmer in meetings, sharper in my thinking, and weirdly — I'm *less tired*, even though I'm doing more. My breath feels like a secret superpower now."

Always prioritize safety with breath-hold training. Never practice in water, while driving, or alone if you have any medical conditions. Progress gradually instead of pushing for dramatic improvements quickly. Slow and steady wins the race!

Bringing It All Together

To maximize the benefits of performance breathing, consistency is key. Here's a simple framework for integrating these practices into your routine:

>> Daily foundation (five to ten minutes)

  - Measure your BOLT score once a week (see Chapter 15).

  - Spend three to five minutes on nasal breathing awareness.

  - Add five to eight gentle carbon dioxide tolerance mini-holds (starting with 50 percent of your BOLT score).

>> Pre-training routine (three to five minutes)

  - To center yourself, do one minute of Physiological Sighs.

  - Do two to three minutes of visualization paired with slow breathing (visualize your ideal performance).

  - Optional: Do 30 seconds of Power Breathing Surge for high-intensity sessions.

>> During-training focus

  - Breathe through your nose as much as possible.

  - Practice your established breathing-to-movement ratio.

  - Let your breath guide your intensity — not the other way around.

>> Dedicated breath training (15 to 20 minutes, two to three times a week)

  - Carbon Dioxide Tolerance Builders

  - Walking Breath Holds

  - Nasal-only cardio sessions

>> Pre-event protocol (five to ten minutes)

  - Begin with Performance Breath Visualization.

  - Do either calming Coherent Breathing or energizing Triple-Pump Primer, depending on your needs.

  - Finish with three grounding Physiological Sighs.

The beauty of these techniques is that they require no special equipment, can be practiced anywhere, and complement any physical training program. They're the hidden performance edge that many elite athletes use but few discuss openly.

Breathwork practitioners all over the world have witnessed the extraordinary transformations in clients who committed to these breathing practices. Beyond measurable performance improvements, they report greater enjoyment of their sports and activities, reduced performance anxiety, and a heightened sense of control during challenging situations.

In my own journey from stressed-out schoolteacher to mindfulness and breathwork teacher, these techniques, along with others in this book, were instrumental in helping me find balance and effectiveness in high-pressure situations. During some of my workshops, I'd experience overwhelming anxiety — until I discovered the power of intentional breathing for performance. Now, teaching groups of hundreds feels natural and energizing rather than draining.

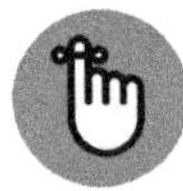

Breathing for performance is a skill that develops with practice. Be patient with yourself, track your progress (the BOLT score is invaluable here), and notice how these practices enhance not just your physical abilities but your overall experience of life's challenges.

Try my guided meditations and breathwork exercises on YouTube (www.youtube.com/@shamashmindful). They're free, and they can be a good avenue into calming breathwork after your performance to calm down.

Chapter **17**

Breathwork Styles for Deeper Exploration

Welcome to the wild and wonderful world of breathwork styles and methods for deeper exploration!

Breathwork styles are the various methodologies that have emerged over the years. They often consist of a set of breathing exercises done one after the other, sometimes with other add-ons like music, community, reflective practice, group sharing, meditation, and more.

Breathwork styles for deeper exploration are like the advanced courses in the university of breathing. The breathing exercises I cover in the previous chapters are like your foundational classes — think of them as Breathing 101. The deeper practices in this chapter can get pretty intense, transformative, and occasionally a bit trippy.

These advanced techniques go beyond simply helping you relax or focus. They're designed to create profound shifts in consciousness, unlock emotional blockages, and sometimes even trigger what practitioners describe as "mystical" or "transcendent" experiences. It's like the difference between taking a gentle stroll through your local park and embarking on a challenging mountain hike — both involve putting one foot in front of the other, but the intensity and destination are quite different.

EXPERIENCING ALTERED STATES OF CONSCIOUSNESS

Breathing can reliably create altered states of consciousness. These states don't mean losing touch with reality. Instead, your perception shifts. Time may feel slower or faster, your awareness may expand, or fresh insights may surface. It's similar to being absorbed in music or a novel. You're still present, just experiencing awareness differently.

Research shows that specific breathwork techniques, especially circular or connected breathing, reduce carbon dioxide levels in the blood, which can trigger these shifts. The effects are often compared to psychedelics, yet they arise purely through intentional breathing.

What makes this so powerful is that the experience isn't just novel — it can be therapeutic, if done safely with a fully qualified professional. Some people report emotional release, greater self-understanding, and a sense of expanded perspective that continues long after the session ends.

REMEMBER

Simpler, more calming breathing exercises can be transformative and deeply healing, too. It's all about finding what's right for you. You don't have to do any of the breathwork styles in this chapter if you don't feel called to do so.

UNDERSTANDING EMOTIONAL RELEASE AND TRAUMA FROM BREATHWORK

One of the most powerful aspects of breathwork is its ability to help people process and release stored emotions and trauma. Now, I know the word *trauma* can sound scary, but remember that trauma doesn't just mean major life-altering events — it can include any experience that overwhelmed your ability to cope at the time.

Our bodies are incredibly smart and have a way of storing unprocessed emotions and experiences. Think of it like having a junk drawer in your house — over time, stuff accumulates, and eventually, you need to clean it out or it becomes dysfunctional. Breathwork can be like that spring-cleaning session for your emotional system.

During intensive breathing sessions, people often experience what's called *emotional release.* This may involve crying, shaking, or other physical expressions of stored emotions. Although this may sound intense (and it can be!), it's generally considered a healthy and healing process when it happens in a safe, supported environment with a trained therapist.

The breathing techniques work by activating the parasympathetic nervous system — your body's "rest-and-digest" response — which can help shift you out of chronic stress patterns. When trauma is stored in the body, people often get stuck in a chronic state of fight-or-flight activation. Breathwork can help reset this system and allow natural healing processes to occur.

Finding the Right Breathwork Style for You

Just as there's no one-size-fits-all approach to exercise or diet, there's no single breathwork style that works perfectly for everyone. Some people thrive on gentle, meditative approaches, while others need something more dynamic and intense to feel the benefits. It's a bit like the difference between people who love gentle yoga versus those who prefer high-intensity interval training (HIIT) — both can be incredibly beneficial, but they appeal to different temperaments and needs.

Discovering breathwork for every temperament or need

Your breathwork preference often reflects your personality and current life circumstances. If you tend to be highly analytical and live mostly in your head, you may benefit from practices that help you drop into your body and emotions. Conversely, if you're naturally very emotional and sensitive, you may prefer practices that help you find calm and stability.

Some people are drawn to breathwork because they're seeking spiritual experiences and expanded consciousness. Others are more interested in practical benefits like stress reduction, better sleep, or improved athletic performance. There's no right or wrong motivation — the key is finding approaches that align with your goals and comfort level.

Finding out why different people prefer different approaches

People gravitate to different breathwork styles based on personality, experience, current needs, and preference. Research shows that breathing patterns evoke distinct emotional states: some energize, others calm. Anxious or overwhelmed individuals often prefer slower, controlled practices, while those feeling stuck may choose more activating ones.

In my case, because I've been practiced mindfulness and meditation for most of my life, I'm naturally drawn to the more calming and centering breathing exercises like 4-6 Breathing (Chapter 2), Ocean Breath (Chapter 8), Coherent Breathing (Chapter 8), Pursed-Lips Breathing (Chapter 11), or the Buteyko Breathing Method (Chapter 9). And these tend to be the exercises I share with my community. They're generally safe, and they currently have more evidence for their benefits than other techniques. You may be different and prefer some of the more vigorous practices in this chapter. These more intense practices should only be done by those in good physical and mental health and with a well-qualified professional.

Doing a self-check to find your favorite approach

Not sure where to start? Use this quick check-in to explore what may suit you best right now. Answer honestly — there are no right or wrong answers, just helpful clues.

1. **How do you usually respond to stress?**

    A. I get caught in overthinking.

    B. I feel overwhelmed with emotion.

    C. I tend to shut down, disconnect, or feel anxious.

    D. I get fidgety or need physical release.

2. **What do you most hope to gain from breathwork?**

    A. Relaxation and calm.

    B. Deep healing or emotional release.

    C. Mental clarity, resilience, or well-being.

    D. Energy, stamina, or better physical health.

3. **How comfortable are you with intense experiences — whether emotional or physical?**

    A. I prefer gentle and gradual practices.

    B. I'm open to intense experiences if they're meaningful.

C. I'm cautious and prefer evidence-based techniques.

D. I enjoy pushing my limits physically and feeling energized.

4. **Which statement sounds most like you?**

A. I love quiet, calming practices like meditation.

B. I'm curious about altered states and inner exploration.

C. I want something practical and backed by research.

D. I'm excited by bold methods and challenges.

Here's how to interpret your results:

>> **Mostly A's:** Try gentle breath practices like Calming Pranayama (Chapter 8), Coherent Breathing (Chapter 8), or Alternate-Nostril Breathing (Chapter 12).

>> **Mostly B's:** Explore deep styles like Holotropic Breathwork or Conscious Connected Breathing (both covered later in this chapter).

>> **Mostly C's;** Consider structured, evidence-based methods like Sudarshan Kriya (SKY; covered later in this chapter) or the Buteyko Breathing Method (Chapter 9).

>> **Mostly D's:** Look into techniques like the Wim Hof Method (covered later in this chapter) or Oxygen Advantage (https://oxygenadvantage.com).

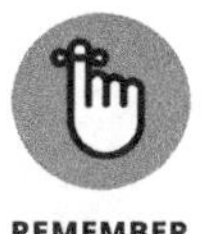

You're not fixed to one style — what helps today may change tomorrow. Start where you feel drawn, and keep exploring.

REMEMBER

Identifying Breathwork Styles to Try

In this section, I introduce you to some breathing styles and approaches that are often used for deeper insight and inner exploration. These aren't the only ones — there are countless methods out there — but they include some of the better-known practices.

Sudarshan Kriya Yoga: The Art of Living's signature style

Sudarshan Kriya Yoga (SKY) is like the modern success story of the breathwork world. Developed by spiritual teacher Sri Sri Ravi Shankar in 1982, it may be one of the most widely practiced and scientifically studied breathing techniques on the planet.

The name *Sudarshan* means "proper vision" in Sanskrit, and *Kriya* refers to a purifying practice.

What makes SKY unique is its systematic approach to rhythmic breathing. The practice involves breathing in specific patterns that range from slow and calming to fast and energizing. It's said to be designed to work with your body's natural rhythms to release stress and tension at the cellular level. Think of it as a complete tune-up for your nervous system.

SKY is taught through the Art of Living Foundation's courses, always with proper instruction rather than from books or videos. The Art of Living says that this ensures that people learn the technique correctly and have support for their practice. The technique has now been taught to millions of people worldwide in more than 150 countries.

What's particularly interesting about SKY is how it bridges ancient wisdom with modern accessibility. Although it's based on traditional yogic principles, it has been adapted and refined for contemporary life. You don't need any previous experience with yoga or meditation to learn and benefit from the practice.

SRI SRI RAVI SHANKAR'S STORY AND SKY BREATHING

In 1982, high up in the hills of southern India, a young man sat in silence for ten days. No phone, no distractions — just stillness. That man was Sri Sri Ravi Shankar. And from that silence emerged something that would go on to transform millions of lives: a breathing practice called Sudarshan Kriya.

But Shankar's story began long before that. Born in 1956, he was a curious and contemplative child. By the age of four, he could already recite entire chapters of the *Bhagavad Gita,* one of India's most sacred texts. He studied both ancient wisdom and modern science — Vedic literature and physics — combining insight with inquiry.

As he grew older, Shankar noticed a growing restlessness in the world: stress, conflict, and disconnection. He believed something as simple and natural as the breath could help. So, he started the Art of Living — a global movement offering tools for inner peace, community well-being, and a stress-free society. At its heart was his unique breathing technique: rhythmic, accessible, and powerful.

A typical session

A full SKY session typically takes about 45 minutes and consists of four distinct breathing stages. The session begins with a few minutes of gentle breath awareness to help you settle in and become present.

The practice is made up of four distinct steps, each one building on the last:

1. **Ujjayi (Victorious Breath or Ocean Breath):** A slow, steady breath where you gently constrict the back of your throat, creating a soft ocean-like sound. You breathe in and out with control — about two to four breaths per minute. This helps to calm both body and mind while keeping you alert and present.

2. **Bhastrika (Bellows Breath):** Here, the breath gets more energized. You inhale and exhale rapidly and forcefully — around 30 breaths per minute. It's a bit like pumping your breath in and out. This creates a wave of energy, followed by a settling calm.

3. **Chanting "Om":** You slow everything down by chanting *Om* three times very slowly. The extended out-breath while chanting helps lengthen your exhalation, soothing the nervous system.

4. **Sudarshan Kriya (Rhythmic Breathing):** Finally, you practice a series of slow, medium, and fast-paced rhythmic breathing cycles. This is the heart of SKY. The varying rhythms help clear mental clutter, balance emotions, and often bring a sense of deep clarity or even joy.

Although it may sound simple, the combination of these four steps can be surprisingly profound — a kind of inner reset through breath.

The evidence

SKY, taught by the Art of Living Foundation, is one of the most widely studied breath-based practices in the world, with more than 100 independent studies conducted across four continents. These studies consistently show that SKY supports both mental and physical health, with measurable improvements across a wide range of areas.

For mental well-being, SKY has been shown to significantly reduce depression, anxiety, stress, and post-traumatic stress disorder (PTSD), with remission from depression seen in about 70 percent of participants, often within just three to four weeks. Benefits include improved emotional regulation, higher self-esteem, better sleep, and increased joy and optimism. Importantly, these effects have been observed even in individuals who did not respond to medication or psychotherapy.

Biologically, SKY has been found to:

>> Normalize brain-wave patterns, shifting the mind from a stressed, high-alert state (beta waves) to calmer, more restorative states (like alpha or theta).

>> Increase *prolactin* (a well-being hormone) after just one session.

>> Reduce *cortisol* (a stress hormone) and other biochemical stress markers.

>> Enhance immune function, antioxidant levels, and even gene expression — showing changes within two hours of practice.

Physically, it improves heart rate, blood pressure, cholesterol, and respiratory function, with increased lung capacity and reduced breath rate over time.

Research shows that SKY has been found to be as effective as antidepressants, but without the side effects.

Safety considerations

SKY is generally considered safe when taught by authorized instructors through the Art of Living Foundation, which follows a structured protocol and offers ongoing support. The breathing stages progress gradually, helping to prevent overwhelm and making the practice accessible for most people.

That said, it's important to approach SKY with care. Those with serious heart or lung conditions, with psychiatric challenges, or who are pregnant should seek medical advice before beginning. One of the strengths of SKY is its self-regulating nature — you can always return to natural breathing if needed. Most people find it both energizing and calming, without the intense emotional waves seen in some other breathwork styles.

Holotropic Breathwork: The psychedelic without the drugs

Holotropic breathwork is a deep breathing technique designed to guide you into a nonordinary state of consciousness (basically, an altered state — but I don't want to make it sound too sci-fi). It was created in the 1970s by two psychiatrists, Stanislav and Christina Grof, who were looking for a legal alternative to LSD for therapeutic and spiritual exploration.

The word *holotropic* means "moving toward wholeness," and that's really the aim — reconnecting with your inner self, your unresolved emotions, your body, your spirit . . . all through your breath.

It's not a technique for your morning commute. This is a big breathwork journey, often used for emotional healing, spiritual awakening, or simply to shake off a sense of stuckness. You may cry. You may laugh. You may see colors. Or you may just yawn a lot. Either way, the idea is: It's all welcome.

A typical session

A Holotropic Breathwork session is a deep and immersive experience, usually lasting several hours. It begins with an opening circle where participants set intentions, receive guidance on the technique and safety, and pair up with a breathing partner. The facilitators create a supportive environment, helping everyone prepare for the journey ahead.

The breathing phase lasts two to three hours and involves lying down with eyes closed while breathing rapidly and continuously through the mouth. Evocative music plays throughout, beginning with rhythmic beats to activate the breath, moving into more emotional or intense phases, and ending with softer sounds to support integration. The music acts as a kind of map for the inner journey.

During this time, people may experience strong emotions, physical sensations, vivid memories, or even visions. Trained facilitators are always present to ensure safety and support. The session ends with a reflective phase — often involving drawing, journaling, or a group sharing circle — helping participants process and make sense of what emerged during the session.

What the research says

Although Holotropic Breathwork hasn't been studied as much as other therapies, the early findings and anecdotal reports are promising for some.

It's tricky to research something like this because the experience is so personal and often intense. People describe it as deeply emotional, spiritual, and sometimes life-changing — not exactly easy to measure in a lab.

That said, many participants report greater self-awareness, emotional release, and a shift in how they see themselves and their life challenges. Some say it helped them move through grief or trauma, while others felt a renewed sense of clarity or purpose.

There are signs that breathwork practices like this can positively influence how the brain processes emotion, pain, and even identity. We don't have all the answers yet, but the science is slowly catching up with what many breathers have been saying for decades: Something powerful seems to happen when you breathe with intention in a safe and supportive space.

Holotropic Breathwork isn't a cure-all, but for some people, it becomes a turning point in their personal growth or healing journey. Just like any deep practice, it's not for everyone — but for the right person at the right time, it can be a real breath of fresh insight.

Safety considerations

Now, let's have a mindful pause and talk safety.

Holotropic Breathwork is powerful, but intense. It's designed to stir up deep physical, emotional, and psychological material. That's why it's not suitable for everyone.

Avoid this practice (or get medical advice first) if any of the following apply to you:

» You have a heart condition, high blood pressure, glaucoma, or epilepsy.

» You've had surgery recently.

» You have acute or chronic hyperventilation.

» You have a psychiatric condition like psychosis or a severe personality disorder, or you're taking a psychiatric medication.

» You're pregnant or breastfeeding.

Even healthy participants may experience strong effects like tingling, cramping, intense emotions, or resurfacing memories. This can be part of the healing — but only in the right environment.

Always practice with a certified facilitator trained in Holotropic Breathwork. They'll keep the space safe, guide you through intense moments, and support your integration afterward. This is definitely not a DIY technique.

Conscious Connected Breathing: Circular breathing for emotional release

Conscious Connected Breathing (CCB) is like the middle child of the breathwork family — not as ancient as pranayama, not as intense as Holotropic Breathwork, but with its own unique personality and powerful effects.

What Conscious Connected Breathing is

CCB is a simple yet powerful breathwork technique where you breathe continuously without any pause between the inhale and exhale. Imagine your breath like a flowing river — no stops, no gaps, just a steady, conscious rhythm. You breathe in through the nose or mouth, and instead of holding or controlling the exhale, you let it go naturally and without effort.

What makes this practice different is the focus on awareness and nonjudgment. You're not just breathing to survive, you're breathing to notice. Over time, this circular breathing pattern can help unlock suppressed emotions, ease tension, and shift your mental state.

It has been used in various forms for decades (sometimes called Rebirthing or Integrative Breathwork). It's increasingly backed by both anecdotal stories and some research. But it isn't a quick fix — it's a practice, one that can be gentle or deep, depending on how it's guided and received.

A typical session

A typical CCB session lasts between 30 minutes and two hours and begins with setting an intention — something simple like "I want to feel more grounded" or "I'm open to letting go." The session is usually guided by a trained facilitator who creates a safe, calm space, often with music and gentle cues.

You'll lie down, close your eyes, and begin breathing in a connected rhythm. That means no pause between inhale and exhale — like a wave that rises and falls. You're encouraged to breathe through your mouth or nose, depending on the style. After around 30 to 45 minutes of continuous breathing, there's usually a phase of integration, where you rest, reflect, and allow any insights or emotions to settle.

Physical sensations (tingling, heat, lightness) or emotional experiences (like tears of sadness or feelings of joy) may arise. All are welcome. It's important to know that you're in control — you can slow down, take a break, or return to normal breathing anytime.

What the evidence says

Although CCB has been practiced since the 1970s, research is still catching up. A recent study explored the effects of CCB and found promising links to emotional release and improved well-being, including reduced anxiety and better mood regulation. Participants often described feeling more "present" and "in touch" with themselves.

However, studies tend to be small and varied in design, making it tricky to draw big, sweeping conclusions. What we do know is that CCB increases awareness of the body, activates the parasympathetic nervous system (the "rest-and-digest" state), and can support emotional processing — especially when facilitated safely.

There's still more to explore in terms of its long-term mental health benefits, but the initial research suggests that CCB can be a helpful complementary approach, particularly for stress and emotional integration. Just bear in mind that it's not a substitute for therapy or medical care.

Safety considerations

CCB is generally considered safer than some intensive breathwork practices, but it's not without potential risks.

Like all strong practices, CCB comes with some safety considerations. This is not just a relaxing breath practice — it can be emotionally intense. That's why it's best done with a trained facilitator, especially if you're new to the practice or have any health conditions.

It's not recommended for anyone with cardiovascular issues, epilepsy, glaucoma, or retinal detachment. It's also not recommended if you've had a surgery recently. If you're pregnant or you have a history of trauma or severe mental health conditions, panic attacks, or chronic hyperventilation, check with a healthcare professional first.

Physically, you may feel lightheaded, experience muscle tension or cramping, or have emotional releases. These can be safe and even healing — but only if you're in the right environment with support available. If in doubt, get guidance.

You can always return to gentle breathing. You're not trying to force a breakthrough — just staying open, curious, and connected, one breath at a time.

Wim Hof Method: The Iceman cometh

Perhaps the most famous teacher of breathwork in the world is Wim Hof, who developed the Wim Hof Method. Let's find out more.

What the Wim Hof Method is

The Wim Hof Method (WHM) is the rockstar of the breathwork world — flashy, popular, and backed by some pretty impressive feats of human endurance. Named after Dutch extreme athlete Wim Hof, also known as "The Iceman," this method combines specific breathing techniques with cold exposure and mental focus. It's like the triathlon of wellness practices.

Hof developed his method through decades of experimentation with cold exposure and breathing techniques. He holds multiple world records for cold endurance, including swimming under ice, climbing mountains in shorts, and sitting in ice baths for extended periods. What makes his achievements scientifically interesting is that he claims they're not due to some genetic superpower, but rather to techniques that anyone can learn.

The breathing component of the WHM involves a specific pattern of hyperventilation followed by breath retention. You take deep, fast breaths, and then exhale and hold your breath for as long as comfortable. This cycle is repeated several times and is often combined with cold exposure. The method also emphasizes mental commitment and gradual progression.

What's particularly fascinating about the WHM is that it appears to allow voluntary control over parts of the nervous system that were previously thought to be impossible. Hof has demonstrated the ability to consciously influence his immune response, body temperature, and stress response through his breathing techniques. This has attracted significant scientific attention and research.

WIM HOF'S STORY AND THE WIM HOF TECHNIQUE

Wim Hof, known as "The Iceman," is a Dutch extreme athlete famous for pushing human limits — like climbing icy mountains in shorts and sitting in freezing water for nearly two hours. But behind the spectacle is a deeper story and a method that's gained global popularity: the Wim Hof Method, a blend of deep breathing, cold exposure, and mental focus.

Hof began experimenting with cold water at 17, drawn to a frozen canal and the rush it gave him. After the tragic loss of his wife in 1995, he turned to breathwork and cold exposure for healing. This personal journey eventually led to international recognition, multiple Guinness World Records, and celebrity followers.

Despite the dramatic headlines, Hof insists his method is about health, resilience, and reconnecting with your inner strength. The breathing involves deep, fast cycles followed by breath holds, and studies show it may influence stress response, immunity, and even brain function. Just remember: Start gently, listen to your body, and don't try it alone in icy waters.

A typical session

The WHM combines breathing, cold exposure, and commitment to help build resilience, focus, and energy. The breathing part is a powerful practice that many people say boosts their mood, sharpens their mind, and even helps them feel more alive.

A typical WHM breathing session usually takes about 15 to 20 minutes. It involves a series of deep, rhythmic breaths, followed by breath holds and recovery breaths. Some people feel tingly or lightheaded during the breathing, and many people report feeling calm, alert, or deeply relaxed afterward.

Because this practice can be quite intense, it's best to learn directly from Wim Hof's recommended approaches — through his official app, his online course, his book *The Wim Hof Method*, or with a certified Wim Hof Instructor. His website is www.wimhofmethod.com.

What the research says

The WHM has certainly caught the world's attention — but does it actually *work*? A systematic review looked at the scientific studies done so far to find out whether WHM really has a positive impact on physical and mental health. The short answer? It may, but we need more high-quality research to be sure.

Here's what we know so far: WHM may help reduce inflammation in the body, thanks in part to the way it affects stress hormones and immune responses. That's promising, especially because chronic inflammation is linked to many modern health problems. There are also early signs that it may boost your mood, help you feel more energized, and improve your ability to cope with stress.

That said, the studies have been small, and the results are mixed — especially when it comes to exercise performance or long-term psychological effects. So, although the WHM *may* help, it's not magic. More independent research is needed to separate fact from hype.

Safety considerations

Before you dive into cold showers and deep breathing, let's have a heart-to-heart about safety. The WHM can be powerful — but like any powerful practice, it comes with some important risks that are easy to overlook in the hype.

The biggest red flag? Never, *ever* do the breathing exercises near water. That includes bathtubs, pools, lakes, and, yes, even the shower. When you combine deep, fast breathing (hyperventilation) with breath holding, it can sometimes cause people to faint. That's dangerous enough on a yoga mat — but underwater, it can be fatal. Sadly, there have been deaths linked to people passing out during breath holds in water, so just don't go there.

The breathing technique can also cause physical side effects like dizziness, tingling, or muscle cramps. These are usually harmless, but in rare cases, seizures have been reported. If you have heart problems, high blood pressure, panic attacks, epilepsy, or any serious health conditions, or if you're pregnant, it's best to speak with your doctor before trying the method.

Also, be cautious of exaggerated claims. Early research is promising (especially around inflammation and stress response), but it's not a miracle cure. Keep your expectations grounded and stay curious, not reckless.

If you're keen to explore the WHM, start slow, stay safe, and learn from a certified instructor if possible. Wim Hof himself built up his practice over decades — so take your time. You don't need to climb a frozen mountain barefoot to enjoy the benefits.

Other breathing styles to consider

The world of breathwork is surprisingly vast — and it's still growing. Beyond the well-known methods I cover earlier in this chapter, several other approaches have popped up over the years. Each one brings its own unique flavor, often blending breath with movement, sound, or even spiritual practice.

Here are a few you may come across:

>> **Transformational Breath** focuses on spotting where your breath may be restricted — often linked to old emotional patterns. Practitioners use breath, bodywork, and sound to help release tension and restore fuller, freer breathing. It's a structured approach that's been used both for physical healing and personal growth.

>> **Rebirthing Breathwork,** developed by Leonard Orr, uses circular breathing to help people explore and release deep early-life experiences, including birth trauma. Some sessions even take place in warm water to simulate the womb. It's certainly a unique angle on healing.

>> **Shamanic Breathwork** takes a more ritualistic path. You'll find elements like drumming, guided visualizations, and references to spirit animals or inner guides. It's not for everyone, but some people find it a powerful way to reconnect with their inner wisdom.

Clarity Breathwork, Integrative Breathwork, the list goes on — all branching off from the core idea of CCB (covered earlier in this chapter). What unites them is a shared belief that the breath isn't just a physical function, but a gateway to healing, insight, and even transformation.

Chapter **18**

Letting Breath Breathe You: Exploring the Deeper Side of Breathing

Breathing exercises are much more than just fancy ways to fill your lungs with air. They offer moments of peace, can melt stress away, and perhaps give a glimpse into something deeper — a sense of connection that goes beyond your individual self or ego.

In this chapter, you explore the most profound aspect of conscious breath: the recognition that breathing is not just something you do, but something you *are*. You discover how your breath connects you to pretty much every living being on Earth, and how this simple act of inhaling and exhaling can lead you home to your truest nature.

Letting Go of Control

"Feelings come and go like clouds in a windy sky. Conscious breathing is my anchor."

—THICH NHAT HANH

Much of this book is about controlling your breath in some way. And most people do need to do that first, to correct bad habits and breathing patterns due to a lifetime of stress. But when you've learned the breathing exercises and they've become second nature, trying to control your breath can be counterproductive.

In this section, you learn why that's the case. You also find out how to take things to the next level with conscious breathing and the gentle art of letting go.

Releasing the need to "do it right"

I remember working with a self-confessed "perfectionist" who came to my breathing workshop absolutely determined to "nail" every technique. She had her notebook out and timed her breaths with military precision, getting frustrated when her mind wandered during meditation. After about 20 minutes of watching her struggle, I gently suggested she close her notebook and just breathe normally. "But I'm not doing it right!" she protested. That's when I shared one of the most liberating truths about breath: There's no such thing as the perfect breath.

The irony of breathing exercises is that the harder you try to control your breath, the more elusive the benefits become. It's like trying to fall asleep — the more effort you put into it, the more awake you become! This is what I call the *effort trap*, and it catches nearly everyone who begins this journey.

Think about it: You've been breathing your entire life without any conscious effort. As a baby, you breathed with complete naturalness — deep, rhythmic, effortless breaths that flowed like gentle waves. Your tiny chest rose and fell, and you never once worried about whether you were "doing it right." But then life happened. Stress, anxiety, social pressures, and the general hustle and bustle of modern living taught you to hold your breath, breathe shallowly, or breathe in ways that create tension rather than ease. On top of that, spending hours hunched over your phone or laptop often causes you to slouch, reducing space for your lungs and making deep, nourishing breaths even harder to take.

The beautiful truth is that through gentle breathing practices, you're not learning something new — you're simply returning to what you already knew.

It's a bit like learning to ride a bicycle. Remember that? At first, it seemed impossible. You wobbled, fell off, got frustrated, and wondered if you'd ever manage to stay upright. But then, almost magically, something clicked. Suddenly, you weren't thinking about balance or pedaling or steering — you were just cycling. The effort dissolved into effortlessness, and what once seemed so difficult became as natural as walking. Learning to breathe better is a bit like that.

Try this simple exercise to get a taste of what letting go feels like. I call it the Art of Effortless Breathing:

1. Sit comfortably and close your eyes.

2. **For the first minute, try to control your breathing.**

   Make it as perfect as you can, count the seconds, focus on getting equal inhales and exhales.

3. **Notice how this feels in your body and mind.**

4. **For the next three minutes, simply observe your breath without changing anything.**

   Let your breath breathe itself while you watch like a curious observer.

5. **Notice the difference in how this feels.**

You may have noticed that being desperate to get your breath perfect had the opposite effect. Sometimes all you need to do is be conscious of your breath, effortlessly, just as it is. It may then naturally deepen, slow down, and correct itself.

Being, not becoming

In our achievement-oriented culture, we're trained to always be working toward becoming something better, different, or more evolved than we are right now. This mindset can easily creep into breathing practice, turning it into another project for self-improvement rather than a celebration of what you already are.

The deepest invitation of breathing practice is to discover the joy of simply being. Not becoming more relaxed, more aware, or more spiritual — just being exactly what you are in this moment. When you can rest in being rather than constantly trying to become, something magical happens: You discover that you're already whole, already complete, already perfect exactly as you are.

This doesn't mean you become passive or stop growing and learning. Instead, any growth or change happens naturally from a place of self-acceptance rather than self-rejection. It's like trying to force a flower to bloom instead of providing the right conditions and allowing the plant to bloom in its own time.

I learned this lesson the hard way during my early years of practice. I was so focused on achieving deep meditative states that I missed the simple beauty of just breathing normally. I was trying so hard to become a "good meditator" that I forgot to enjoy the actual experience of being alive and breathing.

Try this exercise I call the Being Breath. It may give you a glimpse of what it's like to simply enjoy breathing:

1. **Sit comfortably and breathe naturally.**

   Instead of trying to improve or change your breathing, simply celebrate the fact that you're breathing.

2. **With each inhale, silently appreciate "I am here." With each exhale, rest in "This is enough."**

   Let go of any agenda to achieve or become anything. Simply be present with the miracle of being alive and breathing.

3. **Continue for as long as it feels natural.**

   Thoughts will come and go — expect them to. Whenever you remember, go back to repeating the phrases in Step 2, or rest in your feeling of simply being with your breathing as it is. Give yourself full permission to enjoy breathing.

Exploring Choiceless Awareness in breathing

One of my favorite breathing practices doesn't involve controlling the breath at all. Instead, it's about developing what philosopher J. Krishnamurti called Choiceless Awareness — a state of simply observing whatever is present without trying to change or fix anything.

In this approach, your breath becomes your teacher rather than your student. Instead of telling your breath what to do, you learn to listen to what it's already showing you. Is it shallow or deep? Fast or slow? Smooth or irregular? There's no judgment, no attempt to correct or improve — just pure, innocent observation.

This quality of awareness is incredibly healing because it mirrors unconditional acceptance, a feeling you may long for. When you can simply be with your breath exactly as it is, without needing it to be different, you're practicing a form of unconditional love with yourself. And this practice naturally extends into other areas of your life.

This next practice is called Choiceless Awareness. It's a gentle invitation to simply observe whatever arises, without needing to change, fix, or control your experience, including the breath:

1. **Find a comfortable position and gently close your eyes.**

2. **Notice what experiences are arising for you.**

   Sounds, sensations, thoughts, feelings all arise. At some point, you may simply notice that breathing is happening.

   Don't try to breathe in any particular way — just observe.

3. **When you notice yourself trying to control or improve the breath, notice that, too.**

4. **Include everything in your awareness: the temperature of the air, the pause between breaths, any sounds or sensations.**

   There's no right or wrong thing to notice or experience. Just notice *what is.*

5. **Rest in this spacious awareness for five to ten minutes.**

This exercise can be deeply restful. It's less about doing and more about just being.

Letting breath be your teacher

One of the most profound shifts in my own practice came when I stopped trying to use breathing to fix or improve myself and started listening to what my breath was trying to teach me. Your breath is like a wise friend who's always giving you feedback about your internal state and your relationship with life.

When you're stressed, your breath may become shallow and rapid — it's showing you that you're in fight-or-flight mode and you need to slow down. When you're deeply relaxed, your breath naturally becomes slower and deeper. When you're excited or passionate about something, your breathing may become more energized and dynamic.

Instead of immediately trying to change your breathing pattern, you can first listen to what it's communicating. Your breath is a bridge between your conscious and unconscious minds, often revealing things about your emotional state that you may not be fully aware of yet.

But perhaps most important, your breath teaches you about the art of letting go. You can only take your next breath by fully releasing your current one. You can't hold onto breath — it's always flowing, always changing, always letting go into the next moment. This is one of the deepest teachings about life itself.

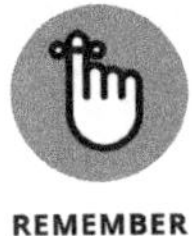

Everything in life follows this same pattern of coming and going. Thoughts arise and pass away. Emotions come and go. Sensations appear and dissolve. Even our lives themselves follow this rhythm of arriving and departing. By learning to let go with each exhale, you're practicing one of the most essential life skills: the ability to release what's no longer needed and remain open to what's arriving.

Breathing like a river flows

Think about a river flowing through a landscape. The river doesn't struggle to flow — flowing is simply its nature. It moves around obstacles, adapts to the terrain, and flows effortlessly toward the sea.

Your breath is like this river. When you watch your breath passively, it tends to find its own natural rhythm and flow. Sometimes it moves quickly, sometimes slowly. Sometimes it's deep and powerful, sometimes gentle and subtle. But it always knows exactly what to do without any interference from your thinking mind.

In Taoism, this quality is called *wu wei* — effortless action or non-doing. It's not about being passive or lazy. It's about aligning with the natural intelligence that's already operating within you. Your body knows how to breathe, just as your heart knows how to beat.

Enjoying a taste of stillness

There's something magical that happens when you stop trying to get somewhere with your breathing and simply rest in what's already here. I call this *the pause that refreshes* — those precious moments when all effort drops away and you taste the stillness that's always been present beneath the surface of your busy mind.

In my own practice, these moments often arise unexpectedly. I may be doing a simple breathing exercise when suddenly the whole thing becomes effortless. There's no sense of "me" trying to breathe, no one concentrating hard on the breath — just a vast, peaceful presence in which breathing is simply happening. These glimpses of stillness are like getting a preview of your deeper nature.

The beautiful thing about these moments is that you can't manufacture them through effort. They're like butterflies — the more you chase them, the more they flutter away. But when you create the right conditions — relaxed attention, gentle curiosity, patient presence — they tend to land on you naturally.

Realizing there's no final step — just this step

I used to think that the goal of breathing practice was to reach some permanent state of enlightenment where I'd never feel stressed or anxious again. What I discovered instead is that the practice itself is the destination. Each breath is complete in itself. Each moment of awareness is whole and perfect exactly as it is.

This realization is incredibly liberating because it takes the pressure off. You don't have to worry about whether you're making "progress" or achieving some imagined ideal state. You simply show up for this breath, right here, right now. And this breath — whether it's calm or agitated, deep or shallow, smooth or choppy — is always enough.

One of my long-term students expressed this beautifully: "I used to feel like I was failing at breathwork because my mind kept wandering and my breathing kept changing. Now I realize that the wandering and changing *is* the practice. I'm not trying to get anywhere anymore — I'm just here with whatever's happening."

Breathing for Self-Discovery

"Let what comes come.

Let what goes go.

Find out what remains."

—RAMANA MAHARSHI

Interestingly, the Latin word *spiritus* means both "breath" and "spirit." Many ancient languages, like Latin, Greek, Sanskrit, and Hebrew, link breath with spirit or life force. This wasn't just poetic language. Our ancestors intuitively understood the deep connection between breathing and our innermost being.

In ancient traditions, breath was seen as the bridge between the physical and spiritual worlds. It's the one bodily function that operates both automatically and consciously, making it the perfect doorway to explore the mystery of consciousness itself.

Remembering that you're not just your body or mind

When you look closely at your experience, you discover that you are not simply your physical body, despite how convincing this identification may feel. The body is constantly changing — cells die and regenerate, sensations come and go, and physical appearance transforms over time.

Yet through all these changes, there remains a consistent sense of "you" that witnesses these bodily transformations. You can observe your body from the inside through sensations of warmth, tension, or relaxation, and you can step back and notice these physical experiences without being completely consumed by them. This observing presence that notices bodily sensations is something deeper and more stable than the ever-changing physical form itself.

Similarly, you are not merely your mind or your thoughts, even though the mental chatter can feel overwhelming. Thoughts arise spontaneously — worries about the future, memories from the past, judgments about the present — but you have the capacity to witness these mental movements without being swept away by every passing idea or emotion.

Just as you can watch clouds moving across the sky without becoming the clouds themselves, you can observe your thoughts and feelings as temporary visitors in the space of your awareness. This witnessing consciousness that notices thoughts, emotions, and mental patterns is more fundamental than any particular mental content that flows through it.

Exploring open, spacious awareness

"You didn't come into this world. You came out of it, like a wave from the ocean. You are not a stranger here."

—ALAN WATTS

During a recent online breathwork session, one of my participants raised his hand with a puzzled expression. "This might sound strange," he said, "but sometimes when I'm doing the breathing exercises, it feels like my body just vanishes. There's breathing happening, but it's like no one is actually doing it." I couldn't help but smile as I told him, "You've just discovered one of the most profound insights in all of mindfulness and breathwork practice!"

What he experienced is something that spiritual teachers have been pointing to for centuries, and modern neuroscience is beginning to understand: Our sense of being a separate person who controls everything may not be as solid as we think.

When you settle into deep, rhythmic breathing, you may notice something fascinating — the clear boundaries between "you" and "your breathing" start to blur and soften.

You don't need to believe in any particular spiritual philosophy to explore this for yourself. It's simply about paying attention to what's actually happening in your direct experience. The next time you're in a calm, relaxed breathing rhythm, try this gentle inquiry: Can you actually locate the "you" who is doing the breathing? Is there really a separate controller managing each inhale and exhale? Or is there simply the natural flow of breath happening within a spacious field of awareness?

What I love about this exploration is that there's no right or wrong answer to discover. Instead, it's about cultivating that wonderful space of not knowing that opens the door to genuine wonder. It's in this beautiful mystery that we often find our deepest insights about who we really are.

YOU'RE THE OCEAN IN A WAVE

Here's one of my favorite metaphors that sums up what this chapter is about.

When you see a wave crashing on the shore, it looks completely separate from the water around it. It has its own shape, its own movement, its own moment of existence. But step back, and you realize something profound: There's no wave without the ocean. The wave is just the ocean dancing, expressing itself in that particular form for that particular moment.

You are that wave. Your breath, your thoughts, your entire sense of being an individual person — these are all just the universe expressing itself as you. In that sense, you're not breathing. The universe is breathing through you. You're not thinking either. Consciousness itself is lighting up the thoughts spontaneously arising in your mind.

Most of us walk around feeling like isolated individuals, cut off from everything else. We feel like we're struggling alone, breathing our own private breath, living our own separate lives. But this is like a wave thinking it's disconnected from the ocean — it's impossible, yet it feels completely real from the wave's perspective.

When you simply observe breathing happening, something extraordinary can happen. The boundaries that seemed so solid begin to dissolve. The sense of being a separate "breather" fades away, and what emerges is the recognition of effortless being.

(continued)

(continued)

This isn't philosophy or theory — it's something you can taste directly. Through breathing practice, the illusion of separation can completely collapse. In that moment, you don't just understand intellectually that you're connected to everything. You become the connection itself. You realize you were never separate to begin with.

The wave discovers it was always the ocean. And the ocean recognizes itself in every wave

This practice, Resting as Awareness, is designed to help you shift from identifying as the one who breathes to recognizing yourself as the awareness in which breathing appears. It's subtle but profound, and it often happens in stages over time.

TRY THIS

1. **Begin with a few minutes of simple breath observation.**

   Notice that there's breathing happening and that you're aware of it.

2. **Now turn your attention toward the awareness itself; ask yourself: "What is aware of the breathing?"**

   Look for this awareness, but don't think about it — simply look.

3. **Notice that you can't actually find awareness as an object.**

4. **Recognize that you *are* the awareness — you're not someone who has awareness.**

5. **From this recognition, simply rest as awareness itself.**

6. **Let breathing happen within this awareness without any effort or control on your part.**

   If you get caught up in thinking, notice that it is also happening in awareness. That's fine. Now gently return to resting as awareness.

7. **Continue for 15 to 20 minutes.**

The beautiful thing about this practice is that it often leads to what are called *flow states* — those delicious experiences where self-consciousness disappears and you feel perfectly aligned with life itself.

There's no need to chase after some special experience. No matter what you experience, even if it's a beautiful experience of being one with your surroundings or a deep sense of flow, it's just another experience, with a beginning and an end. I like to think of myself as the awareness itself. It's not something I need to chase after or attain in the future. It's here and now, no matter what is being experienced — whether it's a traffic jam or my favorite jam on toast!

TIP

Living from Presence, Breathing into Wholeness

"Love says 'I am everything.' Wisdom says 'I am nothing.' Between the two, my life flows."

—NISARGADATTA MAHARAJ

After 20 years of teaching breathing and mindfulness practices, I've learned one of the most important lessons I can share with you: There's no final destination in this work. There's no graduation ceremony where you receive your Advanced Breather certificate and never have to practice again. Instead, there's just this breath, this moment, this step on an endless journey of discovery.

Discovering your shared breath with the planet

This isn't just poetic imagination — it's scientific reality. The Earth's atmosphere is a shared resource. Trees release the oxygen you inhale, and when you exhale carbon dioxide, plants use it to grow and produce more oxygen. We're part of this magnificent breathing dance.

I often share this with clients who feel isolated. It's comforting to realize that we're never truly alone — your exhale becomes someone else's inhale, and theirs becomes yours. We're breathing each other into life.

Even more mind-blowing: The air you breathe out today could circle the globe in just two weeks. That breath may travel through forests, over oceans, into cities, and through the lungs of animals and people around the world.

In a very real sense, we are all breathing the same air. Like cells in the lungs of the Earth, we're part of one global breathing system.

Appreciating that you are nature breathing

I had a profound shift in perspective during a vacation in the Lake District of England a few decades ago, but I can still remember the moment. I was sitting by Lake Windermere, practicing a simple breathing meditation, when it suddenly struck me: I wasn't a separate being sitting in nature — I was nature becoming conscious of itself. My breathing wasn't separate from the wind moving through the trees or the waves lapping on the shore. It was all one seamless expression of the same life force.

BREATH AS A UNIFYING FORCE IN ANCIENT TRADITIONS

The understanding that the breath is a connecting force isn't unique to modern science — it has been at the heart of contemplative traditions around the world for millennia. The word *yoga* comes from the Sanskrit root *yuj,* which means "to unite" or "to join." At its deepest level, yoga is about recognizing the fundamental unity that underlies apparent separation.

Pranayama, the yogic practice of breath regulation, is designed to help practitioners realize this unity experientially. The word breaks down as *prana* (life force) and *yama* (restraint or control), but advanced practitioners understand it as the dissolution of the one who controls into the life force itself. When you practice pranayama deeply, you're not just working with your individual breath — you're connecting with the universal breath that animates all life.

In Chinese tradition, the concept of *qi* or *chi* refers to the vital energy that flows through all things. Breathwork in this tradition is about harmonizing your personal qi with the universal qi, recognizing that your individual life force is part of a much larger energetic web.

Indigenous traditions around the world have similar understandings. Many Native American practices involve breathing with the awareness that you're exchanging spirit with all of creation. In recent years, Indigenous elders have shared breathing techniques that explicitly connect practitioners with the breath of the Earth itself.

This realization transformed my relationship with breathing practice. Instead of seeing it as something I *do* to improve myself or manage my stress (though it certainly does both of those things), I began to experience it as a way of recognizing my fundamental interconnectedness with all life.

When you breathe with this awareness, every inhale becomes a celebration of your participation in the web of life. You're not just drawing air into your lungs — you're welcoming the gift of life itself. And every exhale becomes an offering, a way of sharing your life force with the world around you.

TRY THIS

The One-World breathing practice is a lovely practice to do outdoors, but it works beautifully indoors as well. The key is to cultivate a sense of breathing *with*, rather than merely *in*, the world around you.

1. **Settle into a comfortable position and take a few natural breaths to center yourself.**

2. **Begin to notice that you're not breathing alone — you're part of the Earth's breathing.**

3. **On your next inhale, imagine breathing with all the trees on the planet as they release oxygen.**

4. **On your exhale, breathe with all the plants as they receive your carbon dioxide.**

5. **Inhale with the wind as it moves across the surface of the Earth.**

6. **Exhale with the ocean waves as they breathe onto the shore.**

7. **Breathe in with all the animals, from the tiniest insects to the largest whales.**

8. **Breathe out with all of humanity, sharing in this one planetary breath.**

9. **Let yourself feel held and supported by this vast breathing community.**

10. **Rest in the awareness that you are the Earth breathing.**

Living daily life as breath practice

The real magic of breathing practice happens when you realize that you don't need special cushions, perfect silence, or dedicated meditation time to connect with your breath. Your breath is always with you, which means you always have access to presence and peace, no matter what's happening in your life.

I love teaching people how to weave breath awareness into their daily routines. You can practice mindful breathing while waiting for your coffee to brew, standing in line at the grocery store, or walking from your car to your office. These micro-practices often have a bigger impact on your overall well-being than longer formal sessions because they help you remember that peace is always available.

TRY THIS

Here are some simple daily breath practices to try:

>> Take three conscious breaths before starting your car.

>> Breathe mindfully while your computer starts up each morning.

>> Use red traffic lights as reminders to return to your breath.

>> Take a breathing pause before opening your front door when you come home.

>> Practice breath awareness while waiting for elevators.

>> Breathe consciously while washing dishes or folding laundry.

The key is to start small and be consistent rather than trying to transform your entire life overnight. Pick one or two activities that you do regularly and commit to bringing breath awareness to those moments for a week. You'll be amazed at how quickly these practices become second nature.

Connecting with one breath, one world, one moment

In this very moment, as you take this breath, you are participating in something much larger than your individual life. You are breathing with the entire cosmos.

The oxygen filling your lungs was created by stars billions of years ago. The carbon dioxide you exhale will nourish plants and trees that may live long after you're gone. Your breath connects you to every human being who has ever lived and everyone who is alive right now. In this sense, there is only one breath breathing through all of us, one consciousness aware through all our individual minds, one life living through all our separate stories.

This recognition doesn't diminish your uniqueness — it actually reveals how precious and significant you truly are. You are not separate from the universe. You are the universe becoming conscious of itself through the specific form of your life. Every breath you take is the cosmos breathing. Every moment of awareness you experience is the universe knowing itself through you.

When this understanding moves from being just an idea to being a lived reality, something profound shifts. The anxiety about whether you're breathing "correctly" dissolves because you realize you can't breathe incorrectly — you *are* the breath. The sense of separation that creates so much suffering begins to heal because you remember that you were never actually separate from anything.

REMEMBER

This shift doesn't usually happen all at once. Like learning to ride a bicycle, it's a gradual process of letting go into what you already know how to do. You may experience moments of wobbling, moments of forgetting, moments of trying too hard. But you will also experience moments — perhaps just glimpses at first — when everything feels effortless and flowing, when you remember who you really are.

And in those moments, you'll understand what the ancient traditions have been pointing to all along: that breathing is not just something you do to survive or relax or manage stress. Breathing is a sacred act, a form of prayer, a celebration of the life force that animates all existence. Every breath is an opportunity to remember your true nature and your intimate connection with all of life.

So, as you continue on your breathing journey, remember that you're not trying to get anywhere or become anyone different than who you already are. You're simply coming home to the truth that has been with you all along: You are life itself, breathing through the beautiful, temporary form of your human experience.

In this breath, in this moment, you are already complete. You are already home. You are already one with the world that breathes you into being with each precious inhale and receives you back with each grateful exhale.

Take a moment now to rest in this truth. Feel your breath as it naturally flows. And know that in doing so, you are participating in the most ancient and most sacred practice known to humanity: simply being alive, fully present, breathing as one with all of existence.

5
The Part of Tens

Here you find quick, practical insights to enhance your breathwork practice and resources to find out more.

The part begins with ten simple breathing exercises you can use daily, from relaxation techniques like 4-7-8 breathing to focusing methods like alternate nostril breathing. These exercises are designed to fit into your routine, helping you manage stress, improve focus, and boost overall well-being.

Finally, you discover ten valuable resources to continue your breathwork journey. From books and apps to online courses and in-person retreats, this list guides you to trusted sources for deepening your knowledge and expanding your practice.

Chapter **19**

Ten Quick Breathing Exercises for Every Day (and Night)

ooking for quick breathing exercises that you can do anytime, anywhere? You've come to the right place! In this chapter, I share ten of my favorite breathing techniques that you can easily incorporate into your daily life. Think of these exercises as your portable stress-relief toolkit. No batteries required, always available, and completely free!

When I first learned about breathing exercises, I thought they had to be practiced for an extended period, just in the morning or evening. Boy, was I wrong! Over the years, I've seen clients use these techniques everywhere — in board meetings, while stuck in traffic, before important presentations, and even in the dentist's chair (much to the dentist's confusion!).

The beauty of your breath is that it goes wherever you go. You have a wonderful resource for health, well-being, and success, right under your nose!

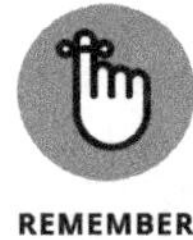

Breathing is one of the only bodily functions that's both automatic and under our conscious control. That's what makes it such a powerful tool for influencing how you feel.

4-7-8 Breathing for Anxiety Relief and Sleep

Ever feel like your mind is a browser with 47 tabs open at once? That's where 4-7-8 Breathing comes in — it's like hitting the refresh button on your nervous system.

This powerful technique, popularized by Dr. Andrew Weil, is what I call the natural tranquilizer for the nervous system. It's based on Pranayama, an ancient yogic practice, but it's packaged in a way that even my tech-obsessed friends can remember.

I discovered the magic of 4-7-8 Breathing during a particularly stressful period when I was due to give a keynote speech at a big conference abroad. The night before, my mind was racing faster than a caffeinated squirrel. Sleep seemed a distant dream. Then I remembered this technique, and within minutes of practicing it, my racing thoughts slowed and I drifted off to sleep. The next morning, I was refreshed and ready to go, and I'm pleased to say the speech was a success!

Turn to Chapter 8 for instructions on how to do 4-7-8 Breathing.

Diaphragmatic Breathing for Health

If breathing techniques were a university, diaphragmatic breathing would be the foundational course everyone is required to take. It's basically breathing the way nature intended — using your diaphragm, not just your chest.

Diaphragmatic breathing (also known as belly breathing, abdominal breathing, or deep breathing) uses your diaphragm fully. You breathe in a relaxed, natural way.

Many people breathe like they're trying to keep their stomachs flat for an Instagram photo — shallow, chest-only breaths that barely let any air in. That's like trying to fill a water balloon through a tiny straw — inefficient and frustrating!

Turn to Chapter 7 for instructions on how to do diaphragmatic breathing.

TIP

Box Breathing for Calm and Focus

If your thoughts are a car speeding down the highway, Box Breathing is like a traffic light turning yellow — it tells everything to slow down and pause for a moment. This technique is so effective that elite military units like the Navy SEALs use it to stay calm under extreme pressure. If it helps in those situations, just imagine how it could help you stay steady during a stressful meeting or a busy day!

Box Breathing gets its name because you visualize tracing a square as you breathe — each side representing one phase of the breath cycle. It's simple, symmetric, and satisfying.

I often teach Box Breathing in my corporate workshops because it's simple, easy to remember, and powerful. During one session with a particularly stressed-out tech team facing a product launch deadline, I introduced this technique. Their manager later told me they had created a silent signal — drawing a square in the air — to remind each other to practice Box Breathing during tense moments. Their deadline crunch became significantly more manageable.

Turn to Chapter 8 for instructions on how to do Box Breathing.

TIP

Alternate-Nostril Breathing for Inner Balance

Ever notice how one nostril is usually more open than the other? That's normal — we naturally cycle between nostrils throughout the day. Alternate-Nostril Breathing (called Nadi Shodhana in yoga) takes advantage of this natural phenomenon to balance your energy.

I like to think of the two nostrils as the gas and brake pedals of the nervous system. Breathing through your right nostril is like gently pressing the gas — energizing and warming. Left-nostril breathing is like tapping the brake — calming and cooling. Alternate-Nostril Breathing helps find that perfect cruising speed.

Some of my clients are coaches and therapists themselves, and they've found Alternate-Nostril Breathing to be a game-changer. Not only do they use it personally to feel more centered and balanced, but they also share it with their clients. They often say the physical nature of the technique helps their clients stay grounded and present — especially when faced with emotionally intense experiences or when their minds start to race.

Turn to Chapter 12 for instructions on how to do Alternate-Nostril Breathing.

Ocean Breath for Peace of Mind

Want to feel like you're at the beach even when you're stuck in a cubicle? The ancient technique of Ocean Breath (called *Ujjayi Pranayama* in yoga), creates a soothing oceanic sound that instantly transports you to a more peaceful state of mind. It's one of my all-time favorites.

This technique involves slightly constricting the back of your throat as you breathe, creating a gentle rushing sound similar to ocean waves. It's like having a white-noise machine built right into your body!

I remember teaching a weekend workshop where the venue was next to a busy road — definitely not the Zen environment I had planned for. Instead of letting the sound of speeding cars disrupt our practice, I taught the group Ocean Breath. The sound of their collective ocean breath not only soothed the noise but created such a focused atmosphere that many participants later said it was the most immersive workshop they'd ever attended.

Turn to Chapter 8 for instructions on how to do Ocean Breath.

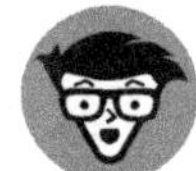

Ocean Breath creates a gentle throat vibration that stimulates the *vagus nerve,* a key player in calming your nervous system. By slightly constricting the back of your throat as you breathe through your nose, you make a soft, wave-like sound. This not only slows and deepens your breath but also activates the vagus nerve, boosting your body's "rest-and-digest" response. The result? A lower heart rate, reduced blood pressure, and a deeper sense of calm. Practicing Ocean Breath regularly can be a simple and powerful way to manage stress.

Humming Breath for Self-Soothing and Serenity

Ever notice how naturally soothing the act of humming is? That's no coincidence. The Humming Breath (called Brahmari Pranayama in yoga) uses the power of vibration to calm your mind and nervous system instantly.

I think of this technique as an internal massage for your brain. The vibration of the humming sound travels through your facial bones, skull, and brain, creating a pleasantly sedative effect. It's like giving your buzzing thoughts a lullaby.

One of my most memorable experiences with this technique involved a client who suffered from chronic migraines. During one of our sessions, she felt a migraine coming on. I guided her through Humming Breath, and after about five minutes, she looked up in amazement. "It's receding," she said. "The pain is actually backing off." Humming Breath wasn't a permanent cure, but it became a valuable tool in her migraine management toolkit.

Turn to Chapter 6 for instructions on how to do Humming Breath.

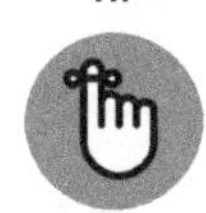

The higher the pitch of your hum, the more energizing the effect. A lower-pitched hum tends to be more calming and grounding. Experiment with different pitches and see what feels best for you.

Coherent Breathing for Heart Health

Coherent Breathing, also called Resonance Frequency Breathing, is what happens when ancient wisdom meets modern science. This technique optimizes *heart-rate variability* (HRV), a key marker of physical and emotional resilience, by synchronizing your breathing with your heart rhythm.

Think of your nervous system as a symphony orchestra. Coherent Breathing is like a skilled conductor, bringing all the instruments into harmony. When your heart, lungs, and brain are playing the same song, magic happens.

In my community, we often finish our breathing sessions with a few minutes of Coherent Breathing. One member, a counselor, told me she uses this technique before entering difficult client situations. "It's like putting on armor," she explained. "But instead of protecting me from others, it protects me from my own stress response so I can better support myself and my clients."

Turn to Chapter 8 for instructions on how to do Coherent Breathing.

Cyclic Sighing for Instant Stress Relief

Feeling overwhelmed or anxious? You've probably noticed that when stress hits, your body naturally lets out a big sigh. That's no accident — it's your nervous system trying to reset itself. Building on this natural reflex is a simple, science-backed technique called Cyclic Sighing (also called the Physiological Sigh). It's a powerful way to calm your mind and body in just a few breaths.

It's done by taking two inhales through your nose — one deep breath followed immediately by a smaller top-up — and then exhale slowly and fully through your mouth. This breathing pattern helps reduce stress by balancing your nervous system and slowing your heart rate. In short, it's nature's reset button — and the best part? You already know how to sigh. Now, you're just doing it on purpose, knowing it's good for you.

Turn to Chapter 3 for instructions on how to do Cyclic Sighing.

1:2 Ratio Breathing for Deeper Sleep and Relaxation

If breathing exercises were desserts, 1:2 Ratio Breathing would be warm milk and honey — simple, comforting, and perfect before bedtime. As the name suggests, you simply make your exhalation twice as long as your inhalation.

This technique works because of a fascinating relationship between your breath and nervous system. Inhaling activates your sympathetic (arousing) nervous system, while exhaling triggers your parasympathetic (calming) nervous system. By extending your exhale, you're essentially pressing the relaxation pedal longer than the activation pedal.

I recommend this technique to anyone suffering from insomnia. One friend, a chronic overthinker, called me and said, "I couldn't sleep last night. Brain won't shut up. Any tips, please!" I guided him through 1:2 Ratio Breathing for just five minutes. A few days later, he reported it was now his nightly ritual, making falling asleep so much easier.

Turn to Chapter 13 for instructions on how to do 1:2 Ratio Breathing.

Inhale using your nose, and exhale with either your nose or your mouth using pursed lips to help slow down that exhale. If you like Ocean Breath, you can combine that with 1:2 Ratio Breathing.

Mini Breath Holds for Calming the Mind and Gentle Energy

Mini breath holds are the breathing equivalent of pressing the pause button on a racing mind. This technique, borrowed from the Buteyko Breathing Method, involves taking brief, controlled pauses after exhaling — creating moments of stillness that can feel remarkably centering.

It works by subtly increasing carbon dioxide levels in the blood, which helps reset breathing rhythm and reduce the "panic reflex" tied to low carbon dioxide. As a result, you can experience a calmer baseline breath and a quieter mind.

During a particularly stressful time, my mind was racing so fast that I couldn't settle into my usual mindful breathing. Then I remembered reading about mini breath holds. Despite feeling counterintuitive, those gentle three- to five-second pauses calmed my thoughts and brought surprising clarity. That experience convinced me to make mini breath holds a regular part of my routine.

Turn to Chapter 9 for instructions on how to do mini breath holds.

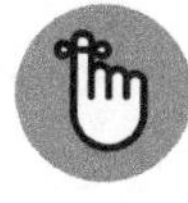

The goal isn't to struggle or strain — these are mini holds for a reason. If three to five seconds feels too long, start with just one to three seconds. You shouldn't feel much or any *air hunger* (a feeling of needing to take a deeper breath) during this practice.

Chapter **20**

Ten Resources to Keep Learning about Breath

Breathing: You've been doing it your whole life, but there's always more to learn! In this chapter, I guide you through ten of my favorite resources to keep your breathwork journey alive and kicking (or, at least, gently inhaling and exhaling). Whether you're a bookworm, an app addict, or a community seeker, there's something here for anyone who wants to breathe better.

Breath by James Nestor

Breath: The New Science of a Lost Art by James Nestor (Riverhead Books) is the book that changed my life. I still remember the day I was browsing in a bookshop in London and my friend said, "Oh, yeah, I've read that book. It's good. Check it out." Just a few pages in, and I realized, despite being a mindfulness and meditation teacher for decades, that I had so much more to learn about breathing. He also offers an excellent online course if you want to go further with him.

The Breathing Cure by Patrick McKeown

Patrick McKeown is the Jedi Master of breathing less. His book *The Breathing Cure: Develop New Habits for a Healthier, Happier, & Longer Life* (Humanix Books) is like a bible for breathing better — a must-read for anyone looking to unlock better health, deeper sleep, enhanced focus, and greater emotional resilience. McKeown blends cutting-edge science with practical exercises in a way that's easy to follow — and surprisingly transformative.

I once had a client who struggled with high blood pressure for years. Medication helped, but only to a point. After I recommended the exercises in *The Breathing Cure* and helped him practice very gentle breath holds and nasal breathing to retrain his respiratory system, his blood pressure readings improved significantly. He said he felt calmer, slept better, and was even able to reduce his reliance on medication — with his doctor's support, of course.

If *The Breathing Cure* is a bit too in-depth for you to read, check out McKeown's other books, like *The Oxygen Advantage* (William Morrow).

The Healing Power of the Breath by Richard P. Brown and Patricia L. Gerbarg

The Healing Power of the Breath (Shambhala Publications) is a practical guide to conscious breathing for health, written by two respected psychiatrists. Drawing on traditions such as yoga, qigong, and Buddhist meditation, the book grounds each technique in modern neuroscience and psychology. It explores coherent breathing and related practices, showing how they can ease stress, anxiety, depression, insomnia, and even trauma. Guided audio practices are also included online so readers can follow along.

Brown and Gerbarg go beyond instructions by explaining the science of why breathwork works and its impact on the nervous system, biochemistry, and emotional regulation. Through real-life stories from trauma survivors and healthcare professionals, they illustrate how regular practice builds resilience and supports lasting healing.

Mind Your Breathing by Sundar Balasubramanian

One book I highly recommend if you're curious to explore the traditional yogic roots of breathwork is *Mind Your Breathing: The Yogi's Handbook with 37 Pranayama Exercises* by Dr. Sundar Balasubramanian (Notion Press). As both a scientist and a trained yoga practitioner, Balasubramanian bridges the ancient wisdom of pranayama with modern research. His approach is grounded, accessible, and refreshingly authentic. He brings not just intellectual depth, but also lived experience. This comes through clearly in the practices he shares.

What I particularly appreciate about this book is how it balances simplicity with substance. Many other pranayama books can be hard to read. In this book, you'll find 37 different breathing techniques, each clearly explained and accompanied by insights into their physical and mental benefits. It's like a practical handbook and a gentle invitation to deepen your relationship with your breath. Whether you're a beginner or an experienced breath explorer, Balasubramanian's work adds value to your breathwork journey. I also recommend his TEDx talk called "The Science of Yogic Breathing," available at https://youtu.be/aIfwbEvXtwo.

Breathing for Warriors by Belisa Vranich and Brian Sabin

Belisa Vranich, a clinical psychologist and founder of The Breathing Class, is renowned for turning breath science into practical tools for performance, posture, and stress management. Her book *Breathing for Warriors* (St. Martin's Essentials) shows how diaphragmatic breathing, rather than shallow chest breathing can enhance core stability, oxygen flow, stamina, clarity, and recovery. Though written for athletes, its lessons apply to everyday life, making efficient breathing a foundation, whether you're training, working, or simply managing stress.

Whether you read the book or not, I also highly recommend you measure your BreathingIQ, developed by Vranich. You can do so at https://mybreathingiq.com. It's one of the few ways to identify your breathing style and get tailored advice on how to improve your breathing patterns if you need to. Learn more about how to do diaphragmatic breathing properly, which she strongly encourages, in Chapter 7.

Take a Deep Breath by Mike Maher

Take a Deep Breath is a YouTube channel by Mike Maher, a passionate breathwork instructor, podcaster, and researcher who's well-versed in many breathing traditions. The channel offers high-quality guided sessions, from five-minute practices to deeper heart-rate variability (HRV) resonance breathwork and bedtime routines. Mike's style is accessible, calm, and reassuring, ideal for anyone wanting a no-fuss, evidence-informed entry into breathing practices. Several videos have more than a million views, showing their wide appeal to beginners and experienced practitioners alike.

Check out the channel at www.youtube.com/c/TAKEADEEPBREATH.

Apps

Let's face it, sometimes you need a little nudge (or a gentle buzz from your phone) to remember to breathe well. Here are a few apps that I currently recommend to clients and friends:

>> **Oxygen Advantage:** An excellent and currently free app by leading expert Patrick McKeown.

>> **Breathing Zone:** I enjoy using this app. I love how I can set my own breathing rate and then listen to the sound of the waves coming in and going out.

>> **iBreathe:** A popular app designed for clarity and simplicity, with a few of the classic breathing exercises on it.

>> **Breathwrk:** A very popular app for breathwork. The animations are well designed. It has guided exercises for energy, sleep, or calm. A paid subscription is required.

>> **Calm, Headspace, and Insight Timer:** These popular apps feature breathwork sessions alongside their meditation content.

Websites

The internet is a treasure trove (and sometimes a rabbit hole) for breathwork. Here are my go-to websites:

>> **My own website, www.shamashalidina.com:** Shameless plug! Here, you'll find free resources, blog posts, and info about my courses and my private community, the Daily Mindfulness Club, in which I offer live and recorded sessions in meditation and calming breathwork at https://dailymindfulnessclub.com.

>> **Buteyko Clinic (https://buteykoclinic.com):** Patrick McKeown's website is packed with articles, videos, and online courses.

>> **Conscious Breathing (www.consciousbreathing.com):** Anders Olsson is the author of the book *Conscious Breathing* and founder of the Conscious Breathing Institute. The site includes articles, online courses, and sells products to rebalance your oxygen and carbon dioxide to healthier levels.

>> **HeartMath Institute (www.heartmath.org):** For those interested in heart coherence and breath.

Online Courses

If you're ready to go deeper, courses are the way to go. Here are a few to consider. I've done most of these courses myself:

>> **My breathing exercise course (https://dailymindfulnessclub.com/breathingcourse):** If you'd like to learn with me, this five-week Breathing for Anxiety and Stress Relief program features concise video trainings designed to enhance your long-term well-being, teaching you how to do a wide range of exercises in this book in video format, and more.

Alternatively, I have a free ten-day email course sharing tips, audio tracks, and the latest research-backed exercises, which is a nice place to start for beginners at https://shamashalidina.com/breath.

>> **Oxygen Advantage Online Course by Patrick McKeown (https://oxygenadvantage.com/online-breathing-course):** This two-hour online course, led by Patrick McKeown, teaches science-backed practices like nasal breathing, the Body Oxygen Level Test (BOLT), and rhythmic breath drills. You'll learn to breathe more efficiently for better oxygen delivery, stress resilience, sleep, focus, and performance. McKeown offers many other courses as well.

>> **Art of Living (www.artofliving.org):** Learn Sudarshan Kriya, a time-honored powerful breathing technique rooted in ancient traditions and other breathing exercises, including Pranayama. There's good evidence to show the benefits of this technique.

>> **Breath Body Mind** (`www.breath-body-mind.com`): Drs. Brown and Gerbarg, authors of *The Healing Power of the Breath*, created Breath Body Mind (BBM), a course blending coherent breathing, movement, and somatic techniques to support healing of both body and mind. You can do their course with a live teacher online.

Their nonprofit, the Breath Body Mind Foundation, brings Breath Body Mind to vulnerable communities worldwide.

Online Communities

We're stronger together. If you're looking for ways to connect with others online, and maybe even share a few mindful breaths, here are some great places to start:

>> **Daily Mindfulness Club — Guided Morning Breathwork and Meditation** (`www.dailymindfulnessclub.com`): Run by yours truly, this is an online community where we meet live every morning for a 30-minute guided mindfulness session, with a dedicated mindful breathwork session once a week. It's a supportive space for starting your day calmly and with intention. Whether you're new to breathing exercises or looking for consistency, the Daily Mindfulness Club offers gentle structure and kind connection.

>> **Insight Timer — Breathwork Courses & Community** (`www.insighttimer.com`): Perfect for beginners dipping their toes into mindful breathing. Insight Timer has hundreds of free guided breathwork sessions, from calming to energizing. You can leave comments under each session and connect with others on the same journey.

>> **The Oxygen Advantage Community** (`www.facebook.com/groups/290807441400098`): If you're curious about the science of breath and how it affects sleep, anxiety, and performance, this group is a fantastic resource. Based on the work of Patrick McKeown, it's ideal for those wanting practical, research-based techniques.

Index

Feather Flying technique, 264–265

fight-or-flight response. *See* sympathetic nervous system

Figure-Eight Breath. *See* Infinity Breath technique

Fitbit, 61

Five-Finger Breathing, 277

flow states, 23–24, 342

focus

Alternate-Nostril Breathing *(Nadi Shodhana)*, 225–226

and box breathing, 127, 353

and breathing, 49–52

breathing exercises for enhancing, 38–39, 50–52

daytime, and sleep-focused breathwork, 238–239

impact of oxygen on, 304

mindful breathing for enhancing, 70, 82

pre-event, 310–311

of teenagers, 270–272

Focused Breath Awareness, 199

food, 99, 138

Forest Breath, 228–229

Friendship Breathing, 282

full system reset, 218

functional breathing, 56

G

games

biofeedback, 63

for children, 259, 264–265, 268–270, 281

virtual reality, 63

gentle Buteyko Breathing Method, 253–254

Gentle Rain Breath, 269

Gerbarg, Patricia L., 121, 360, 364

Gevirtz, Richard, 120

glymphatic system, 238, 239

Gradual Breath Extension exercise, 198

Gregorian chants, 121

Grof, Christina, 325

Grof, Stanislav, 325

H

Hand Breathing technique, 299

Hand on Heart, Hand on Belly technique, 15

headaches, 199–201, 355

Headspace (app), 62, 362

Healing Power of the Breath, The (Brown and Gerbarg), 360

Heart Blossom Breath, 279

heart rate, 33, 105, 121

heart rate variability (HRV), 59–61

and Coherent Breathing, 121, 123, 355

and immune function, 196

and mindful breathing, 166

heart-rate variability biofeedback breathing. *See* Coherent Breathing

HeartMath, 59, 61, 363

hemoglobin, 35, 40, 141, 304

high-altitude exposure, 104, 314

hiking, 313–314

Hof, Wim, 329, 330, 331

Holotropic Breathwork, 325–327

Homework Helper technique, 282

HRV. *See* heart rate variability

Huberman, Andrew, 51

huff coughing, 192–193

humming

for loosening of diaphragm, 108

and nitric oxide production, 91

for relaxation in children, 267–268

Humming Bee Breath (Bhramari Pranayama), 121, 241, 355

hydration, 95, 212

hyperventilation. *See* over-breathing

hypnagogic state, 237

hypocapnia, 139

I

iBreathe (app), 62, 362

Iceman, The. *See* Hof, Wim

immune system, 29, 86

boosting immune function, 195–196

About the Author

Shamash Alidina, MEng, MA(Ed), PGCE, is a teacher and trainer specializing in mindfulness, Acceptance and Commitment Training (ACT), and mindful breathwork, based in North London, UK. He has trained specifically in breathwork with James Nestor, Patrick McKeown, Dr. Richard Brown, Dr. Patricia Gerbarg, and more.

Since 2010, he has dedicated his career to helping individuals and organizations cultivate mindfulness, creativity, resilience, and well-being through evidence-based techniques. He delivers keynote talks, workshops, and events, and is the author of *Mindfulness For Dummies* and *Relaxation For Dummies* (both published by John Wiley & Sons), *The Mindful Way Through Stress* (The Guilford Press), and several other books on mindfulness and self-care. He also runs the Daily Mindfulness Club (`https://dailymindfulnessclub.com`), a live online meditation and breathwork community, offering daily guided sessions.

Shamash's journey into breathwork started with mindfulness, but it wasn't until he explored the science of breathing — drawing insights from leading experts — that he fully realized its transformative power. This discovery led him to integrate breathwork into his teaching, helping people harness the breath for better health, focus, and well-being.

Outside of teaching and writing, Shamash enjoys walking, making art, diving into nondual Eastern philosophy, and creating ways to make mindfulness fun and accessible for all.

You can learn more about his work at `www.shamashalidina.com`. You can try his free breathwork challenge at `www.shamashalidina.com/breathwork-challenge`. Finally, feel free to reach out to Shamash anytime via email at `info@shamashalidina.com` and let him know how this book has helped you. He'd love to hear from you!

Dedication

To everyone who's ever felt breathless — not just physically, but emotionally or spiritually — this book is for you. To my community, friends, family, and all who've sat and breathed with me, thank you for your presence, your curiosity, and your support. Finally, to anyone who's ever searched "how to breathe properly" and thought, "Wait, am I doing this right?" — this is for you.

Author's Acknowledgments

Writing this book has been an incredible journey, and I couldn't have done it without the support, generosity, and wisdom of some truly remarkable people.

First and foremost, a huge thank you to James Nestor for his groundbreaking *New York Times* bestseller, *Breath* (Riverhead Books). Despite having practiced meditation for more than 20 years, I had never fully grasped the immense power of breathing correctly and breathwork until reading his book. His research and storytelling opened my eyes to the deeper potential of breathwork, and I'm incredibly grateful for the insights he has shared with the world.

A massive thank-you also goes to Patrick McKeown, who generously wrote the foreword for this book. His expertise in breathwork, particularly through his Buteyko Breathing Method, has profoundly influenced my understanding of optimal breathing. Our conversation on my podcast and his instruction in the Buteyko method, as well as his dedication to teaching others, have been invaluable. Completing his training was a game-changer for me, and I deeply appreciate his generosity and knowledge.

To all my friends and family, thank you so much for your unwavering support and patience as I've taken the rather unusual path of becoming a full-time teacher and trainer in mindfulness, ACT, and breathwork since 2010. Your encouragement has kept me going, and I am forever grateful for the love and understanding you've shown me on this journey.

A big thank-you to the many people working behind the scenes to turn my script into something far more interesting and informative for you to read. A big thank-you to my editor, Elizabeth Kuball, for her attention to detail and for turning my rambling words into the coherent and polished version you read today. Thanks to Tracy Boggier for her belief in my ability to turn this idea into a book. And thank you to Catherine Bane, the technical editor and breathwork expert, who made so many insightful points that were added to this book.

And finally, thank you to you, dear reader, for trusting me to be your guide, and for being curious enough to explore the potential of your own breath. I hope this book serves as a valuable companion on your journey to better breathing and a more mindful life.

Publisher's Acknowledgments

Managing Editor: Ajith Kumar

Executive Editor: Tracy Boggier

Editor: Elizabeth Kuball

Technical Editor: Catherine Bane, PhD

Production Editor: Bharaneedharan Murthy

Cover Images: © Inside Creative House/
Getty Images, © PeopleImages/Getty Images

Special Help: Carmen Krikorian, Kristie Pyles